Examining the Development, Regulation, and Consumption of Functional Foods

Sailas Benjamin
University of Calicut, India

A volume in the Advances in Environmental Engineering and Green Technologies (AEEGT) Book Series

IGI GLOBAL
DISSEMINATOR OF KNOWLEDGE
www.igi-global.com

Published in the United States of America by
IGI Global
Medical Information Science Reference (an imprint of IGI Global)
701 E. Chocolate Avenue
Hershey PA 17033
Tel: 717-533-8845
Fax: 717-533-8661
E-mail: cust@igi-global.com
Web site: http://www.igi-global.com

Library of Congress Cataloging-in-Publication Data

Names: Benjamin, Sailas, 1966- editor.
Title: Examining the development, regulation, and consumption of functional foods / Sailas Benjamin, editor.
Description: Hershey PA : Medical Information Science, [2017] | Includes bibliographical references and index.
Identifiers: LCCN 2016042237| ISBN 9781522506072 (hardcover) | ISBN 9781522506089 (ebook)
Subjects: | MESH: Functional Food
Classification: LCC RA784 | NLM QU 145.5 | DDC 613.2--dc23 LC record available at https://lccn.loc.gov/2016042237

This book is published in the IGI Global book series Advances in Environmental Engineering and Green Technologies (AEEGT) (ISSN: 2326-9162; eISSN: 2326-9170)

British Cataloguing in Publication Data
A Cataloguing in Publication record for this book is available from the British Library.

Advances in Environmental Engineering and Green Technologies (AEEGT) Book Series

ISSN: 2326-9162
EISSN: 2326-9170

Mission

Growing awareness and an increased focus on environmental issues such as climate change, energy use, and loss of non-renewable resources have brought about a greater need for research that provides potential solutions to these problems. Research in environmental science and engineering continues to play a vital role in uncovering new opportunities for a "green" future.

The **Advances in Environmental Engineering and Green Technologies (AEEGT)** book series is a mouthpiece for research in all aspects of environmental science, earth science, and green initiatives. This series supports the ongoing research in this field through publishing books that discuss topics within environmental engineering or that deal with the interdisciplinary field of green technologies.

Coverage

- Electric Vehicles
- Cleantech
- Policies Involving Green Technologies and Environmental Engineering
- Alternative Power Sources
- Biofilters and Biofiltration
- Renewable Energy
- Air Quality
- Contaminated Site Remediation
- Pollution Management
- Radioactive Waste Treatment

IGI Global is currently accepting manuscripts for publication within this series. To submit a proposal for a volume in this series, please contact our Acquisition Editors at Acquisitions@igi-global.com or visit: http://www.igi-global.com/publish/.

The Advances in Environmental Engineering and Green Technologies (AEEGT) Book Series (ISSN 2326-9162) is published by IGI Global, 701 E. Chocolate Avenue, Hershey, PA 17033-1240, USA, www.igi-global.com. This series is composed of titles available for purchase individually; each title is edited to be contextually exclusive from any other title within the series. For pricing and ordering information please visit http://www.igi-global.com/book-series/advances-environmental-engineering-green-technologies/73679. Postmaster: Send all address changes to above address.

Titles in this Series

For a list of additional titles in this series, please visit: www.igi-global.com

Applying Nanotechnology for Environmental Sustainability
Sung Hee Joo (University of Miami, USA)
Information Science Reference • copyright 2017 • 558pp • H/C (ISBN: 9781522505853) • US $225.00 (our price)

Exploring the Nutrition and Health Benefits of Functional Foods
Hossain Uddin Shekhar (University of Dhaka, Bangladesh) Zakir Hossain Howlader (University of Dhaka, Bangladesh) and Yearul Kabir (University of Dhaka, Bangladesh)
Medical Information Science Reference • copyright 2017 • 523pp • H/C (ISBN: 9781522505914) • US $200.00 (our price)

Smart Cities as a Solution for Reducing Urban Waste and Pollution
Goh Bee Hua (National University of Singapore, Singapore)
Information Science Reference • copyright 2016 • 362pp • H/C (ISBN: 9781522503026) • US $190.00 (our price)

Food Science, Production, and Engineering in Contemporary Economies
Andrei Jean-Vasile (Petroleum-Gas University of Ploiesti, Romania)
Information Science Reference • copyright 2016 • 473pp • H/C (ISBN: 9781522503415) • US $240.00 (our price)

Smart Grid as a Solution for Renewable and Efficient Energy
Ayaz Ahmad (COMSATS Institute of Information Technology, Pakistan) and Naveed Ul Hassan (LUMS School of Science & Engineering, Pakistan)
Information Science Reference • copyright 2016 • 415pp • H/C (ISBN: 9781522500728) • US $220.00 (our price)

Biologically-Inspired Energy Harvesting through Wireless Sensor Technologies
Vasaki Ponnusamy (Universiti Tunku Abdul Rahman, Malaysia) Noor Zaman (King Faisal University, Saudi Arabia) Tang Jung Low (Universiti Teknologi Petronas, Malaysia) and Anang Hudaya Muhamad Amin (Multimedia University, Malaysia)
Information Science Reference • copyright 2016 • 318pp • H/C (ISBN: 9781466697928) • US $200.00 (our price)

Handbook of Research on Waste Management Techniques for Sustainability
Ulas Akkucuk (Bogazici University, Turkey)
Information Science Reference • copyright 2016 • 438pp • H/C (ISBN: 9781466697232) • US $240.00 (our price)

Table of Contents

Detailed Table of Contents

One of the key areas in animal husbandry is to improve the quality (nutritional value) of dairy and meat products by enriching them with Conjugated Linoleic Acids (CLAs) like (cis-9, trans-11)- and (trans-10, cis-12)-octadecadienicacids; the former (rumenic acid) predominates all the CLAs. Though Vaccenic Acid (VA) is the immediate precursor of rumenic acid, dietary unsaturated fatty acids like Oleic Acid (OA), Linoleic Acid (LA) and α-Linolenic Acid (ALA) are the distant precursors of CLAs; and that CLA and VA are formed as intermediates during the biohydrogenation of the dietary OA, LA and ALA into fully saturated stearic acid. The mutual inter-relationship of rumen microbiota encompassing bacteria, protozoa and fungi facilitates the biohydrogenation process. Thus, this chapter critically evaluates the knowledge accumulated during the past four decades on the precursor of CLAs, micro-organisms involved in the production of CLA, the mechanism of biohydrogenation, and chemical synthesis of CLA, coupled with the rationale for biohydrogenation and factors affecting the production of CLA.

This chapter mainly summarizes the sources of dietary fibers and how they act as functional food for benefiting the human health. Dietary fibers could be soluble and insoluble in water and the major sources are fruits, vegetables, nuts and whole grains. Dietary fibers play role in the control of various disorders like cardiovascular diseases, digestive disorders, diabetes, obesity and colonic cancer. Dietary fibers benefit the human health by acting through various mechanisms in the gastrointestinal tract. According to the WHO recommendations at least 25 g of dietary fiber per day should be consumed. Effect of food processing practices on the physiochemical and functional properties of dietary fibers is also covered in this chapter.

Phytotherapy re-emerged in the latest years as a healing system accepted and spread worldwide, and different molecules have been investigated due to their benefits to health. Nutraceutical formulations, which allow the intake of phytonutrients (generally in low levels in plant food) in concentrations that are enough to achieve the desired outcomes, represent feasible alternatives to improve general health and to prevent and treat varied diseases. Notwithstanding the incompleteness of an evidence-based clinical use of nutraceuticals, many questions remain unanswered regarding their global effects in humans and animals. Thus, the aim of this chapter is to provide recent evidence on chemical and pharmacological features of the main phytonutrients explored in nutraceutical formulations, focusing antimicrobial, antioxidant and antiproliferative potentials. Also, some insights on drug-phytonutrients interactions will be discussed.

Millets are small grained cereals belonging to the family Gramineae and they include major millets and minor millets. Millets are quite important from the point of food and nutritional security at regional and house hold level. In India's dry lands, they play a significant role in meeting food and fodder requirements of farming communities. Millets are found to have high nutritive value comparable and even superior to major cereals with respect to protein, energy, vitamins and minerals. They are also rich sources of phytochemicals and micronutrients. Since millet is gluten-free, it is an excellent option for the people who are suffering from atherosclerosis, diabetics and heart disease. In the face of increasing population and stagnant wheat and rice production, millets can be a promising alternative in solving the problem of food insecurity and malnutrition, because of their sustainability in adverse agro-climatic conditions. These crops have substantive potential in broadening the genetic diversity of the food basket and ensuring improved food and nutrition security.

In recent years, multiple drug resistance has been developed due to indiscriminate use of existing drugs in the treatment of infectious diseases. One such herbal drug is Coriandrum Sativum L that possesses potential pharmaceutical activities and used in several ayurvedic formulations. Keratitis caused by bacteria, viruses, fungi and parasites. The main goal of this study is to evaluate the antibacterial, antifungal activity, anti-oxidant activity and anti-inflammatory activity of Coriandrum Sativum L leaves and seeds using various organic solvent of plant extract against keratitis disease. The present study carried out the effect on various organic solvents extract of leaves and seeds of Corindrum sativum not only on the bacterial and fungal populations isolated from the conjunctivitis infected eyes but also to screen the phytochemical, anti-inflammatory and in vitro antioxidant potential of the leaf and seed extracts.

Rice (Oryza sativa L.) which belongs to the family poaceae, is the life and the prince among cereals as this unique grain helps to sustain two thirds of the world's population. India have traditionally been used or rice cultivation due to availability of water and conductive soil (Nadesa panic). Rice was grown in 155.30 million hectares and around 600 million tonnes of rice harvested each year globally. About 114 countries produce rice with China and India supporting 50 per cent of total production. India stands first in area under cultivation (41.85 mha) and ranks second in production, where as China ranks first in production with just half of the area. India's production is 89.13 million tonnes with a productivity of 2130 kg/ha. Among the rice producing states of India, Tamil Nadu ranks sixth in production (6.53 million tonnes) and second in productivity of 3918 kg/ha with an area of 20.16 lakh ha. Local farmers in such farming systems retain the traditional varieties based on their knowledge of the quality of the rice varieties and their adaptation to varying agro-ecological situations created by diverse seasons and land situations. Among the major micronutrient deficiencies common in rice consuming countries, iron and zinc deficiencies ("hidden hunger"), affect over three billion people worldwide, mostly in developing countries.

In the recent years, there has been a great deal of attention in investigating the disease preventive properties of functional foods. Particularly, impact of the antioxidant property of functional foods in reducing the risk or progression of chronic diseases has gained considerable interest amongst researchers and practitioners. Free radicals such as reactive oxygen species are generated in the body by exposure to a number of physiochemical or pathological mechanisms. It is imperative to preserve a balance between the levels of free radicals and antioxidants for routine physiological function, a disparity of which would accelerate oxidative stress. Increased oxidative stress and associated consequences in metabolic disorders such as obesity, cardiovascular diseases and diabetes has warranted the need for exogenous antioxidant concentrates derived from natural foods to alleviate the adverse effects. This chapter provides an overview on the efficacy of functional foods in reducing free radical-mediated damage in metabolic syndrome.

In retrospect to the rise in the occurrence of ageing related disorders and the everlasting desire to overcome ageing, exploring the causes, mechanisms and therapies to curb ageing becomes relevant. Reactive Oxygen Species (ROS) are commonly generated during normal growth and development. However abiotic and biotic stresses enhance the level of ROS which in turn pose the threat of oxidative stress. Ability to perceive ROS and to speedily commence antioxidant defenses is crucial for the survival as well as longevity of living cells. Therefore living organisms are bestowed with antioxidants to combat the damages caused by oxidative stress. This chapter aims to elucidate an overview of the process of ageing, generation and enhancement of reactive oxygen species, damages incurred by oxidative stress, its amelioration strategies, therapeutic and biotechnological potentials of antioxidants and various sources of bioactive compounds significant in retardation of aging process.

Taken into account data from which is considered a product not safe, estimate the safe level of a contaminant on food, for example, always have many unavoidable uncertainties. It cannot be overemphasized enough, that this also happens as in any other human activity. In most cases, we hope, to define as clearly as possible the eventual risk associated with particular conditions of exposure to a given substance in food. There are numerous toxic compounds that reside naturally in certain foods that unable these to be consumed above certain limits or even are fully prohibited in some other countries. Chapter starts with a clear explanation of differences and relationships between food allergy and food poisoning, continued with main allergens in food and main toxics. Finally, authors summarize different origins of toxins and allergens (natural from foods, from additives, pollutants and food processing).

Functional foods are recently introduced to assure superior nutritional quality; contain biologically active compounds in defined amounts. These foods have to be effectively packaged and stored in order to prevent microbial spoilage and risk of food borne infections. Recently, food technologists and scientists are formulating the Essential Oil (EOs) containing functional foods. The antibacterial, antifungal, antioxidant and anti-carcinogenic properties of EOs have been proved by a number of researchers. Health conscious consumers prefer natural additives, hence these volatile oils due to their green image can be safely used as a replacement of synthetic preservatives. The shelf life of functional foods can be improved by antimicrobial packaging incorporating EOs and their derivatives in the edible films and coatings. EOs can be easily fabricated as microencapsules and nanoparticles, which increases their stability and solubility. Hence EOs are considered as the most usable additives in future functional foods.

Preface

Medical and functional foods are getting increased momentum in the health and allied sector. Medical foods are specially formulated for the dietary management of a disease that demands distinctive nutritional support, which cannot be met or supplemented by normal diet alone; while apart from nutritional value, a functional food provides *additional or supplementary function* for the human health management (often one related to health-promotion or disease prevention) by adding new ingredients or more of existing ingredients. Functional food is a *natural* or *processed food* that contains known biologically-active compounds - which when in defined qualitative and quantitative amounts - provides a clinically proven and documented health benefit; and thus, it serves as an important source in the prevention, management and treatment of chronic diseases (especially of lifestyle) of the modern age.

The principal objective of this endeavor is to bring together the knowledge accumulated on the fundamental and applied aspects of scientific research on functional foods into a handy module as *Examining the Development, Regulation, and Consumption of Functional Foods*. This book looks to discuss and address the *Functional foods* with the perspectives of dietary supplements, phytonutrients, micronutrients, vitamins, minerals, probiotics, *etc*. It covers the crucial issues related to the efficacy and safety of bioactive compounds and other functional food constituents and characterization of functional foods with reference to product development; preparation of natural and synthetic ingredients for use in foods, supplements or premixes and improvement of ingredient quality; effects of processing (including packaging, storage, *etc*.) on functionality and improvement of product quality; verification, quality control and traceability of natural and synthetic functional food ingredients and products; improvement of the quality of foods with inherent health benefits; development and commercialization of specific functional food products, and the regulatory aspects of functional foods and related issues, *e.g*., labeling, substantiation of health claims.

Regarding contents, this book embodies ten chapters dedicated to different aspects of functional foods. It starts with "biosynthesis of conjugated linoleic acids"; followed by "dietary fibers and their role as functional food for human health: food fibers and human health"; "phytonutrients of nutraceutical importance"; "millets as an integral part of nutritional diet in India"; "analysis of bioactive compounds in *Coriandrum sativum* L. against microbial keratitis"; "breeding for improving human nutrition and grain quality through biofortification of traditional land races and improved cultivars of rice (*Oryza sativa*)"; "antioxidants as functional foods in metabolic syndrome"; "exploring the potentials of antioxidants in retarding ageing"; "food allergy and food poisoning: toxicology on culinary science"; and finally "development of functional foods and antimicrobial packaging containing essential oils".

"Biosynthesis of conjugated linoleic acids" critically evaluates the knowledge accumulated during the past four decades on the precursor of conjugated linoleic acids, micro-organisms involved in the production of conjugated linoleic acid, the mechanism of biohydrogenation mechanism, and chemical synthesis of conjugated linoleic acid, coupled with the rationale for biohydrogenation and factors affecting the production of conjugated linoleic acid. "Dietary fibers and their role as functional food for human health: food fibers and human health" summarizes the sources of dietary fibers and how they act as functional food for benefiting the human health by alleviating cardiovascular diseases, digestive disorders, diabetes, obesity and colonic cancer; coupled with the effect of dietary fibers in food processing practices on the physiochemical and functional properties. "Phytonutrients of nutraceutical importance" addresses recent evidence on chemical and pharmacological features of the main phytonutrients explored in nutraceutical formulations, focusing antimicrobial, antioxidant and antiproliferative potentials along with drug-phytonutrients interactions will be discussed. The chapter "millets as an integral part of nutritional diet in India" discusses the higher nutritive value of millets comparable and even superior to major cereals with respect to protein, energy, vitamins and minerals. "Analysis of bioactive compounds in *Coriandrum sativum* L. against microbial keratitis" evaluates the antibacterial, antifungal, antioxidant and anti-inflammatory activities of the leaves and seeds of *Coriandrum sativum* L using various organic solvent against keratitis. "Breeding for improving human nutrition and grain quality through biofortification of traditional land races and improved cultivars of rice (*Oryza sativa*)" deals with quality breeding of rice for improved iron and zinc contents - their deficiency would lead to hidden hunger.

"Antioxidants as functional foods in metabolic syndrome" provides an overview on the efficacy of functional foods in reducing free radical-mediated damage in metabolic syndrome. "Exploring the potentials of antioxidants in retarding ageing" gives an overview of the process of ageing, generation and enhancement of reactive oxygen species, damages incurred by oxidative stress, its amelioration strategies, therapeutic and biotechnological potentials of antioxidants and various sources of bioactive compounds significant in retarding the aging process. "Food allergy and food poisoning: toxicology on culinary science" provides clear explanation on the differences and relationships between food allergy and food poisoning, main allergens in food and main toxics; in addition to providing different origins of toxins and allergens (from foods, additives, pollutants and food processing). "Development of functional foods and antimicrobial packaging containing essential oils" deals with importance of essential oils as natural additives, in improving the shelf life of functional food.

Thus, it is expected that policy makers, academicians, researchers, medical practitioners, advanced-level students, technology developers, and government officials would find this text useful in furthering their research exposure to pertinent topics in electronic government and assisting in furthering their own research efforts in this field.

Furthermore, the assistance rendered by Dr. M.K. Sarath Josh – former research scholar at my laboratory – during the initial stages of this book project is gratefully acknowledged.

Sailas Benjamin
University of Calicut, India

Chapter 1
Biogenesis of Conjugated Linoleic Acids

Sailas Benjamin
University of Calicut, India

Kizhakepowathil Nair Unni
University of Calicut, India

Prakasan Priji
University of Calicut, India

Andre-Denis Girard Wright
University of Arizona, USA

ABSTRACT

One of the key areas in animal husbandry is to improve the quality (nutritional value) of dairy and meat products by enriching them with Conjugated Linoleic Acids (CLAs) like (cis-9, trans-11)- and (trans-10, cis-12)-octadecadienicacids; the former (rumenic acid) predominates all the CLAs. Though Vaccenic Acid (VA) is the immediate precursor of rumenic acid, dietary unsaturated fatty acids like Oleic Acid (OA), Linoleic Acid (LA) and α-Linolenic Acid (ALA) are the distant precursors of CLAs; and that CLA and VA are formed as intermediates during the biohydrogenation of the dietary OA, LA and ALA into fully saturated stearic acid. The mutual inter-relationship of rumen microbiota encompassing bacteria, protozoa and fungi facilitates the biohydrogenation process. Thus, this chapter critically evaluates the knowledge accumulated during the past four decades on the precursor of CLAs, micro-organisms involved in the production of CLA, the mechanism of biohydrogenation, and chemical synthesis of CLA, coupled with the rationale for biohydrogenation and factors affecting the production of CLA.

DOI: 10.4018/978-1-5225-0607-2.ch001

INTRODUCTION

Conjugated linoleic acids (CLAs, the 18:2 octadecadienoic acids with *cis-cis, cis-trans, trans-cis, trans-trans* conjugated double bond system between 6 to 16 C along the acyl chain), the supposed health-promoting fatty acid (FA), are a mixture of biologically active positional and geometric isomers of linoleic acid [LA, 18:2 (*cis*-9,*cis*-12)-octadecadienoic acid] with two conjugated (adjacent) double bonds (Benjamin & Spener, 2009). Naturally, CLAs are found predominantly in milk and milk products, meat and meat products of ruminants. It is generally formed as an intermediate during the biohydrogenation of C_{18}unsaturated FAs like oleic acid [OA, 18:1(*cis*-9)-octadecenoic acid], LA and α-linolenic acid [ALA, 18:3 (*cis*-9,*cis*-12,*cis*15)-octadecatrienoic acid] in the rumen of ruminants to saturated 18:0 stearic acid (SA) (Dawson &Kemp, 1969; Aii et al., 1999; Dhiman et al., 2000; Hristov et al., 2005) or by the Δ^9-desaturase mediated endogenous conversion of vaccenic acid [18:1 VA, (*trans*-11)-octadecenoic acid)] in the mammary (lactation) and adipose (growth) tissues of mammals (Bartlett & Chapman, 1961; Bauman et al., 1999;Grinari et al., 2000; Turpinen et al, 2002; Kuhnt et al., 2009). As CLAs are supposed to be associated with various health benefits like anti-carcinogenic, anti-artherogenic, anti-diabetic and anti-adipogenic effects, these minor lipid nutrients may impart some benefits toward improving health (Benjamin & Spener, 2009; Benjamin et al., 2013). As a result, CLA gained significant attention in various research domains, especially the food and health industry in particular.

Ruminal biohydrogenation of unsaturated FAs into CLA is unequivocal. However, a comprehensive analysis of the literature on CLA pertaining to various aspects of the biogenesis of CLA is missing. Hence, this review is designed to address the sources of FAs and the microorganisms involved in biohydrogenation, including the mechanisms and the rationale behind of biohydrogenation, and the factors affecting CLA production.

CHEMISTRY OF CLA, THE OMEGA PARADIGM

Very often, CLAs are erroneously classified as *omega*-6 (abbreviated as ω-6) FAs. In fact, CLA is a class of FAs comprising as many as 56 isomers with conjugated (neighboring) double bond pairs (*i.e.*, at positions 6,8-; 7,9-; 8,10-; 9,11-; 10,12-; 11,13-; 12,14-; and 13,15- with *cis-cis, cis-trans, trans-cis* or *trans-trans* geometric configurations) varying along the acyl chain of LA (Dobson, 2003). From this, it is evident that only the isomers with the conjugated double bonds on carbon positions

Figure 1. Major ω fatty acids with their common names, structures, and systemic names

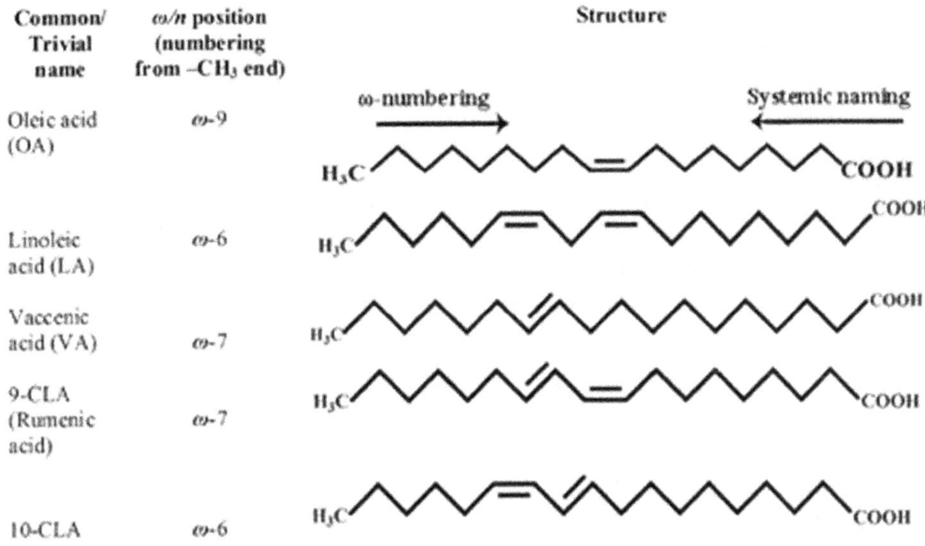

starting at 10 (from –COOH terminus) have indeed their first C-C double bond at the ω-6 position, while counting from the methyl (CH_3-) terminus (*i.e.* from the last or *omega*-C on the acyl chain) (Figure 1). Thus, *trans*-10, *cis*-12-CLA (designated as 10-CLA) is a typical ω-6 CLA; while the biologically active and predominantly (natural) occurring *cis*-9, *trans*-11-CLA (designated as 9-CLA, the rumenic acid) is a typical ω-7 FA (Benjamin & Spener, 2009; Benjamin et al., 2015). Though, LA is devoid of conjugated double bonds, it is also an ω-6 FA, while counting the double bond position from the methyl terminus of the FA chain (Figure 1).

During biohydrogenation of monounsaturated FA (MUFA, *e.g.* OA) and polyunsaturated FAs (e.g., LA and ALA) to SA; 9-CLA is formed as the predominant isomer, followed by 10-CLA (very less concentration) and other isomers in traces; *i.e.*, all are the intermediates formed during the course of action, and they escape from the biohydrogenation cascade without terminating as SA. The 9-CLA represents 80 to 90% of the total CLA in milk fat, but its proportion in meat fat is less; *i.e.*, under certain dietary conditions, the proportion of the 10-CLA isomer increases. Thus, dietary factors also alter the direction of the biohydrogenation pathways in the rumen (Daley et al., 2010).

In fact, to meet the commercial needs, CLAs are synthesized either chemically or biologically, and chemical synthesis predominates over biosynthesis.

THE PRECURSOR OF CLA

The uniqueness of CLA in ruminant fat relates to the biohydrogenation of dietary unsaturated FAs by rumen bacteria. Plant-derived FAs like OA, LA and ALA are shown as the distant precursors for the microbial production of CLA (Figure 2). Concentration of CLA in dairy and meat products is highly correlated with the dietary intake of either LA or ALA or both (Aii et al, 1999; Dhiman et al., 2000). However, LA is generally used for the microbial production of CLA. Now-a-days, new and advanced methods have been developed for the recognition of biohydrogenation mechanism occurring on the precursor FAs. Earlier studies were performed with the help of radioactive isotopes, but of late, it was accomplished by stable isotopes (Mosley et al., 2006). Wallace et al. (2007) used deuterium oxide (D_2O)-containing buffer to examine CLA production from LA. They showed that pure cultures of *Butyrivibrio fibrisolvens* and *Clostridium proteoclasticum* produced mostly 9-CLA with minor quantities of other 9,11 isomers, all labeled at C_{13}. In contrast, a ruminal isolate of *Propionibacterium acnes* produced 10-CLA and other 10,12 isomers that were minimally labeled (Wallace et al., 2007). Thus, isomer-specific microbial production of CLA is made possible.

Figure 2.

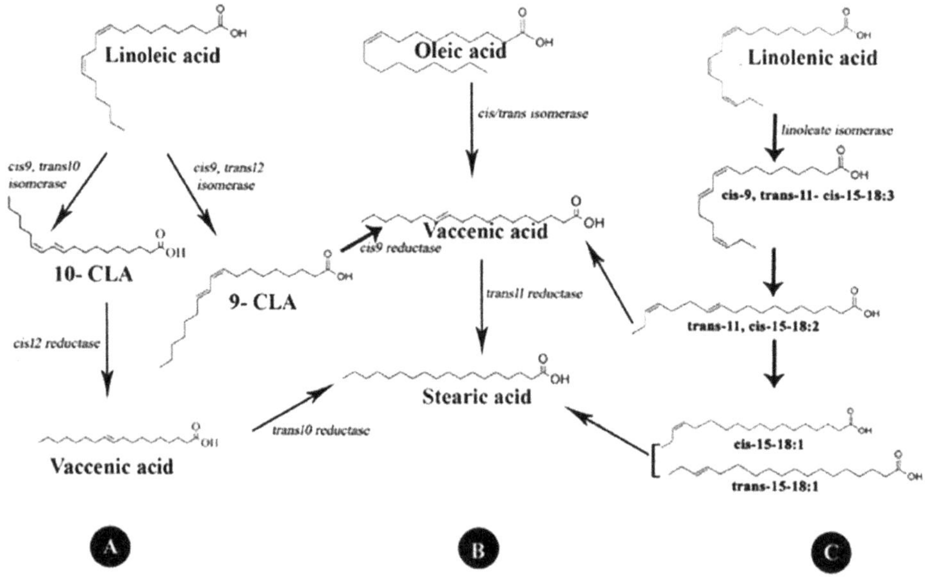

FEED AND LIPID PROFILE

Feed is a major component of variable costs associated with dairy systems (Pryce et al., 2014). The FA profile of the feed depends on the nature of forage or silage (conserved forage) with or without supplements to augment the nutritional quality of the feed. Generally, the energy content of mature forage is lower than that of vegetative (immature) forage, of which grasses offer superior nutritional values. Thus, more concentrates (cereal grains, oil seeds, pulses, bone meal, *etc.*) will be required in rations (daily feed), based on mature forages or silage (Eastridge, 2006). The energy demand of the cattle increases with increase in milk production and that the quantity of concentrate required in the ration is higher for a high-yielding cow, than for a low-yielding one. Thus, based on the activity of cattle, the proportion of concentrate may vary between 0 to 60%. A dry (non-lactating) cow should eat a ratio of about 90 to 100% forage (+ 0 to 10% concentrate), *i.e.*, a lactating cattle needs more concentrates in the daily rations. The crude protein needed in the concentrate mix depends on the type of forage in the ration. Forage with high crude protein contents such as legumes, can be combined with a concentrate mix of low protein content, and *vice versa* – so as to make a balanced diet.

Leaves are the major store house of lipids, which comprises about 30% of the dry matter (DM), while lipid fraction in normal plant tissues constitutes 3-10% of DM, and that the lipid content will be higher in grasses (Mir et al., 2006). In plants, lipids are mainly embedded in the membranes as galactolipids - a mixture of glycerol, unsaturated FAs, one or more galactose units, and in some cases, either a hydroxyl or a sulfonic acid group is attached as an extra moiety (Schmid et al., 2002; Van Meer et al., 2008). Five major FAs are seen in forage plants [plamitic acid (C16:0), SA (C18:0), OA, LA and ALA)], which constitute up to 95% of their total FAs content (Arvidsson, 2009). The FAs associated with galactolipids contain higher proportions of LA and ALA (Van Soest, 1994). The chloroplasts constitute the most abundant membranes (as thylakoids) in green leaves, comprising up to 70% of the lipids in green tissue. Thus, the galactolipids dominate the lipids in photosynthetic tissues (Taiz & Zeiger, 2002). So, leaves are rich in ALA (between 60% and 75% of total FAs), LA and C16:0 (6% - 20%), while OA is a minor component (less than 5%). The concentration of galactolipids declines with age and varies with the proportion of leaves to stems and other metabolically active plant tissues (Arvidsson, 2009). Importantly, biohydrogenation of unsaturated C_{18} FAs in the rumen is higher on grass-based diets, which might result in decreased levels of CLAs in the milk (*i.e.*, the intermediate CLA is not retained as a by-product), which may adversely affect the expected nutritional properties of diary and meat products imparted by CLA

(Daley et al., 2010; Lejonklev et al., 2013). However, olive leaf forage was found more efficient to enhance the concentration of 9-CLA and ALA in milk. Apart from nutritional value, it may help ruminal biohydorgenation at several steps (Abbeddou et al., 2011).

OLEIC ACID (OA)

Share of OA in the lipid profile of leafy food is comparatively less (1-5%). Compared to LA and ALA, OA is less significant to serve as a precursor of CLA. However, being an unsaturated FA, it undergoes biohydrogenation in the rumen toward SA. Forty-five years ago, Dawson & Kemp (1969) incubated (39 ^{o}C) OA directly with rumen content collected from sheep and demonstrated that by hydrogenation, OA was completely converted into SA. This conversion rate was evaluated using ^{14}C-labeled substrate and rumen fluid (mixed population of bacteria and protozoa), and SA formed at 15, 30 and 60 min was 35, 50 and 62%, respectively. In addition, using ^{13}C-labeled OA, Abughazaleh et al. (2005) examined whether any connection existed between the effect of pH and dilution rate of rumen content on the biohydrogenation of OA. The conversion rates (biohydrogenation intermediates) of OA were determined by using ruminal micro-organisms grown in continuous culture at pH 5.5 and 6.5, and dilution rates were 0.05 and 0.10/h, respectively. They concluded that the ruminal microbiota are able to convert OA to a variety of *trans*-$C_{18:1}$ positional isomers, when the ruminal environment reached at pH 6.5 and 0.10/h dilution treatment. Also, at low pH and dilution rate, the biohydrogenation of OA to *trans*-C18:1 still occurred.

The biohydrogenation of OA by mixed ruminal micro-organism involves the arrangement of several positional isomers of *trans*-monoenes, rather than merely through biohydrogenation to form SA (Morvan & Joblin, 2000). It also suggests that the capacity to hydrate OA may be a property of many lactic acid bacteria, such as *Lactobacillus lactis* and *Leuconostoc dextranicum* in anaerobic cultures, and that there was no evidence to prove the direct conversion of OA to SA. From this, it is evident that OA may be distorted to be a variety of lipid species (like 10-hydoxy SA and 10-keto SA) (Jenkins et al., 2006). Thus, the biohydrogenation of OA by mixed ruminal microbes involves the formation of several positional isomers of *trans* monoenes (18:1) rather than only direct biohydrogenation to form SA; which span from C_6 to C_{16} along the acyl chain including VA, the immediate precursors of CLA (Grinari et al., 2000; Turpinen et al., 2002; Mosley et al., 2002).

LINOLEIC ACID

LA serves as the predominant precursor of CLA in the rumen (Figure 2). One of the first conclusive studies in this regard demonstrated that upon incubation with LA in D_2O, 9-CLA was produced with a single deuterium atom at C_{13} (Kepler & Tove, 1967). Apart from 9-CLA, an additional CLA isomer reported to arise during the biohydrogenation of LA was 10-CLA (in comparison to 9-CLA, the concentration of 10-CLA was very less or even negligible).

Species belonging to the genera *Butyrivibrio (B)*, *Bifidobacterium (Bif)*, *Lactobacillus (Lb)* and *Propionibacterium (P)* are the common bacteria used for biohydrogenation studies with LA. Like *B. fibriosolvens*, *Bifidobacterium* spp. have also been shown to possess high efficiency for converting LA to CLA isomers (Table 1 in the Appendix). Production of CLA by *Bifidobacterium* spp. exhibited considerable interspecies variations: *Bif. breve* and *Bif. dentium* are the most efficient producers of CLA, with *Bif. breve* converting up to 65% of LA to 9-CLA when grown in 0.55 mg/ml LA (Coakely et al., 2003). Strains of *Lactobacillus*, *Lactococcus (Lc)*, *Pediococcus (Pc)* and *Bifidobacterium* showed considerable variations with respect to their sensitivity to LA (Coakely et al., 2003). Of the various strains of lactic acid bacteria, *Lb. plantarum* was shown as the best producer of CLA from LA, which could produce up to 40 mg 9-CLA/ml reaction mixture containing 12% LA (w/v) in 120 h incubation, mostly in cell-bound form (Kishino et al., 2002). *Lactobacillus plantarum* strain lp15 isolated from naturally fermented Chinese pickle showed up to 26% conversion (75% of the CLA isomers were 9-CLA) with the best tolerance (up to 600 μg/ml) of LA in the medium (Liu et al., 2011), while *Lactobacillus* spp. showed the maximum production of CLA (80.14 to 131.63 μg/ml) at 24 h of incubation in broth containing 0.02% of free LA (Alonso et al., 2003). *Propionibacterium freudenreichii*, a commonly used bacterium in dairy starter cultures showed the extracellular production of CLA (2.65mg/ml), of which 70% represented 9-CLA (Jiang et al., 1999).

ALPHA-LINOLENIC ACID (ALA)

Owing to the health benefits of ALA, it is popularly known as vitamin F (Burr & Burr, 1930). Over 3 decades ago, it was demonstrated that ALA, the major FA of grass lipids could be biohydrogenated to SA through the mediation of various FAs, including VA, by mixed rumen bacteria dominated by *Butyrivibrio* spp. (Kemp & Lander, 1983). Compared to insignificant biohydrogenation activities of pure culture like *Streptococcus faecalis, Escherichia coli, Clostridium perfringens,* and coliforms isolated from sheep faeces, the conversion rate of ALA to VA by *B. fibrisolvens* was better (Wilde & Dawson, 1966). *Butyrivibrio hungatei* isolated from the rumen of a grazing cow could efficiently convert ALA into SA *via* CLA, LA and VA, which indicates that mixed *trans*-positional isomers are intermediate in the biohydrogenation of *cis*-FAs to SA (Vossenberg & Joblin, 2003).

In fact, compared to LA, ruminal biohydrogenation of the essential ALA is not fully understood. Nevertheless, Dhiman et al. (2000) demonstrated that CLA content in the milk fat could be enhanced by four-folds (up to 2.08% of total FAs), if the cows are fed with the diet enriched by soybean oil (4% w/w), which is rich in ALA. However, it was not conclusive whether this effect was due to LA or ALA present in the oil. Therefore, information on the routes involved in biohydrogenation of LA and ALA in the rumen and subsequent endogenous metabolism of related biohydrogenation products needs to be made clear (Destaillats et al., 2005). Lactic acid bacteria could produce conjugated trienoic FAs from α- and γ-linolenic acids; the trienoic FAs produced from ALA were *cis*-9,*trans*-11,*cis*-15- and *trans*-9,*trans*-11,*cis*-15-octadecatrienoic acids (18:3) (Kishino et al., 2009). The presence of (*cis*-9,*trans*-11,*cis*-15)-octadecatrioenic acid and (*cis*-9,*trans*-13,*cis*-15)-octadecatrioenic acid (isorumenic acid) in the milk fat were observed by the biohydrogenation of ALA. Therefore, it appears that 9-CLA found in milk fat could be partially formed by both ruminal biohydrogenation of ALA through the reduction of isorumelenic acid, and the rest by endogenous Δ^9-desaturation of VA (Destaillats et al., 2005). However, under *in vivo* conditions, the normal biohydrogenation may be hindered by the dietary factors, for instance, tannins inhibited the biohydrogenation of ALA to SA (Khiaosa-Ard et al., 2009). Khiaosa-Ard et al. (2009) also showed that the concentration of VA can be enhanced by suppressing the population of protozoa, and enhancing the bacterial population in the rumen; thus removing potential microbes involved in biohydrogenation and increasing competition between bacteria involved in biohydrogenation and others.

Chemical Synthesis

Chemical synthesis is the major route for CLA production because it is simple and does not require sophisticated equipment, or expensive enzymes. Conventional alkali isomerization methods (in organic solvents like ethylene glycol, propylene glycol, dimethyl sulfoxide or dimethyl formamide) are used for producing CLA from oils like sunflower, safflower, and soybean, which are rich in LA (Table 2 in the Appendix). In fact, most of the commercially available CLAs are produced by the alkaline isomerization of oils, and tend to contain an equimolar mixture of 9- and 10-CLAs, together with a mixture of variable quantities (up to 30%) of other geometrical and positional isomers of CLA, and that 100% pure CLA isomer is not available on the market (Christie, 2003). Therefore, the primary focus of all mechanistic, preclinical and clinical studies pertaining to CLA were on 9- and 10-CLAs – especially a mixture of both or rarely one of these two isomers (with others isomers as impurities) (Benjamin et al., 2005; Benjamin et al., 2013; Benjamin et al., 2015).

Photoisomerization of vegetable oils with iodine as a catalyst seems to be a simple step of producing CLA in laboratory without high-energy input or expensive enzymes and microorganisms (Gangidi & Proctor, 2004). Jain et al. (2008) showed that ultraviolet irradiation of soy oil could yield up to 16.4% CLA; and LA from soy oil in static mode could yield up to 22% of total CLA content in the presence of 0.35% iodine (catalyst) in a 0.5 cm thick oil layer on reflective surfaces maintained at 48 °C for 12 h. In soy oil medium, metals like Ruthenium and Nickel showed the best isomerization activity, while lead favored the double bond hydrogenation. Chemisorbed hydrogen amplified the conversion rate of the reaction, but with decreased isomerization selectivity (Bernas et al., 2003). The isomerization property of LA was checked by the Na-zeolites (i.e., microporous, aluminosilicate minerals commonly used as commercial adsorbents and catalysts) and its acid modified types (H^+, Ni^{2+}), the rate of conversion of LA to CLA was increased in the excess quantity of weak-moderate acid centers coupled with convenience of the acid sites (Cardó et al., 2012). Pakdeechanuan et al. (2010) performed alkylene isomerization for CLA production in propylene glycol solvent system. It could be done by blending sunflower oil with propylene glycol at different proportions, and that a 2:1 ratio (oil: propylene) for 80 min would be effective. CLA can be produced from castor oil by dehydration in the presence of dehydrating agents [(Potassium hydroxideor 1,8- diazabicyclo- (5.4.0)- undec- 7- ene (DBU)]. Potassium hydroxidefacilitated 77% conversion at 80 °C, while DBU catalyzed the reaction with 88% conversion efficiency (Yang et al., 2002). Though various methods as above are applied successfully for the commercial production of CLA, biological production is a thrust area for many researchers.

BIOSYNTHESIS OF CLA

The rumen is the major site for the biosynthesis of CLA in ruminant animals. The rumen microbial ecosystem is well established for its capacity to biohydrogenate unsaturated MUFAs and PUFAs in the feed into SA. Ruminants consume lignocellulosic agricultural by-products such as tree foliage, sugarcane bagasse (i.e., the fibrous matter that remains after sugarcane is

crushed to extract its juice), cereal straws, cake oil seeds (like coconut, groundnut, cotton, mustard and soybean), *etc*., which are rich in OA, LA, ALA. Szolloskei et al. (2005) demonstrated three kinds of oil-based diets such as sunflower oil, soybean oil and fish oil, which were incubated in rumen-fistulated adult ewes. After the incubation period, sunflower and soybean oils containing the LA ratio were decreased significantly due to an increased quantity of 9-CLA. Apart from soybean oil, vegetable oils like cottonseed and corn oils supplemented diets also increased the formation of CLA, coupled with improvement in the milk production (Zheng et al., 2005). A possible route for the biosynthesis of CLA is shown in Figure 2.

Generally speaking, the enrichment of cattle feed is intended for enhancing the quantity and quality (*e.g.*, by enriching CLA and VA) of milk. For instance, Bu et al.(2007) fed Holstein dairy cows a diet containing 59% forage (control) or a basal diet supplemented with either 4% soybean oil (rich ion LA), 4% flaxseed oil (rich in ALA) or 2% soybean oil plus 2% flaxseed oil on a DM basis. Total FAs in the diet were: 3.27, 7.47, 7.61, and 7.50 g/100 g in control, soybean oil, flaxseed oil and combination of these two oils, respectively. The proportions of VA were increased by 318% (soybean), 105% (flaxseed), and 206% (soybean and flaxseed) in milk fat from cows compared with the control group. Similarly, concentration of 9-CLA was also increased 273% (soybean), 150% (flaxseed) and 183% (soybean and flaxseed). From this, it is evident that oils rich in LA are better for biohydrogenation than ALA-rich oils (Bu et al., 2007).

CLA PRODUCTION: PLANTS, MICROBES, AND MAMMALS

Plants produce the precursor FAs for the bio- and chemical synthesis of CLAs. Plants such as sunflower, soybean, groundnut, coconut, safflower, oil palm are the major sources of edible oils (Table 2) (Anonymous, 2014). These oils contain high nutritional values because it contains essential FAs (*i.e.*, LA and ALA). Food products such as high CLA salad oils, CLA rich potato chips, yogurts, and dairy products meet the daily requirements of CLA isomers. However, no plants are known to produce CLA.

Microbial Production

Ruminal microorganisms hydrogenate MUFAs and PUFAs present in forages. Therefore, the direction of biohydrogenation determines the concentration of CLA in meat and milk (Maia et al., 2007). The rumen microbial ecosystem is comprised of a diverse consortium of microorganisms, consisting of over 1000 species of bacteria (10^{10} to 10^{12}cells/ml), over 100 species of methanogenic archaea (10^{7} to 10^{9}cells/ml), over 25 genera of rumen protozoa (10^{4} to 10^{6}/ml), at least5 genera of anaerobic fungi (10^{3} to 10^{6} zoospore/ml), and 10^{9} to 10^{10}viruses/ml (Wright & Klieve, 2011). Of this, bacteria play the pivotal role in biohydrogenation.

Bacterial CLA Production

A number of CLA producing bacteria have been isolated from the gastro-intestinal (GI) tract (especially rumen) of ruminants, they mainly belong to the genera *Bifidobacterium, Butyvibrio, Lactobacillus, Lactococcus* and *Propionibacterium* (Table 1). *Lactobacillus acidophilus, Lactobacillus delbrueckii* subsp.*bulgaricus, Lactobacillus delbrueckii* subsp.*lactase, Lactobacillus lactis* subsp. *cremoris,*and *Lactobacillus lactase* subsp.*lactis,* are the prominent CLA producing lactobacilli (Ogawa et al., 2001; Coakley et al., 2003; Lin et al., 2005; Lin, 2006; Liu et al., 2011). Different species of *Bifidobacteria (e.g., B. brevi, B. lactis, B. delactis* and *B. dentium*) produce relatively higher quantities of CLA (Coakley et al., 2003; Hennessy et al., 2012; O'Shea et al., 2012; Bogsan et al., 2013). *Propionibacterium freudenreichii* subsp.*freudenreichii, P. freudenreichii* ssp. *Shermanii* (Jiang et al., 1998; McKain et al., 2010; Cousin et al., 2011), *B. fibrisolvens, B. hungatei* (Kepler et al., 1966; Devillard et al., 2007), *Megasphaera elsdenii* (Kim et al., 2002), *C. proteoclasticum* (Wallace et al., 2007), and *Pediococcus* sp. (Dubey et al., 2012) have also been shown to produce CLA. In 1966, Kepler et al. studied the biohydrogenation of LA in to CLA isomers by *B. fibrisolvens,* and demonstrated that the first reaction in the biohydrogenation of LA by *B. fibrisolvens* is the isomerization of LA to 9-CLA, along with the formation of different octadecadienoic (18:2) and monoenoic(18:1) acids. Since *B. fibriosolvens* has a greater CLA producing capacity than other ruminant bacteria, it has often been used as the model bacterium for CLA production *in vitro.*

The main focus of microbial CLA production has been on 9-CLA. However, if the normal feed is enriched. Then the ruminal production of CLA can be reversed. For instance, Kim et al. (2002) showed that *M.elsdenii* strain YJ4, isolated from the ruminal content of cow fed with lactate and trypticase enriched grains, catalized LA to 10-CLA (7 μg/mg protein)*via* biohydrogenation. *Propionibacterium acnes* isomerized LA to 10-CLA, *B. proteoclasticus* carried out substantial conversion of 18:1 substrates to 18:0, *P. acnes* hydrated OA and VA to 10-OH-18:0, which was further oxidized to yield 10-O-18:0 (McKain et al., 2010). The ability of lactic acid bacteria (especially *Lb. plantarum*) to produce CLA from ricinoleic acid (12-OH-9-*cis*-octadecenoic acid) has been demonstrated (Ando et al., 2003). The CLA produced (in the free FA form) consisted of a mixture of two CLA isomers, 9-CLA (21% of total CLA) and *trans*-9,*trans*-11-octadecadienoic acid (79% of total CLA), and accounted for 72% of the total FA obtained

Role of Protozoa

Rumen protozoa, like *Dasytricha ruminantium, Isotricha prostoma, Eremoplastron dilobum, Entodinium caudatum, Ophryoscolex purkinjei,* and *Polyplastron multive-*

siculatum are known to contribute to the production of various CLA isomers (Williams & Coleman,1997; Or-Rashid et al., 2008; Khiaosa-Ard et al., 2009, Wright, 2009). Towne et al. (1990) showed that bacteria alone or bacteria in association with protozoa could produce various CLA isomers from LA, and finally to SA by the reduction of $C_{18:1}$ FA. In fact, protozoa *per se* are incapable of biohydrogenating LA, but in comparison to the independent biohydrogenation activity of bacteria, in conjunction with protozoa, enhanced the rate of biohydrogenation of LA significantly (Or-Rashid et al., 2011).

Rumen protozoa are shown to have viable bacteria within (intracellular) and or attached to the surface (extracellular) of the protozoa (Williams & Coleman, 1997). Although protozoa are rich in CLA and VA, they appear to lack the ability to form these two FAs from LA or SA. The flow of CLA and VA across the duodenum is intimately associated with the protozoal population in the rumen. The most likely explanation to this is that protozoa preferentially incorporate CLA and VA (formed by bacteria), and that the flow of unsaturated FAs, including CLA and VA, from the rumen could depend on the flow of protozoa rather than bacteria (Devillard et al., 2006; Yanez-Ruiz et al., 2006; Váradyová et al., 2007).The balance between the protozoal and bacterial communities in the rumen decides the predominance of a particular intermediate of the biohydrogenation (Khiaosa-Ard et al., 2009). It clearly indicates a symbiotic association between ruminal bacteria and protozoa. Thus, removing potential microbes involved in biohydrogenation and increasing competition between ruminal bacteria and prototoa specific isomers of CLA can be produced.

Role of Fungi

Apart from bacteria and protozoa, ruminal anaerobic fungi like *Piromonas communis, Neocallimastix frontalis,* and *Orpinomyces* spp., also contribute to CLA production (Nam & Garnsworthy, 2007). Approximately 10^3-10^5 zoospore/ml (Phycomycetes) anaerobic fungi are present in the rumen fluid. Recently, Ando et al. (2009) showed that non ruminal fungi (species of *Mortierella* and *Delacroixia*) and yeast (*Pichia farinose, P. wickerhamii* and *Saccharomyces rouxii*) could produce CLA from VA. Of them, *Delacroixia coronata* IFO 8586 selectively produced 9-CLA (98% of total CLA) from VA by Δ^9-desaturase activity, mainly in the form of triacylglycerols (69% of total CLA).Selective production of 10-CLA (5.9% total FA) was achieved in glucose medium by the heterologous expression of LA-isomerase gene from *P. acnes* in the oleaginous yeast, *Yarrowia lipolytica* (Zhang, et al., 2012)

Figure 3.

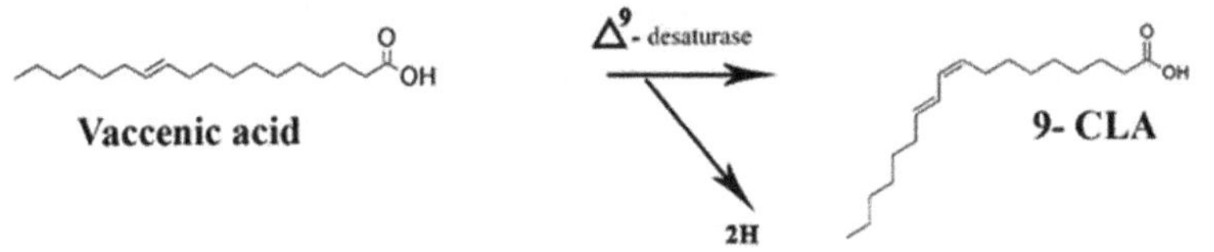

CLA PRODUCTION IN MAMMALS

Apart from the ruminal microbial biosynthesis, CLA is formed by the endogenous conversion at the tissue level from the dietary VA (Griinari et al., 2000; Turpinen et al., 2002). The Δ^9-desaturase inserts a double bond in *cis*-configuration on the VA, thereby 9-CLA is formed (Figure 3). Apart from VA, it was shown that microorganisms dwelling in the gastrointestinal tract of humans can also produce CLA from VA, just as in rumen biohydrogenation. Rosberg-Cody et al. (2004) collected fecal material from 24 neonates aged between 3 days and 2 months in a neonatal unit (Erinville Hospital, Cork, Ireland). A total of 46 isolates from six neonates were confirmed to be *Bifidobacterium* spp. (Rosberg-Cody et al., 2004). They showed that the most efficient producers belonged to *Bif. breve*, which converted up to 27% of the free LA to the 9-CLA/μgdry cells. In addition, a strain of *Bif. bifidum* showed a conversion rate of 18%/μg dry cells. The use of lactic acid bacteria like *Lb. acidophilus* and *Lb. casei* isolated from human intestine synthesized 9-CLA in skim milk supplemented with 0.02% free LA. In this medium, the total quantity of free CLA after 24 h of incubation ranged from 54.31 to 116.53 μg/ml (Alonso et al., 2003). *Ruberia* spp. isolated from intestine (Devillard et al., 2007) could efficiently produce 9-CLA from LA, probably though the mediation of VA (in tissues) or 10-hydroxy octadeceinoic acid.

MODULATORS OF MICROBIAL CLA PRODUCTION

Microbial PUFA production is discussed mainly as a typical example for single cell oils (Sakuradani et al., 2010). A wide range of plant bioactive components (phytochemicals like saponins, tannins and essential oils, *etc.*) have been identified as having potential to modulate the processes of fermentation in the rumen. The use of plants or plant extracts as natural feed additives has become a subject of interest. Tannins seem to be a good means to modulate the FA profile of rumen bacteria, favouring the accumulation of VA during *in vitro* rumen fermentation (Buccioni et al., 2011), probably by changing ruminal microbial populations (Vasta et al., 2010). Recently, it was concluded that the cumin seed extract had the potential to enhance CLA and PUFA content of milk in lactating goat (Miri et al., 2013). Further investigations are necessary to assess the mode of action of cumin in the rumen and to explore the effect of cumin on the activity of Δ^9-desaturase activity (Miri et al., 2013).

FACTORS AFFECTING BIOHYDROGENATION

Numerous factors can affect the biohydrogenation process. *In vitro* studies show that the main factors like pH, type of FA (feed), incubation time, microorganisms and aeration decide the biohydrogenation process. Park et al (2009) studied the effect of pH, aeration (anaerobic or aerobic condition), and incubation time for CLA production, and concluded that pH is a significant factor. They also found that the maximum CLA production could be reached at around pH 5.5 under anaerobic condition in 24h of incubation, and production reduced subsequently at higher or lower pH level. Many reports reveal inhibitory role of high FA concentration in the biohydrogenation mechanism. For instance, CLA production was inhibited when the LA concentration in the medium reached above 0.5mg/ml (Coakely et al., 2003). An in vitro pH around 6.0 would be better for the concomitant production of 9-CLA and VA (Martin& Jenkins, 2002). *Lactobacillus plantarum* showed a higher yield of CLA (80% molar yield to LA) with 2.6% (wt/vol) LA as the substrate in 96 h (*i.e.*, 20 mg/mL reaction mixture). However, the molar yield was reduced to 33% when the LA concentration was increased to 12% (wt/vol) (Kishino et al., 2002). Lactose and fructose are suggested for use in maintaining a high CLA level when lactic acid bacteria are employed for the production of CLA (Lin, 2000). While growing *P. freudenreichii* subsp. *shermanii,* the inhibitory effect of FA on CLA was overcome by using a detergent like polyoxyethylene sorbitanmonooleate (LA:detergent ratio, 1:15) (Rainio et al., 2001). Though rumen biohydrogenation is occurring anaerobically, most of the bacteria are aerotolerant (i.e., facultative aerobes) can also be used for CLA production. Interestingly,various studies show that bacteria efficiently produce CLA in vitro under aerobic (Lin, 2000; Choi et al., 2005) or micro-aerobic (Wang et al., 2007) conditions.

IS RUMINAL BIOHYDROGENATION A DEFENSIVE MECHANISM?

The rumen diet typically contains PUFAs, which are toxic to many rumen microorganisms. To protect themselves against these toxins, certain rumen microorganisms have evolved the ability to hydrolyze and biohydrogenate these dietary lipids into a saturated form; resulting in the formation of CLA (Kemp et al., 1984). Based on the reaction and end product of biohydrogenation, these bacteria are grouped into two groups: Group A bacteria are able to hydrogenate LA and ALA to VA (i.e., the major end product), and Group B bacteria are able to utilize VA as one of the main substrates with SA being the end product (Kemp et al., 1984).

Cellulolytic bacteria did not grow in the presence of any PUFA at 50 μg/ml concentration, nor did some butyrate-producing bacteria, including the SA producer *C. proteoclasticum, B.hungatei* and *Eub. ruminantium* (Maia et al., 2007). PUFA also inhibited the growth of the cellulolytic ruminal fungi like *N. frontalis* (Maia et al., 2007). Thus, the toxicity imparted by unsaturated FAs to the ruminal microbes compels them to unsaturated (to detoxify) the FAs to (VA); during the process, CLA is produced as a by-product. Unsaturated FAs may act as true inhibitors of bacterial conjugation, thereby genetic variability is debarred (Fernandez-Lopez et al., 2005). Conjugation inhibitors may provide a means to control the spread of antibiotic resistance (Fernandez-Lopez et al., 2005). CLAs may inhibit the hyphal growth in *C. albicans* by modulating Ras1p and down regulating TEC1 expression (Shareck et al., 2011). Briefly, microorganisms have evolved the ability to unsaturate FAs, and the energy derived during the process enables them to survive in their micro ecological niche (i.e, the rumen).

CONCLUSION

Research on CLA spanning four decades suggests that grass-based diets can significantly improve the FA composition and antioxidant content of beef, albeit with variable impacts on overall palatability. Bio-hydrogenation of C_{18} unsaturated FAs in the rumen occurs rapidly, but the range of hydrogenation is quite varying, and dependent on the degree of unsaturation and configuration of FAs, microbial type and the experimental condition. A consortium of rumen microorganisms is more efficient for the *in vitro* production of CLA, than individual cultures, which indicates the significance of mutualism between bacteria and protozoa in the rumen. It further shows that protozoa are incapable of producing CLA, but augment CLA production in conjunction with the bacteria. Although there has been an unprecedented resurgence in the area of microbial production of CLA, a viable strategy for its production at commercial level is yet to be developed.

CONFLICT OF INTEREST

The authors declare that there exists no conflict of interest.

ACKNOWLEDGMENT

The authors gratefully acknowledge the Department of Biotechnology (DBT), Ministry of Science and Technology, Government of India, for a research grant (No. BT/PR 12714/FNS/20/411/2009).

REFERENCES

Abbeddou, S., Rischkowsky, B., Richter, E. K., Hess, H. D., & Kreuzer, M. (2011). Modification of milk fatty acid composition by feeding forages and agro-industrial byproducts from dry areas to Awassi sheep. *Journal of Dairy Science*, *94*(9), 4657–4668. doi:10.3168/jds.2011-4154 PMID:21854938

AbuGhazaleh, A. A., Riley, M. B., Thies, E. E., & Jenkins, T. C. (2005). Dilution rate and pH effects on the conversion of oleic acid to trans C 18: 1 positional isomers in continuous culture. *Journal of Dairy Science*, *88*(12), 4334–4341. doi:10.3168/jds.S0022-0302(05)73120-9 PMID:16291625

Aii, T., Tamaki, M., Shimabukuro, H., Hayasawa, H., Shimizu, T., & Ishida, S. (1999). Conjugated linoleic acid content in milk fat of the cows fed a large amount of linseed. *Animal Science Journal*, *70*(6), 535–541.

Alonso, L., Cuesta, E. P., & Gilliland, S. E. (2003). Production of free conjugated linoleic acid by Lactobacillus acidophilus and Lactobacillus casei of human intestinal origin. *Journal of Dairy Science*, *86*(6), 1941–1946. doi:10.3168/jds.S0022-0302(03)73781-3 PMID:12836928

Ando, A., Ogawa, J., Kishino, S., & Shimizu, S. (2003). CLA production from ricinoleic acid by lactic acid bacteria. *Journal of the American Oil Chemists' Society*, *80*(9), 889–894. doi:10.1007/s11746-003-0790-1

Ando, A., Ogawa, J., Sugimoto, S., Kishino, S., Sakuradani, E., Yokozeki, K., & Shimizu, S. (2009). Selective production of cis-9, trans-11 isomer of conjugated linoleic acid from trans-vaccenic acid methyl ester by Delacroixia coronata. *Journal of Applied Microbiology*, *106*(5), 1697–1704. doi:10.1111/j.1365-2672.2008.04139.x PMID:19226396

Anonymous. (n.d.). Retrieved 1 July 2014 from: http://thepaleodiet.com/vegetable-oil-fatty-acid-composition/

Arvidsson, K. (2009). *Factors affecting fatty acid composition in forage and milk*. (Doctoral Thesis). Swedish University of Agricultural Sciences.

Bartlet, J. C., & Chapman, D. G. (1961). Butter adulteration, detection of hydrogenated fats in butter fat by measurement of cis-trans conjugated unsaturation. *Journal of Agricultural and Food Chemistry*, *9*(1), 50–53. doi:10.1021/jf60113a015

Bauman, D. E., Everett, R. W., Weiland, W. H., & Collier, R. J. (1999). Production responses to bovine somatotropin in northeast dairy herds. *Journal of Dairy Science*, *82*(12), 2564–2573. doi:10.3168/jds.S0022-0302(99)75511-6 PMID:10629802

Benjamin, S., Flotho, S., Börchers, T., & Spener, F. (2013). Conjugated linoleic acid isomers and their precursor fatty acids regulate peroxisome proliferator-activated receptor subtypes and major peroxisome proliferator responsive element-bearing target genes in HepG2 cell model. *Journal of Zhejiang University. Science. B.*, *14*(2), 115–123. doi:10.1631/jzus.B1200175 PMID:23365010

Benjamin, S., Hanhoff, T., Börchers, T., & Spener, F. (2005). An improved molecular test system for the screening of human PPAR transactivation by conjugated linoleic acid isomers and their precursor fatty acids. *European Journal of Lipid Science and Technology*, *107*(10), 706–715. doi:10.1002/ejlt.200401041

Benjamin, S., Prakasan, P., Sreedharan, S., Wright, A. D. G., & Spener, F. (2015). Pros and cons of CLA consumption: An insight from clinical evidences. *Nutrition & Metabolosm*, *12*(1), 4. doi:10.1186/1743-7075-12-4 PMID:25972911

Benjamin, S., & Spener, F. (2009). Conjugated linoleic acids as functional food: An insight into their health benefits. *Nutrition Metabolism*, *6*(1), 36. doi:10.1186/1743-7075-6-36 PMID:19761624

Bernas, A., Kumar, N., Mäki-Arvela, P., Kul'kova, N. V., Holmbom, B., Salmi, T., & Murzin, D. Y. (2003). Isomerization of linoleic acid over supported metal catalysts. *Applied Catalysis A, General*, *245*(2), 257–275. doi:10.1016/S0926-860X(02)00646-4

Bogsan, C. S., Florence, A. C. R., Perina, N., Hirota, C., Soares, F. A. S. M., Silva, R. C., & Oliveira, M. N. (2013). Survival of Bi fi dobacterium lactis HN019 and release of biogenic compounds in unfermented and fermented milk is affected by chilled storage at 4 C. *Journal of Probiotics and Health*, *4*(1).

Bu, D. P., Wang, J. Q., Dhiman, T. R., & Liu, S. J. (2007). Effectiveness of oils rich in linoleic and linolenic acids to enhance conjugated linoleic acid in milk from dairy cows. *Journal of Dairy Science*, *90*(2), 998–1007. doi:10.3168/jds.S0022-0302(07)71585-0 PMID:17235178

Buccioni, A., Minieri, S., Rapaccini, S., Antongiovanni, M., & Mele, M. (2011). Effect of chestnut and quebracho tannins on fatty acid profile in rumen liquid-and solid-associated bacteria: An in vitro study. *Animal*, *5*(10), 1521–1530. doi:10.1017/S1751731111000759 PMID:22440342

Burr, G. O., & Burr, M. M. (1930). On the nature and role of the fatty acids essential in nutrition. *The Journal of Biological Chemistry*, *86*(2), 587–621.

Cardó, X., Bergadà, O., Cesteros, Y., & Salagre, P. (2012). Effect of catalyst acidity and porosity on the catalytic isomerization of linoleic acid to obtain conjugated linoleic acids (CLAs). *Chemical Engineering Journal*, *183*, 459–465. doi:10.1016/j.cej.2011.12.088

Choi, N. J., Imm, J. Y., Oh, S., Kim, B. C., Hwang, H. J., & Kim, Y. J. (2005). Effect of pH and oxygen on conjugated linoleic acid (CLA) production by mixed rumen bacteria from cows fed high concentrate and high forage diets. *Animal Feed Science and Technology*, *123*, 643–653. doi:10.1016/j.anifeedsci.2005.04.054

Christie, W. W. (2003). Analysis of conjugated linoleic acid: An overview. *Advances in Conjugated Linoleic Acid Research*, *2*, 1–12.

Coakley, M., Ross, R. P., Nordgren, M., Fitzgerald, G., Devery, R., & Stanton, C. (2003). Conjugated linoleic acid biosynthesis by human-derived *Bifidobacterium* species. *Journal of Applied Microbiology*, *94*(1), 138–145. doi:10.1046/j.1365-2672.2003.01814.x PMID:12492934

Cousin, F. J., Mater, D. D., Foligne, B., & Jan, G. (2011). Dairy propionibacteria as human probiotics: A review of recent evidence. *Dairy Science & Technology*, *91*(1), 1–26.

Daley, C. A., Abbott, A., Doyle, P. S., Nader, G. A., & Larson, S. (2010). A review of fatty acid profiles and antioxidant content in grass-fed and grain-fed beef. *Nutrition Journal*, *9*(1), 10. doi:10.1186/1475-2891-9-10 PMID:20219103

Dawson, R. M., & Kemp, P. (1969). The effect of defaunation on the phospholipids and on the hydrogenation of unsaturated fatty acids in the rumen. *The Biochemical Journal*, *115*(2), 351–352. doi:10.1042/bj1150351 PMID:5378385

Destaillats, F., Trottier, J. P., Galvez, J. G., & Angers, P. (2005). Analysis of α-linolenic acid biohydrogenation intermediates in milk fat with emphasis on conjugated linolenic acids. *Journal of Dairy Science*, *88*(9), 3231–3239. doi:10.3168/jds.S0022-0302(05)73006-X PMID:16107413

Devillard, E., McIntosh, F. M., Duncan, S. H., & Wallace, R. J. (2007). Metabolism of linoleic acid by human gut bacteria: Different routes for biosynthesis of conjugated linoleic acid. *Journal of Bacteriology*, *189*(6), 2566–2570. doi:10.1128/JB.01359-06 PMID:17209019

Devillard, E., McIntosh, F. M., Newbold, C. J., & Wallace, R. J. (2006). Rumen ciliate protozoa contain high concentrations of conjugated linoleic acids and vaccenic acid, yet do not hydrogenate linoleic acid or desaturate stearic acid. *The British Journal of Nutrition*, *96*(04), 697–704. PMID:17010229

Dhiman, T. R., Satter, L. D., Pariza, M. W., Galli, M. P., Albright, K., & Tolosa, M. X. (2000). Conjugated linoleic acid (CLA) content of milk from cows offered diets rich in linoleic and linolenic acid. *Journal of Dairy Science*, *83*(5), 1016–1027. doi:10.3168/jds.S0022-0302(00)74966-6 PMID:10821577

Dobson, G. (2003). Gas chromatography-mass spectrometry of conjugated linoleic acids and metabolites. *Advances in Conjugated Linoleic Acid Research*, *2*, 13–36.

Dubey, V., Ghosh, A. R., & Mandal, B. K. (2012). Appraisal of conjugated linoleic acid production by probiotic potential of *Pediococcus* spp. GS4. *Applied Biochemistry and Biotechnology*, *168*(5), 1265–1276. doi:10.1007/s12010-012-9855-9 PMID:22971829

Eastridge, M. L. (2006). Major advances in applied dairy cattle nutrition. *Journal of Dairy Science*, *89*(4), 1311–1323. doi:10.3168/jds.S0022-0302(06)72199-3 PMID:16537963

Fernandez-Lopez, R., Machón, C., Longshaw, C. M., Martin, S., Molin, S., Zechner, E. L., & de la Cruz, F. et al. (2005). Unsaturated fatty acids are inhibitors of bacterial conjugation. *Microbiology*, *151*(11), 3517–3526. doi:10.1099/mic.0.28216-0 PMID:16272375

Gangidi, R. R., & Proctor, A. (2004). Photochemical production of conjugated linoleic acid from soybean oil. *Lipids*, *39*(6), 577–582. doi:10.1007/s11745-004-1266-7 PMID:15554158

Griinari, J. M., Corl, B. A., Lacy, S. H., Chouinard, P. Y., Nurmela, K. V. V., & Bauman, D. E. (2000). Conjugated linoleic acid is synthesized endogenously in lactating dairy cows by Δ9-desaturase. *The Journal of Nutrition*, *130*(9), 2285–2291. PMID:10958825

Hennessy, A. A., Barrett, E., Ross, R. P., Fitzgerald, G. F., Devery, R., & Stanton, C. (2012). The production of conjugated α-linolenic, γ-linolenic and stearidonic acids by strains of *bifidobacteria* and *propionibacteria*. *Lipids*, *47*(3), 313–327. doi:10.1007/s11745-011-3636-z PMID:22160449

Hristov, A. N., Kennington, L. R., McGuire, M. A., & Hunt, C. W. (2005). Effect of diets containing linoleic acid-or oleic acid-rich oils on ruminal fermentation and nutrient digestibility, and performance and fatty acid composition of adipose and muscle tissues of finishing cattle. *Journal of Animal Science*, *83*(6), 1312–1321. PMID:15890808

Jain, V. P., Proctor, A., & Lall, R. (2008). Pilot-scale production of conjugated linoleic acid-rich soy oil by photoirradiation. *Journal of Food Science*, *73*(4), 183–192. doi:10.1111/j.1750-3841.2008.00718.x PMID:18460128

Jenkins, T. C., AbuGhazaleh, A. A., Freeman, S., & Thies, E. J. (2006). The production of 10-hydroxystearic and 10-ketostearic acids is an alternative route of oleic acid transformation by the ruminal microbiota in cattle. *The Journal of Nutrition*, *136*(4), 926–931. PMID:16549452

Jiang, J., Björck, L., & Fonden, R. (1998). Production of conjugated linoleic acid by dairy starter cultures. *Journal of Applied Microbiology*, *85*(1), 95–102. doi:10.1046/j.1365-2672.1998.00481.x PMID:9721660

Jiang, J., Wolk, A., & Vessby, B. (1999). Relation between the intake of milk fat and the occurrence of conjugated linoleic acid in human adipose tissue. *The American Journal of Clinical Nutrition*, *70*(1), 21–27. PMID:10393134

Kemp, P., & Lander, D. J. (1983). The hydrogenatrion of Gamma-linoleic acids by pure culture of two rumen bacteria. *The Biochemical Journal*, *216*(2), 519–522. doi:10.1042/bj2160519 PMID:6318740

Kemp, P., Lander, D. J., & Gunstone, F. D. (1984). The hydrogenation of some cis- and trans-octadecenoic acids to stearic acid by a rumen *Fusocillus* sp. *The British Journal of Nutrition*, *52*(01), 165–170. doi:10.1079/BJN19840083 PMID:6743636

Kemp, P., Lander, D. J., & Holman, R. T. (1984). The hydrogenation of the series of methylene-interrupted cis, cis-octadecadienoic acids by pure cultures of six rumen bacteria. *The British Journal of Nutrition*, *52*(01), 171–177. doi:10.1079/BJN19840084 PMID:6743637

Kepler, C. R., Hirons, K. P., McNeill, J. J., & Tove, S. B. (1966). Intermediates and products of the biohydrogenation of linoleic acid by *Butyrivibrio fibrisolvens*. *The Journal of Biological Chemistry*, *241*(6), 1350–1354. PMID:5936712

Kepler, C. R., & Tove, S. B. (1967). Biohydrogenation of unsaturated fatty acids III. Purification and properties of a linoleate Δ12-cis, Δ11-trans-isomerase from Butyrivibrio fibrisolvens. *The Journal of Biological Chemistry*, *242*(24), 5686–5692. PMID:5633396

Khiaosa-Ard, R., Bryner, S. F., Scheeder, M. R. L., Wettstein, H. R., Leiber, F., Kreuzer, M., & Soliva, C. R. (2009). Evidence for the inhibition of the terminal step of ruminal α-linolenic acid biohydrogenation by condensed tannins. *Journal of Dairy Science*, *92*(1), 177–188. doi:10.3168/jds.2008-1117 PMID:19109277

Kim, Y. J., Liu, R. H., Rychlik, J. L., & Russell, J. B. (2002). The enrichment of a ruminal bacterium (Megasphaera elsdenii YJ-4) that produces the trans-10, cis-12 isomer of conjugated linoleic acid. *Journal of Applied Microbiology*, *92*(5), 976–982. doi:10.1046/j.1365-2672.2002.01610.x PMID:11972704

Kishino, S., Ogawa, J., Omura, Y., Matsumura, K., & Shimizu, S. (2002). Conjugated linoleic acid production from linoleic acid by lactic acid bacteria. *Journal of the American Oil Chemists' Society*, *79*(2), 159–163. doi:10.1007/s11746-002-0451-4

Kishino, S., Ogawa, J., Yokozeki, K., & Shimizu, S. (2009). Microbial production of conjugated fatty acids. *Lipid Technology*, *21*(8-9), 177–181. doi:10.1002/lite.200900044

Kuhnt, K., Flotho, S., Benjamin, S., Boerchers, T., Schubert, R., Jahreis, G., & Spener, F. (2009). Gene expression after dietary intervention with trans fatty acids (trans-11/trans-12 18: 1) in humans. *European Journal of Lipid Science and Technology*, *111*(5), 442–450. doi:10.1002/ejlt.200800217

Lejonklev, J., Storm, A. C., Larsen, M. K., Mortensen, G., & Weisbjerg, M. R. (2013). Differences in rate of ruminal hydrogenation of C18 fatty acids in clover and ryegrass. *Animal*, *7*(10), 1607–1613. doi:10.1017/S1751731113001286 PMID:23842207

Lin, T. Y. (2000). Conjugated linoleic acid concentration as affected by lactic cultures and additives. *Food Chemistry*, *69*(1), 27–31. doi:10.1016/S0308-8146(99)00218-6

Lin, T. Y. (2006). Conjugated linoleic acid production by cells and enzyme extract of *Lactobacillus delbrueckii* ssp. *bulgaricus* with additions of different fatty acids. *Food Chemistry*, *94*(3), 437–441. doi:10.1016/j.foodchem.2004.11.032

Lin, T. Y., Hung, T. H., & Cheng, T. S. (2005). Conjugated linoleic acid production by immobilized cells of *Lactobacillus delbrueckii* ssp. *bulgaricus* and *Lactobacillus acidophilus*. *Food Chemistry*, *92*, 23–28. doi:10.1016/j.foodchem.2004.07.003

Liu, P., Shen, S. R., Ruan, H., Zhou, Q., Ma, L. L., & He, G. Q. (2011). Production of conjugated linoleic acids by *Lactobacillus plantarum* strains isolated from naturally fermented Chinese pickles. *Journal of Zhejiang University. Science. B.*, *12*(11), 923–930. doi:10.1631/jzus.B1100072 PMID:22042657

Maia, M. R., Chaudhary, L. C., Figueres, L., & Wallace, R. J. (2007). Metabolism of polyunsaturated fatty acids and their toxicity to the microflora of the rumen. *Antonie van Leeuwenhoek*, *91*(4), 303–314. doi:10.1007/s10482-006-9118-2 PMID:17072533

Martin, S. A., & Jenkins, T. C. (2002). Factors affecting conjugated linoleic acid and trans-C18: 1 fatty acid production by mixed ruminal bacteria. *Journal of Animal Science*, *80*, 3347–3352. PMID:12542176

McKain, N., Shingfield, K. J., & Wallace, R. J. (2010). Metabolism of conjugated linoleic acids and 18: 1 fatty acids by ruminal bacteria: products and mechanisms. *Microbiology*, *156*(2), 579–588. doi:10.1099/mic.0.036442-0 PMID:19926650

Mir, P. S., Bittman, S., Hunt, D., Entz, T., & Yip, B. (2006). Lipid content and fatty acid composition of grasses sampled on different dates through the early part of the growing season. *Canadian Journal of Animal Science*, *86*(2), 279–290. doi:10.4141/A05-050

Miri, V. H., Tyagi, A. K., Ebrahimi, S. H., & Mohini, M. (2013). Effect of cumin (Cuminum cyminum) seed extract on milk fatty acid profile and methane emission in lactating goat. *Small Ruminant Research*, *113*(1), 66–72. doi:10.1016/j.smallrumres.2013.01.015

Morvan, B., & Joblin, K. N. (1999). Hydration of Oleic Acid by Enterococcus gallinarum, Pediococcus acidilactici andLactobacillus sp. Isolated from the Rumen. *Anaerobe*, *5*(6), 605–611. doi:10.1006/anae.1999.0306

Mosley, E. E., McGuire, M. K., Williams, J. E., & McGuire, M. A. (2006). Cis-9, trans-11 conjugated linoleic acid is synthesized from vaccenic acid in lactating women. *The Journal of Nutrition*, *136*(9), 2297–2301. PMID:16920844

Mosley, E. E., Powell, G. L., Riley, M. B., & Jenkins, T. C. (2002). Microbial biohydrogenation of oleic acid to trans isomers in vitro. *Journal of Lipid Research*, *43*(2), 290–296. PMID:11861671

Nam, I. S., & Garnsworthy, P. C. (2007). Factors influencing biohydrogenation and conjugated linoleic acid production by mixed rumen fungi. *Journal of Microbiology (Seoul, Korea)*, *45*(3), 199. PMID:17618224

O'Shea, E. F., Cotter, P. D., Stanton, C., Ross, R. P., & Hill, C. (2012). Production of bioactive substances by intestinal bacteria as a basis for explaining probiotic mechanisms: Bacteriocins and conjugated linoleic acid. *International Journal of Food Microbiology*, *152*(3), 189–205. doi:10.1016/j.ijfoodmicro.2011.05.025 PMID:21742394

Ogawa, J., Matsumura, K., Kishino, S., Omura, Y., & Shimizu, S. (2001). Conjugated linoleic acid accumulation via 10-hydroxy-12-octadecaenoic acid during microaerobic transformation of linoleic acid by *Lactobacillus acidophilus*. *Applied and Environmental Microbiology*, *67*(3), 1246–1252. doi:10.1128/AEM.67.3.1246-1252.2001 PMID:11229917

Or-Rashid, M. M., AlZahal, O., & McBride, B. W. (2008). Studies on the production of conjugated linoleic acid from linoleic and vaccenic acids by mixed rumen protozoa. *Applied Microbiology and Biotechnology*, *81*(3), 533–541. doi:10.1007/s00253-008-1690-0 PMID:18797866

Or-Rashid, M. M., AlZahal, O., & McBride, B. W. (2011). Comparative studies on the metabolism of linoleic acid by rumen bacteria, protozoa, and their mixture in vitro. *Applied Microbiology and Biotechnology*, *89*(2), 387–395. doi:10.1007/s00253-010-2865-z PMID:20865258

Pakdeechanuan, P. S., Salaemae, A., & Odpiban, S. (2010). Effect of reducing propylene glycol content on conjugated linoleic acid production from sunflower oil. *KKU Science Journal*, *38*, 532–543.

Park, H. G., Cho, S. D., Kim, J. H., Lee, H., Chung, S. H., Kim, S. B., & Kim, Y. J. et al. (2009). Characterization of conjugated linoleic acid production by *Bifidobacterium breve* LMC 520. *Journal of Agricultural and Food Chemistry*, *57*(16), 7571–7575. doi:10.1021/jf9014813 PMID:20349924

Pryce, J. E., Wales, W. J., De Haas, Y., Veerkamp, R. F., & Hayes, B. J. (2014). Genomic selection for feed efficiency in dairy cattle. *Animal*, *8*(01), 1–10. doi:10.1017/S1751731113001687 PMID:24128704

Rainio, A., Vahvaselkä, M., Suomalainen, T., & Laakso, S. (2001). Reduction of linoleic acid inhibition in production of conjugated linoleic acid by *Propionibacterium freudenreichii* ssp. *shermanii*. *Canadian Journal of Microbiology*, *47*(8), 735–740. doi:10.1139/cjm-47-8-735 PMID:11575500

Rosberg-Cody, E., Ross, R. P., Hussey, S., Ryan, C. A., Murphy, B. P., Fitzgerald, G. F., & Stanton, C. (2004). Mining the microbiota of the neonatal gastrointestinal tract for conjugated linoleic acid-producing bifidobacteria. *Applied and Environmental Microbiology*, *70*(8), 4635–4641. doi:10.1128/AEM.70.8.4635-4641.2004 PMID:15294796

Sakuradani, E., Ogawa, J., Kishino, S., Ando, A., Yokozeki, K., & Shimizu, S. (2010). Oils, microbial production. Encyclopedia of Industrial Biotechnology.

Schmid, B., Einsle, O., Chiu, H. J., Willing, A., Yoshida, M., Howard, J. B., & Rees, D. C. (2002). Biochemical and structural characterization of the cross-linked complex of nitrogenase: Comparison to the ADP-AlF4--stabilized structure. *Biochemistry*, *41*(52), 15557–15565. doi:10.1021/bi026642b PMID:12501184

Shareck, J., Nantel, A., & Belhumeur, P. (2011). Conjugated linoleic acid inhibits hyphal growth in *Candida albicans* by modulating Ras1p cellular levels and downregulating TEC1 expression. *Eukaryotic Cell*, *10*(4), 565–577. doi:10.1128/EC.00305-10 PMID:21357478

Szöllőskei, G., Wagner, L., Németh, S., & Husvéth, F. (2005). In sacco studies of conjugated linoleic acid production from various oils in the rumen of sheep. *Acta Veterinaria Hungarica*, *53*(4), 411–423. doi:10.1556/AVet.53.2005.4.2 PMID:16363143

Taiz, L., & Zeiger, E. (2002). *Plant physiology* (3rd ed.). Sinauer Associates Inc Publishers.

Towne, G., Nagaraja, T. G., Brandt, R. T., & Kemp, K. E. (1990). Ruminal ciliated protozoa in cattle fed finishing diets with or without supplemental fat. *Journal of Animal Science*, *68*(7), 2150–2155. PMID:2117004

Turpeinen, A. M., Mutanen, M., Aro, A., Salminen, I., Basu, S., Palmquist, D. L., & Griinari, J. M. (2002). Bioconversion of vaccenic acid to conjugated linoleic acid in humans. *The American Journal of Clinical Nutrition*, *76*(3), 504–510. PMID:12197992

Van Meer, G., Voelker, D. R., & Feigenson, G. W. (2008). Membrane lipids: Where they are and how they behave. *Nature Reviews. Molecular Cell Biology*, *9*(2), 112–124. doi:10.1038/nrm2330 PMID:18216768

Van Soest, P. J. (1994). *Nutritional Ecology of the Ruminant* (2nd ed.). Ithaca, NY: Cornell University Press.

Váradyová, Z., Kisidayova, S., Siroka, P., & Jalc, D. (2007). Fatty acid profiles of rumen fluid from sheep fed diets supplemented with various oils and effect on the rumen ciliate population. *Czech Journal of Animal Science*, *52*(11), 399.

Vasta, V., Yáñez-Ruiz, D. R., Mele, M., Serra, A., Luciano, G., Lanza, M., & Priolo, A. (2010). Bacterial and protozoal communities and fatty acid profile in the rumen of sheep fed a diet containing added tannins. *Applied and Environmental Microbiology*, *76*(8), 2549–2555. doi:10.1128/AEM.02583-09 PMID:20173064

Vossenberg, J. L. C. M., & Joblin, K. N. (2003). Biohydrogenation of C18 unsaturated fatty acids to stearic acid by a strain of *Butyrivibrio hungatei* from the bovine rumen. *Letters in Applied Microbiology*, *37*(5), 424–428. doi:10.1046/j.1472-765X.2003.01421.x PMID:14633116

Wallace, R. J., McKain, N., Shingfield, K. J., & Devillard, E. (2007). Isomers of conjugated linoleic acids are synthesized via different mechanisms in ruminal digesta and bacteria. *Journal of Lipid Research*, *48*(10), 2247–2254. doi:10.1194/jlr.M700271-JLR200 PMID:17644775

Wang, L. M., Lv, J. P., Chu, Z. Q., Cui, Y. Y., & Ren, X. H. (2007). Production of conjugated linoleic acid by *Propionibacterium freudenreichii*. *Food Chemistry*, *103*(2), 313–318. doi:10.1016/j.foodchem.2006.07.065

Wilde, P. F., & Dawson, R. M. C. (1966). The bihydrogenation of alpha- linoleic and oleic acid by rumen micro- organisms. *The Biochemical Journal*, *98*(2), 469–475. doi:10.1042/bj0980469 PMID:4287407

William, A. G., & Coleman, G. S. (1997). The rumen protozoa. In The rumen microbial ecosystem (pp. 73-139). Springer.

Wright, A. D. G. (2009). The rumen ciliates. In R. Röttger, R. Knight, & W. Foissner (Eds.), *Protozoological Monographs* (Vol. 4, pp. 202–210). Shaker Verlag Achen, Germany.

Wright, A. D. G., & Klieve, A. V. (2011). Does the complexity of the rumen microbial ecology preclude methane mitigation? *Animal Feed Science and Technology*, *166*, 248–253. doi:10.1016/j.anifeedsci.2011.04.015

Yanez-Ruiz, D. R., Scollan, N. D., Merry, R. J., & Newbold, C. J. (2006). Contribution of rumen protozoa to duodenal flow of nitrogen, conjugated linoleic acid and vaccenic acid in steers fed silages differing in their water-soluble carbohydrate content. *The British Journal of Nutrition*, *96*(05), 861–869. doi:10.1017/BJN20061927 PMID:17092374

Yang, L., Huang, Y., Wang, H. Q., & Chen, Z. Y. (2002). Production of conjugated linoleic acids through KOH-catalyzed dehydration of ricinoleic acid. *Chemistry and Physics of Lipids*, *119*(1), 23–31. doi:10.1016/S0009-3084(02)00052-X PMID:12270670

Zhang, B., Rong, C., Chen, H., Song, Y., Zhang, H., & Chen, W. (2012). De novo synthesis of trans-10, cis-12 conjugated linoleic acid in oleaginous yeast *Yarrowia lipolytica*. *Microbial Cell Factories*, *11*(1), 51. doi:10.1186/1475-2859-11-51 PMID:22545818

Zheng, H. C., Liu, J. X., Yao, J. H., Yuan, Q., Ye, H. W., Ye, J. A., & Wu, Y. M. (2005). Effects of dietary sources of vegetable oils on performance of high-yielding lactating cows and conjugated linoleic acids in milk. *Journal of Dairy Science*, *88*(6), 2037–2042. doi:10.3168/jds.S0022-0302(05)72880-0 PMID:15905434

APPENDIX

Table 1. Important bacteria producing 9- and 10-CLA isomers from linoleic acid

Strain	Type of CLA	Reference
B. breve NCFB 2258	9-CLA & *trans*-9, *trans*-11- CLA	Coakely et al.2003
B. dentum NCFB 2243	9-CLA & *trans*-9, *trans*-11- CLA	Coakely et al.2003
B. lactis Bb12	9-CLA & *trans*-9, *trans*-11-CLA	Coakely et al.2003
B. fibriosolven A38	9-CLA	Kepler et al. 1966
L. acidophilus AKU 1137	9-CLA or *cis*-11-18:2 & *trans*-9, *trans*-11-18:2	Kishno et al. 2002
L. brevi IAM 1082	9-CLA, *trans*-9, *trans*-11-18:2, *cis*-11-18:2	Kishno et al. 2002
Lac. casei E5	9-CLA	Alonso et al. 2003.
*Lac. casei*E10	9-CLA	Alonso et al. 2003.
L. paracesi subsp. *paracesi* IFO 12004	9-CLA or *cis*-11-18:2 & *trans*-9, *trans*-11-18:2	Kishno et al. 2002
*L. plantarum*AKU 1009	9-CLA, *trans*-9,*cis*-11 or *trans*- 9, *trans*-11	Kishno et al. 2002
L. rhamnosus AKU 1124	9-CLA, *trans*-9, *trans*-11-18:2 or *cis*-11-18:2	Kishno et al. 2002
M. elsdenii YJ - 4	10-CLA	Kim et al. 2002
P. freudenreichiis subsp. *shermanii* PFS 9093	9-CLA	Jiang et al. 1998
P. shermanii AKU 1254	9-CLA or *cis*-11-18:2 & *trans*- 9, *trans*-11-18:2	Kishno et al. 2002

Table 2. Composition of CLA precursor fatty acids in commercially available oil/ vegetable seeds (units: grams fatty acids per 100 grams oil)

Seed	Oleic Acid	Linoleic Acid	α-Linolenic Acid
Almond	69.4	17.4	-
Apricot Kernel	58.5	29.3	-
Avocado	**67.9**	12.5	0.96
Canola	56.1	20.3	**9.3**
Coconut	5.8	1.8	-
Corn	27.3	53.5	1.2
Cotton	17	51.5	0.2
Flax	20.2	12.7	**53.3**
Grape	15.8	**69.6**	0.1
Hazelnut	**77.8**	10.1	-
Mustard	11.6	15.3	5.9
Oat	34.9	39.1	1.8
Olive	**72.8**	9.2	0.2
Palm	33.6	9.1	0.2
Peanut	44.8	32	-
Rice bran	39.1	33.4	1.6
Safflower	14.4	**74.6**	-
Sesame	39.3	41.3	0.3
Soybean	22.8	51	6.8
Sunflower	19.5	**65.7**	-
Walnut	22.2	52.9	**10.4**
Wheat germ	14.6	54.8	6.9

Chapter 2

Dietary Fibers and their Role as Functional Food for Human Health:

Food Fibers and Human Health

Murlidhar Meghwal
Jain University, India

Ravi-Kumar Kadeppagari
Jain University, India

ABSTRACT

This chapter mainly summarizes the sources of dietary fibers and how they act as functional food for benefiting the human health. Dietary fibers could be soluble and insoluble in water and the major sources are fruits, vegetables, nuts and whole grains. Dietary fibers play role in the control of various disorders like cardiovascular diseases, digestive disorders, diabetes, obesity and colonic cancer. Dietary fibers benefit the human health by acting through various mechanisms in the gastrointestinal tract. According to the WHO recommendations at least 25 g of dietary fiber per day should be consumed. Effect of food processing practices on the physiochemical and functional properties of dietary fibers is also covered in this chapter.

DOI: 10.4018/978-1-5225-0607-2.ch002

INTRODUCTION

Ancient Greek physicians had some knowledge of prevention of constipation by using food items that had bulked excretions (British Nutrition Foundation, 1990). Fibers are the components of plant material that resist the human digestive enzymes. According to the Institute of Medicine which contains the dietary fiber can be defined as the non-digestible carbohydrates and lignin that are intrinsic and intact in plants; whereas the functional fiber consists of isolated, non-digestible carbohydrates that have beneficial physiological effects in humans and total fiber is the sum of both. According to the American Association of Cereal Chemists the dietary fiber is the edible parts of plants or analogous carbohydrates that are resistant to digestion and absorption in the human small intestine with complete or partial fermentation in the large intestine and as per this association the dietary fiber includes polysaccharides, oligosaccharides, lignin and associated plant substances. Dietary fibers promote beneficial physiological effects including laxation, blood cholesterol attenuation and blood glucose attenuation. The codex committee on nutrition and foods for special dietary uses defines dietary fiber (adopted as Codex definition, July 2009) as carbohydrate polymers with ten or more monomeric units that are not hydrolyzed by the endogenous enzymes in the small intestine of humans. They are classified into the following categories (Daniel, 2006; Lupton, 2010):

1. Edible carbohydrate polymers naturally occurring in the food.
2. Carbohydrate polymers which have been obtained from raw food material by physical, enzymatic or chemical means.
3. Synthetic carbohydrate polymers. The indigestible portion of food derived from plants is termed as dietary fiber (roughage) and it has two main components, soluble fiber and insoluble fiber.

Where patients are on hospital stay, post-operation, bedridden, pain medication control, etc constipation should be watched to prevent unwanted complications such as bowel impaction, vitals instability, hemorrhoids or even death as a result of straining and consequent vagal stimulation. Easy way to prevent those complications is through anticipatory interventions like high fiber diet. Such dietary fiber helps in keeping intestinal and bowel health in good condition. Hence the current chapter deals with major sources of dietary fiber, major health benefits of dietary fiber, recommendations and guidelines for the dietary fiber intake and effects of various food processing operations on the quality of dietary fiber (Daniel, 2006).

SOURCES OF DIETARY FIBERS

Eating of significant quantity of dietary fiber will help to keep the good health. Man, women and children will need different amount of fiber in their food. Main sources of fibers are plants and fibers are classified into two types: soluble and insoluble. Both kinds of fibers are important for optimal health (Association of Official Analytical Chemists, 1980; Indian Standard Institution, 1985). Fruits, vegetables and whole grains are rich sources of fiber and can be eaten directly or can be used to make supplements and fiber-rich processed foods. It was observed that fiber content in the meat is negligible compared to the plant sources. The Academy of Nutrition and Dietetics, USA recommends for the consumption of variety of fiber-rich foods. Some of the fibers are listed in the Table 1.

Soluble fiber is found in varying quantities in all plant sources. Some examples are legumes (peas, soybeans, lupins, lentils and other beans); oats, rye, chia, barley, oat bran and psyllium husk; fruits like (figs, avocados, plums, prunes, berries, ripe bananas and the skin of apples, quinces and pears); vegetables such as broccoli, carrots, jerusalem artichokes and ladies finger; root tubers and root vegetables such as sweet potatoes and onions (skins of these are sources of insoluble fiber also);

Table 1. Major fibers and their sources

Sr No.	Fiber	Solubility	Source
1	Cellulose	Water insoluble	Cereals, fruit and vegetables
2	Chitin	Water insoluble	Fungi, exoskeleton of insects and crustaceans
3	Hemicellulose	Water insoluble	Cereals, bran, timber and legume
4	Hexosane	Water insoluble	Wheat and barley
5	Pentosane	Water insoluble	Rye and oat
6	Lignin	Water insoluble	Stones of fruits, vegetables and cereals
7	Xanthan	Water insoluble	Bacteria (*Xanthomonas*)
8	Fructans	Water soluble	Plants that store starch
9	Inulin	Water soluble	Plants like Topinambour, chicory etc
10	Pectin	Water soluble	Fruit skin (apples and quinces) and vegetables
11	Carrageen	Water soluble	Red algae
12	Alginates	Water soluble	Algae
13	Raffinose	Water soluble	Legumes
14	Polydextrose	Water soluble	Synthetic polymer
15	Lactulose	Water soluble	Synthetic disaccharide

psyllium seed husks (a mucilage soluble fiber) and flax seeds and nuts with almonds being the highest source of dietary fiber.

Foods having higher insoluble dietary fibers are listed below. Brown rice, whole wheat and wheat bran; seeds and nuts; vegetables like green leafy vegetables, cabbage, tomato, cauliflower, zucchini (courgette) and celery; legumes such as beans and peas; fruits including avocado and unripe bananas and skins of some fruits including kiwifruit, grapes and tomatoes. Fiber supplements do not have the same health benefits as naturally occurring high-fiber foods. People should eat more natural fiber which is found in whole grains, fruits, vegetables, seeds and nuts as listed above rather than taking fiber supplements. Besides fiber, whole food contains nutrients including antioxidants and other biological active components which can offer more

Figure 1. Gaur gum

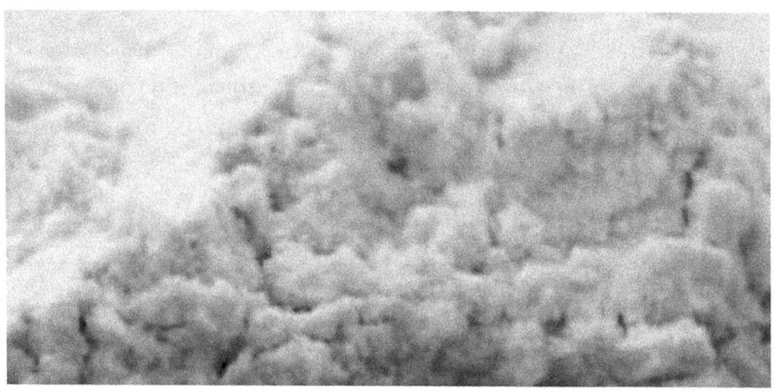

Figure 2. Acacia senegal gum

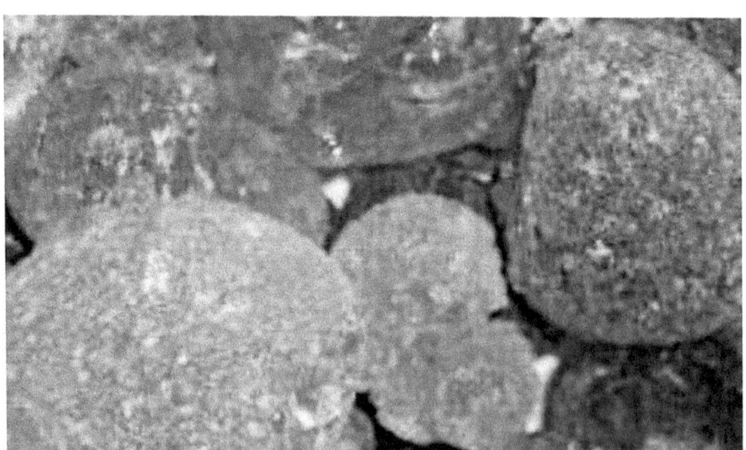

Figure 3. Major health benefits of dilatory fiber

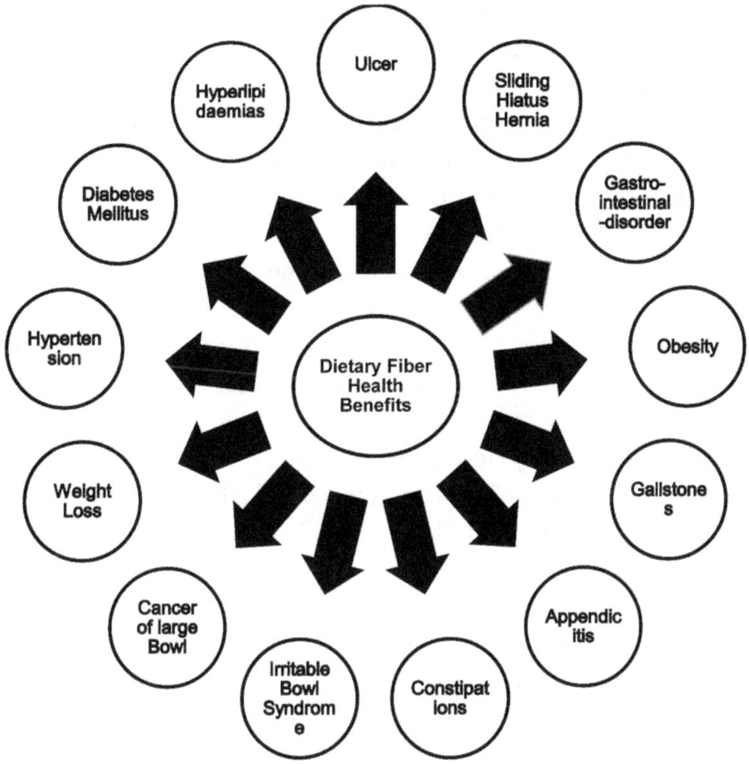

protection against chronic diseases. Vegetable gum fibers are available as powder or solid. They can be easily dissolved into water. Parisi et al. (2002) reported their effectiveness for the treatment of irritable bowel syndrome. Guar gum (Figure 1) and *Acacia senegal* gum (Figure 2) are examples of vegetable gum fibers (Figure 3).

DETERMINATION OF THE TOTAL FIBER CONTENTS

The standard gravimetric method can be used for the determination of total dietary fiber after the enzymatic digestion of the given food sample. The fat and moisture free food sample will be enzymatically digested to solubilize starch and protein and the residue remained behind is estimated gravimetrically as insoluble fraction of food fiber. The soluble fiber complex is precipitated from the enzyme digest and separated. The total dietary fiber content of the food sample is the sum of the insoluble and soluble fractions. This value will be expressed as grams per 100 g of the dry weight of the original food sample.

The sample taken for the determination should represent the entire lot. The sample of food grains should be milled to a particle size of 0.5 - 1 mm in a mill or grinder. The moist foodstuffs such as fruits and vegetables should be sliced and homogenized before drying. The dry matter content of all the samples will be determined as the weight after drying for 5 h at 105°C. For foodstuffs containing more than 5 percent of lipids, lipids will be soxlet extracted for 5 h by using chloroform methanol mixture. This system removes the free, bound and polar lipids and also facilitates the subsequent removal of free sugars by ethanol extraction. If required lipid content in the sample will be quantified and lipid free residue will be used for further treatment. Free sugar in the sample will be removed by treating with 80% ethanol and if the free sugar content of the sample is to be estimated then the ethyl alcohol extract will be collected quantitatively. Then the sample will be digested with enzymes and soluble and insoluble fractions of dietary fiber will be estimated. Fifty milliliter of water will be added to the sample residue and autoclaved at 120°C for 20 minutes in order to gelatinize the starch. After cooling pH will be adjusted to 1.5 by using 5M HCl and 50 mg pepsin and 200 ul of chloroform will be added and incubated at 37°C for 20 hours. Then pH will be adjusted to 6.0 with 3 N NaOH and added 25 ml of phosphate buffer, 100 mg of pancreatin, 20 mg of glucoamylase and a few crystals of thymol and Incubated at 37°C for 18 h and centrifuged at 3000 g for 30 minutes. Supernatant will be collected and residue will be washed three times with water and the washings will be added to the supernatant. Then the residue will be used for the estimation of insoluble fraction of the dietary fiber and supernatant will be used for the determination of soluble fraction of dietary fiber (Indian Standard Institution, 1985; Ranganna, 1995). For determining insoluble fraction of dietary fiber residue will be washed three times with acetone and then with ether and then dried to a constant weight in a hot air oven or vacuum oven. This remnant represents the insoluble fraction of the dietary fiber. In order to find soluble fraction of the dietary fiber, the supernatant will be diluted with four volumes of ethanol and centrifuged at 3000 g for 30 minutes and collected the residue. The residue will be washed three times each with ethanol and acetone and then with diethyl ether and dried to a constant weight. This remnant will represent the soluble fraction of the dietary fiber. The total percentage of dietary fiber in the food sample will be calculated as below (Indian Standard Institution, 1985; Ranganna, 1995).

% total dietary fiber = [(Mass of soluble fraction + Mass of insoluble fraction) X 100]/ Mass of the sample

Table 2. Dietary fibers and their effects

Fiber	Effect
Soluble	Lowers total and LDL cholesterol and reduce the risk of cardiovascular disease; slows emptying of the stomach and intestinal transit time, shielding carbohydrates from enzymes delays absorption of glucose, lowers variance in blood sugar levels
Insoluble	Adds bulk to the stool and alleviates constipation, regulates blood sugar, reduce glucose and insulin levels in diabetic patients, facilitates regular defecation;
Soluble and insoluble	Balances intestinal pH, stimulates intestinal fermentation and production of short-chain fatty acids; increases food volume without increasing caloric content, provide satiety and may reduce appetite.

HEALTH BENEFITS OF DIETARY FIBERS

Dietary fibers will play a role in the improvement of different disease conditions as shown in the Table 2 and Figure 3. They can be broadly categorized into the following headings:

1. Cardiovascular and associated diseases,
2. Digestive disorders,
3. Diabetes,
4. Obesity,
5. Colonic cancer.

Cardiovascular and Associated Disorders

The American Dietetic Association (ADA) has published a systematic review on the health implications of dietary fiber. According to this review there is a fair evidence that dietary fiber from whole foods will lower blood pressure, improve serum lipids and reduce inflammation. Other recent studies reported a range of cardiovascular benefits associated with dietary fiber. Flint et al. (2009) reported that cereal fiber was associated with reduced blood pressure in adults.

Dietary fiber appears to affect cholesterol metabolism by different means and some ways discussed here: An important action of some fibers is to reduce the re-absorption of bile acids in the ileum and hence the amount and type of bile acid and fats reaching the colon. Reduction in the reabsorption of bile acid from the ileum has several direct effects like bile acids will be trapped within the lumen of the ileum due to a high luminal viscosity or due to their binding to a dietary fiber; water-soluble bile acids e.g. deoxycholic and lithocholic acids are adsorbed to dietary fiber and an increased fecal loss of sterols dependent in part on the amount and type of fiber; an increase in the bacterial mass and activity in the ileum as some fibers (e.g. pectin) are digested by bacteria; As the bacterial mass increases the cecal bacterial activity increases; the enteric loss of bile acids results in increased synthesis of bile acids from cholesterol which in turn reduces body cholesterol (Nagengast, 1992).

The fibers that are most effective in influencing sterol metabolism are fermented in the colon. Hence, it is unlikely that the reduction in body cholesterol is due to then adsorption of cholesterol to this fermented fiber in the colon. There might be alterations in the end-products of bile acid bacterial metabolism or the release of short chain fatty acids which are absorbed from the colon and return to the liver and modulate either the synthesis of cholesterol or the catabolism of cholesterol in to bile acids. The prime mechanism whereby fiber influences cholesterol metabolism is through bacteria binding bile acids in the colon after the initial deconjugation and dehydroxylation. Fermentable fibers like pectin will provide a medium for bacterial growth thereby increasing the bacterial mass in the colon. Bile acids excreted in feces. Other fibers like gum arabic act as stabilizers and cause a significant decrease in serum cholesterol without increasing fecal bile acid secretion.

Digestive Disorder

Dietary fiber increases the weight of stools and softens. The stool passes through the intestinal tract easily thus reduces the strained bowel movements. This helps to maintain bowel health and to avoid constipation. In addition, insoluble fiber decreases the transit time of food waste through the intestinal tract. This reduces the contact period of potentially harmful substances in the food waste with the intestinal wall. Soluble fiber may help to lower total cholesterol levels. Fiber appears to help bile acids which are made of cholesterol to pass through the intestine as waste. Flourie (1992) reported that fibers and fiber derivatives can exert acute and chronic effects on the bioavailability of carbohydrates from the gastro-intestinal tract. Contributing factors for the slow absorption of carbohydrates after the consumption of viscous fibers are reduced rate of gastric emptying, altered enzyme-substrate interactions and motility in the small intestine, poorer mixing of digesta in the gut lumen, slower diffusion from the gut to the epithelial cells, etc. Viscous fibers do not appear to exert these effects by acting on secretory function, hydrolytic processes and transport; rather they act by modifying the physical characteristics of gastro-intestinal contents. The higher viscosity would spread the absorption across a longer time-span and this would explain the flat glucose tolerance curves seen after viscous fiber ingestion. Long term use of high fibre or fibre supplemented diets may be accompanied by lower postprandial glucose levels that result from events occurring within the gastro-intestinal tract and long term improvement in glucose metabolism (changes in hepatic glucose metabolism and enhanced tissue sensitivity to insulin). To prove the possibility that fibers induce adaptive changes in the gastrointestinal tract with respect to carbohydrate digestion and absorption further studies need to be conducted in the humans (Flourie, 1992).

Non-starch polysaccharides and lignin in the foods do not have any nutritionally significant effect on mineral and trace element absorption, while substances associated with dietary fiber and present in fiber-rich foods are important antagonists or enhancers for the uptake of these nutrients. A strong negative effect on zinc and iron absorption has consistently been shown for phytate, inositol hexaphosphate and some of its degradation products. For iron, the antagonizing of absorption is pronounced even at low levels of phytate. Some of the phenolic compounds present in vegetables impair iron absorption. However, some fiber-rich foods also contain potential enhancers for iron absorption such as ascorbic acid and other organic acids. The absorption of minerals depend on the total composition of the meal. Strictly vegetarian diets based on unrefined cereals and possibly also some legume-based diets will result in low absorption of zinc and iron. However, the utilisation of zinc and iron and probably other minerals can be improved by food processes such as fermentation or soaking and malting which decrease the phytate content. Fiber rich foods would then become good sources of iron and zinc as the content of these minerals will be high in these foods (Read and Eastwood, 1992; Rossander et al., 1992).

In the colon, bacterial fermentation of some dietary fibers takes place which will lead to an increase in bacterial mass and thereby increase in bacterial enzyme activity. After fermentation there will be changes in the water-holding capacity of the fiber residue. Enlargement of the cecum is a common finding when some dietary fibers are fed and this is now believed to be normal physiological adjustment. Some non-absorbed carbohydrates like pectin, gum arabic, oligosaccharides and resistant starch are fermented to short chain fatty acids (mainly acetic, propionic and n-butyric), carbon dioxide, hydrogen and methane. The cecal fermentation of 40–50 g of complex polysaccharides will yield 400–500 mmol total short-chain fatty acids, 240–300 mmol acetate and 80–100 mmol of both propionate and butyrate. Almost all of these short-chain fatty acids will be absorbed from the colon. The production of short-chain fatty acids has several possible actions on the gut mucosa. All the short chain fatty acids are readily absorbed by the colonic mucosa, but only acetic acid reaches the systemic circulation in appreciable amounts. Butyric acid appears to be used as a preferred energy source for the colonic cells.

Diabetes

Soluble fiber reduces the rate of the release of sugars from digested food into the bloodstream, thus preventing a rapid rise in blood sugar levels which will help in the control of diabetes mellitus. Calorimetric studies showed that foods that contained significant amounts of crude fiber increased fecal energy losses and suggested that crude fiber did not contribute metabolizable energy to the body (Atwater, 1900). As mentioned earlier long term consumption of fiber rich diets will lower postprandial sugar levels in the blood which could be due to the improvement in the hepatic glucose metabolism and tissue sensitivity to the insulin.

Obesity

Dietary fiber helps in the energy intake control and managing obesity. The dietary fiber enriched food helps to have earlier satiation and prolonged satiety. Fiber rich diets have a reduced energy density compared with high fat diets. This is related to fiber's ability to add bulk and weight to the diet. The relationship of body weight status and fiber effect on energy intake suggests that obese individuals may be more likely to reduce food intake with dietary fiber inclusion (Britt et al., 2013). Since fibers will be fermented to short- chain fatty acids, which will be absorbed from the colon and utilized for metabolism, the concept that dietary fiber contributes no energy is wrong. But, determining the caloric value of dietary fiber is complex. The best estimate of energy yield generated by fiber fermentation in humans is between 6.2 and 10.4 kJ/g (1.5 and 2.5 kcal/g) (Institute of Medicine USA, 2002) compared to 16.7 kJ/g (4.0 kcal/g) for starch (Slavin, 2013). High fiber foods generally require a longer time to chew. This slows down and may make us eat less. On the other hand, with the added bulk, they help us feel full for a longer period. People should eat a variety of high-fiber foods in order to control obesity related problems.

Colonic Cancer

The incidence of colorectal cancer is high in Western countries and is related to dietary habits (Hill, 1985). It is assumed that dietary factors modulate a genetic susceptibility (Bruce, 1987). In epidemiological observations the consumption of animal fat is positively related to the incidence of colon cancer and the intake of fiber is negatively related to this incidence. However, inconsistencies exist. One thing that has always to be kept in mind is the reciprocal relation between fat and fiber intake. An interesting substance that has drawn more attention but whose role in colonic carcinogenesis is far from clear is "resistant starch". In a case-control study it was found that a high starch diet reduced the relative risk of colonic cancer to 0.82 (Tuyns et al., 1988). There are several possible explanations for the protective effects of fiber and starch. The most important ones are, the stool-bulking effect, the acceleration of gut transit time, the binding of bile acids and the fermentation of parts of the fiber and probably most of the starch to short chain fatty acids thereby reducing the formation of secondary bile acids and enhancing the production of butyrate which has antineoplastic properties in vitro. In most animal experiments a protective effect of fiber on colonic carcinogenesis has been shown. However, controversies too exist in this regard (Castleden 1977; Fleiszer et al., 1978).

RECOMMENDATION AND GUIDELINES FOR DIETARY FIBER INTAKE

The United States National Academy of Sciences and Institute of Medicine (USA), recommended the consumption of 20-35 g of dietary fiber per day for adults (Fiber, 2015). The Academy of Nutrition and Dietetics, USA suggest a minimum consumption of 20–35 g per day for a healthy adult based on calorie intake (Nugent, 2005) and for children fiber intake should equal to age in years plus 5 g per day. Patients with constipation, vomiting and abdominal pain should take as per the suggestions of the physician. Certain bulking agents are not commonly recommended with the prescription of opioids because they may lead to severe constipation, pain or obstruction. The British Nutrition Foundation has recommended a minimum fiber intake of 18 g per day for healthy adults (British Nutrition Foundation, 2014). According to the WHO report (2003) at least 25 g per day should be provided to the humans from fruit, vegetable and wholegrain foods. This recommendation was based on the evidence linking high intake of dietary fiber from fruit, vegetables and wholegrain foods with decreased risk of weight gain. European Food Safety Authority (EFSA) (2010) considers a fiber intake of 25 g/day to be adequate for normal laxation in adults. The EFSA Panel notes that there is evidence that in adults health benefit is associated with consumption of diets having fiber greater than 25 g per day, for example reduced risk of coronary heart disease and type-2 diabetes and improved weight maintenance. Such evidences should be considered when formulating food based dietary guidelines. A fiber intake of 2 g/MJ is considered adequate for normal laxation in children from the age of one year. Although EFSA mentions one intake quantity, the effects of different fiber types on fecal weight show marked differences like 5.4 g stool/g fiber from wheat bran, 4.9 g/g fiber from fruit and vegetables, 3 g/g fiber from isolated cellulose and 1.3 g/g fiber from isolated pectin (Cummings, 1993). Therefore, the EFSA recommendation may also be seen as being in favor of consumption of fruit, vegetables and wholegrain products. The Institute of Medicine (2005) and the Health Council of Netherlands recommended 3.4 g fiber/MJ for adults corresponding to 25 to 40 g fiber/day, depending on the energy delivered in the daily diet. This higher level (compared with those recommended by WHO and EFSA) was chosen taking into account not only laxation but also the reduced risk for coronary heart diseases. The Health Council of Netherlands did not issue a dietary reference intake level for fiber, but given a guideline mentioning that the recommended level refers to intake of fiber as present in (non-enriched) food products such as fruits, vegetables and whole grain products and this approach was chosen since observational studies showed that beneficial effects may be obtained from the consumption of such foods which contain both fiber and bioactive co- passengers. A healthy male of age groups 14-50 years old is suggested to consume 38 g food fiber daily whereas a healthy females of 9-50 years old age group is suggested to include 25 g of dietary fiber into their daily diets. On average human requires about 14 g of fiber per 1000 calories. If enough fruits, vegetables, nuts and whole grains are included in the diet then body's required fiber will be easily received.

EFFECT OF FOOD PROCESSING PRACTICES ON FIBERS

Most of the dietary fibers are consumed in processed form thus studying the effect of food processing practices on the physic-chemical and functional properties of food fibers is very important (Thibault et al, 1992). Heller et al (1977) and Caprez et al (1986) reported that there will be lower level of insoluble dietary fiber in the milled bran compared to coarse bran. Grinding and milling might affect the hydration characteristics of food fibers. The chemical treatments can solubilize some of the constituents of fibers like pectin and lignin (Thibault et al.,1992). The treatment of alkaline hydrogen peroxide with wheat straw, corn stalk, cereal bran, vegetable and fruit pulp will remove the lignin and resulted fibers will able to absorb more water (Gould et al., 1989). The sugar beet fibers treated with acid and alkaline solutions were found to be having altered hydration properties and increased cation exchange capacity (Bertin et al., 1988). The thermal treatment of food can result in to Maillard reaction rather than changing food fiber into insoluble compounds and resistant starch (Thibault et al., 1992). In one study, the fiber content of wheat products was found to be increased with intensity of extrusion cooking (Bjorck et aI, 1984; Asp et al, 1986). Extrusion cooking can increase the amount of water soluble pectin (Ralet et al, 1991). Wet thermal processing of fruit and vegetable fibers will increase the amount of soluble fiber by partially degrading the pectic polysaccharides. The degree of the various heat treatments will decide the change in the physic- chemical properties of fibers. Heating may lower fiber content or modify the fiber distribution between water soluble and insoluble fractions by degrading components into smaller compounds (Anderson and Clydesdale, 1980; Varo et al, 1984; Arrigoni et al, 1986; Asp et al, 1986; Caprez et al, 1986).

Increasing the dietary fiber too fast can cause abdominal cramping, bloating and gas. Hence, intake should be increased slowly with 5 g per week and also consumption of fluids (about 8-10 cups per day) should be increased. Too much inclusion of dietary fiber can bind some minerals and decrease their absorption. However, if mineral intake is adequate then a recommended dietary fiber intake will not compromise mineral balance. Consuming a diet that provides a variety of nutrients is the key. Scanning electron microscopy results showed the two processing methods yielded fiber that had a much greater surface area, as reflected by increased furrowing and cracking on the surface of the heat treated fiber (Chang & Morris 2007).

CONCLUSION

The detailed review of dietary fibers is given in this chapter. Various sources of dietary fibers and the health benefits of dietary fibers are discussed. The appropriate intake of dietary fiber appear to lower the risk of developing coronary heart disease, stroke, hypertension, diabetes, obesity and certain gastrointestinal disorders. Fiber intake reduces the blood pressure and serum cholesterol levels. Recommended intake of soluble fiber improves the glycemia and insulin sensitivity in the diabetic patients. Fiber supplementation can help in obesity management. Suggested dietary fiber intake will help in controlling the gastrointestinal disorders such as gastroesophageal reflux disease, duodenal ulcer, diverticulitis, constipation and hemorrhoids. Some fiber like cellulose inhibits induced colon cancer. In addition, the effect of various food processing operations on the dietary fiber is also discussed. Daily recommended doses were discussed and it will be more appropriate to consult the dietician or physician for individual requirements (Read and Eastwood, 1992).

REFERENCES

Anderson, N. E., & Clydesdale, F. M. (1980). Effects of processing on the dietary fiber content of wheat bran, pureed green beans and carrots. *Journal of Food Science*, *45*(6), 1533–1537. doi:10.1111/j.1365-2621.1980.tb07556.x

Arrigoni, E., Caprez, A., Amado, R., & Neukom, H. (1986). Chemical composition and physical properties of modified dietary fibre sources. *Food Hydrocolloids*, *1*(1), 57–64. doi:10.1016/S0268-005X(86)80007-8

Asp, N. G., Bjorck, I., & Nyman, M. (1986). Effects of processing on dietary fibre. In R. Amado & T. F. Schweizer (Eds.), *Nahrungsfasem dietary fibres* (pp. 177–189). London: Academic Press.

Association of Official Analytical Chemists. (1980). *Official methods of analysis* (11th ed.). Washington, DC: AOAC.

Atwater, W. O. (1900). *Discussion of the terms digestibility, availability and fuel value*. Twelfth Annual Report of the Storrs Agricultural Experimental Station.

Bertin, C., Rouau, X., & Thibault, I. F. (1988). Structure and properties of sugar beet fibres. *Science of Food and Agriculture*, (44), 15-29.

Bjorck, I., Nyman, M., & Asp, N. G. (1984). Extrusion-cooking and dietary fiber. I. Effects on dietary fiber content and on degradation in the rat intestinal tract. *Cereal Chemistry*, *61*, 74–179.

British Nutrition Foundation. (1990). *Complex carbohydrates in foods*. London: Chapman and Hall.

Britt, B., Freeman, A., & Amgen, C. (2013). Incorporated, thousand oaks, Dietary Composition and Obesity. *Digestive Diseases and Sciences*, *4*(3), 16–24.

Caprez, A., Arrigoni, E., Amado, R., & Neukom, H. (1986). Influence of different type of thermal treatment on the chemical composition and physical properties of wheat bran. *Journal of Cereal Science*, *4*(4), 233–239. doi:10.1016/S0733-5210(86)80025-X

Chang, M. C., & Morris, W. C. (2007). The Effect of Heat Treatments on Dietary Fiber as Assessed by Scanning Electron Microscopy. *Journal of Food Processing and Preservation*, *14*(5), 335–343. doi:10.1111/j.1745-4549.1990.tb00138.x

Daniel, D. G. (2006). *Dietary Fiber*. Washington, DC: ILSI Press.

Flint, A. J., Hu, F. B., Glynn, R. J., Jensen, M. K., Franz, M., Sampson, L., & Rimm, E. B. (2009). Whole grains and incident hypertension in man. *The American Journal of Clinical Nutrition*, *90*(3), 493–498. doi:10.3945/ajcn.2009.27460 PMID:19571218

Flourie, B. (1992). The Influence of Dietary Fibre on Carbohydrate Digestion and Absorption. In T. F. Schweizer et al. (Eds.), *Dietary Fibre - A Component of Food* (pp. 40–54). Springer-Verlag London Limited. doi:10.1007/978-1-4471-1928-9_10

Gould, J. M., Jasberg, B. K., Dexter, L. B., Hsu, J. T., Lewis, S. M., Fahey, G. C. (1989). High fiber, non-caloric flour substitute for baked food properties of alkaline peroxide-treated lignocellulose. *Cereal Chemistry*, (66), 201-205.

Heller, S. N., Rivers, J. M., & Hackler, L. R. (1977). Dietary fiber: The effect of particle size and pH on its measurement. *Journal of Food Science*, *42*(2), 436–439. doi:10.1111/j.1365-2621.1977.tb01517.x

Indian Standard Institution (ISI). (1985). Method for Estimation Of total Dietary Fibre in Foodstuffs. Author.

Lupton, J. R. (2010). Codex definition of dietary fibre and issues requiring resolution. In Dietary fibre: new frontiers for food and health. Texas A&M University.

Nagengast, F. M. (1992). Dietary Fibre and Bile Acid Metabolism. Academic Press.

Nugent, A. P. (2005). Health properties of resistant starch. *Nutrition Bulletin*, *30*(1), 27–54. doi:10.1111/j.1467-3010.2005.00481.x

Parisi, G. C., Zilli, M., Miani, M. P., Carrara, M., Bottona, E., Verdianelli, G., & Leandro, G. et al. (2002). High-fiber diet supplementation in patients with irritable bowel syndrome (IBS): A multicenter, randomized, open trial comparison between wheat bran diet and partially hydrolyzed guar gum (PHGG). *Digestive Diseases and Sciences*, *47*(8), 1697–1704. doi:10.1023/A:1016419906546 PMID:12184518

Ralet, M. C., Thibault, J. F., & Della, V. G. (1991). Solubilisation of sugar beet cell wall polysaccharides by extrusion-cooking. *Lebensmittel-Wissenschaft + [i.e. Und] Technologie. Food Science + Technology. Science + Technologie Alimentaire*, *24*, 107–112.

Ranganna, S. (1995). *Handbook of Analysis and Quality control for fruit and vegetable project*. New Delhi: McGraw-Hill.

Read, N. W., & Eastwood, M. A. (1992). Gastro-intestinal physiology and function. In T. F. Schweizer et al. (Eds.), *Dietary Fibre - A Component of Food* (pp. 40–54). Springer-Verlag London Limited. doi:10.1007/978-1-4471-1928-9_5

Rossander, L., Sandbergv, A. S., & Sandstrom, B. (1992). The influence of dietary fibre on mineral absorption and utilization. In T. F. Schweizer et al. (Eds.), *Dietary Fibre - A Component of Food* (pp. 40–54). Springer-Verlag London Limited. doi:10.1007/978-1-4471-1928-9_11

Slavin, J. (2013). Health aspects of dietary fiber. In J. Slavin (Ed.), *Fibre- rich and wholegrain foods* (pp. 234–239). New York: Woodhead Publishing Limited. doi:10.1533/9780857095787.1.61

Thibault, J. F., Lahaye, M., & Guillon, F. (1992). Physico-chemical properties of food plant cell walls. In T. F. Schweizer et al. (Eds.), *Dietary Fibre - A Component of Food* (pp. 40–54). Springer-Verlag London Limited. doi:10.1007/978-1-4471-1928-9_2

Varo, P., Veijalainen, K., & Koivistoinen, P. (1984). Effect of heat treatment on the dietary fibre contents of potato and tomato. *Journal of Food Technology*, *19*(4), 485–492. doi:10.1111/j.1365-2621.1984.tb00372.x

W.H.O. (2003). *Diet, nutrition and the prevention of chronic diseases*. Report of a Joint WHO/FAO Expert Consultation. WHO Technical Report Series 916.

KEY TERMS AND DEFINITIONS

Crude Fiber: The fiber that remains unchanged even after food is digested with alkali and acid, but generally alkali and acid destroys all soluble and some insoluble fiber.

Edible Fiber/Dietary Fiber: Indigestible roughage portion of food received from plants. It has two parts (1) Soluble (2) Insoluble.

Fiber: Substance that is resistant to the action of digestive enzymes since it has some resistant filamentous thread like structured substances. Examples are cellulose, lignin, pectin, etc.

Functional Food: A modified food which gives an additional health promoting and disease preventing function.

Insoluble Fiber: Dietary fibers that are insoluble in water and indigestible in human intestine. This fiber increases bulk to the stool and seem to help in quicker movement of food through the stomach and intestine. Wheat bran, vegetables, and whole grains are the major sources of insoluble fiber.

Prebiotics: Indigestible food ingredients which enhances the growth of beneficial microorganisms in the human intestine. Examples of some prebiotics are fructooligosaccharide, isomaltooligosaccharide, inulin, fiber, xylooligosaccharide, oligomate, palatinose, pyrodextrin and raftiline.

Probiotics: The microorganisms which are found to be health benefiting when consumed by humans or animals. Some of the examples are lactic acid bacteria, yeasts.

Soluble Fiber: This fiber is soluble in water and becomes gel like or gummy or viscous during digestion. It will slow down the digestion. It will promote the excretion of fatty substances and help to regulate the body's use of sugars. Oat bran, barley, nuts, seeds, beans, lentils, peas and psyllium are common sources for soluble fiber.

Chapter 3
Phytonutrients of Nutraceutical Importance: Exploring Antimicrobial, Antiproliferative, and Antioxidant Activities

Marcus Vinícius Dias-Souza
Federal University of Minas Gerais, Brazil

Renan Martins dos Santos
Federal University of Minas Gerais, Brazil

ABSTRACT

Phytotherapy re-emerged in the latest years as a healing system accepted and spread worldwide, and different molecules have been investigated due to their benefits to health. Nutraceutical formulations, which allow the intake of phytonutrients (generally in low levels in plant food) in concentrations that are enough to achieve the desired outcomes, represent feasible alternatives to improve general health and to prevent and treat varied diseases. Notwithstanding the incompleteness of an evidence-based clinical use of nutraceuticals, many questions remain unanswered regarding their global effects in humans and animals. Thus, the aim of this chapter is to provide recent evidence on chemical and pharmacological features of the main phytonutrients explored in nutraceutical formulations, focusing antimicrobial, antioxidant and antiproliferative potentials. Also, some insights on drug-phytonutrients interactions will be discussed.

DOI: 10.4018/978-1-5225-0607-2.ch003

INTRODUCTION

The rapidly increasing knowledge on nutrition, pharmacology and plant biotechnology has changed some concepts about food and health. Epidemiologic studies from the latest 50 years have provided evidence of an inverse association between the dietary intake of fruit and vegetables and occurrence of varied illness such as diabetes, osteoporosis, cancers, cardiovascular and infectious diseases. This protective effect obtained in food intake has been assigned to plant secondary metabolites; specifically, phytomolecules with nutritional properties, the phytonutrients. In a few words, phytonutrients can be defined as plant-derived compounds with nutritive properties that can have also curative or preventive effects over diseases (Michels et al., 2000). These phytomolecules are thought to be responsible for most of the health benefits observed in individuals that adopted long-time diets rich in fruits, vegetables, beans, cereals, and plant-based beverages such as tea and wine. The correlation between observed effects and the type or concentration of some phytomolecules has been described, such as Lycopene and Resveratrol, for instance, in cancer prevention. In plants, several phytomolecules of nutraceutical interest are part of defense mechanisms against environmental challenges such as damage due to ultraviolet light exposure and natural predators such as insects and other plagues (Hecht, 2000; Sharma et al., 2009).

The low bioavailability of phytomolecules is an important limitation on their use to prevent or treat diseases. The often low concentration found in plasma has led to some skepticism in this sense; however, in spite of their low bioavailability, varied studies in the latest years have provided evidence of their beneficial effects in humans and animals. To overcome the issue of low levels of phytonutrients in fruits and vegetables, pharmaceutical and nutritional companies have developed several pharmaceutical dosage forms of nutraceutical formulations and other dietary plant-based supplementary products. This becomes even more relevant considering that nutraceutical formulations provide adequate concentrations of phytomolecules and thus, different beneficial effects to health can be expected. Moreover, nutraceutical formulations make the use of phytonutrients feasible in a clinical perspective (McCullough et al., 2003; Key et al., 2004; Yang et al., 2010). Examples of Nutraceuticals are presented in Table 1.

The Dietary Supplement Health and Education Act, adopted by the American Association of Clinical Endocrinologists (Mechanick et al., 2003), provides adequate definitions of dietary supplements and nutraceuticals, which will be adopted and slightly adapted in this chapter for a better comprehension by non-specialist readers. According to Mechanick et al. (2003), dietary supplements comprise five main groups of ingredients/elements:

Table 1. Examples of phytomolecules-based nutraceutical formulations

Formulation Brand	Phytomolecules	Manufacturer	Indications
Inneov Solar®	β-carotene, Lycopene, tocopherols and *Polypodium leucotomos* extract	Loreal and Nestlé	Oral photoprotection
Lauricidin®	Lauric acid	Med-Chem	Stimulation of the immune system
Extra-Strength Broccoli Extract with Glucosinolates®	Glucosinolates of broccoli extract	Green Foods	ROS/RNS scavenger, protection of the cardiovascular system
Flavonoid 1000®	Hisperidin, rutin, bromelin and citric bioflavonoids (200, 50, 50, 1000 mg, respectively)	DaVinci	Relief on varicose veins, reduction of inflammatory processes associated to pain, metabolism booster.

ROS: Reactive oxygen species; RNS: Reactive nitrogen species.

1. Vitamins or minerals;
2. General phytomolecules;
3. Amino acids;
4. Other substances that increase the total dietary intake such as enzymes;
5. Byproducts such as metabolites and constituents, or even extracts of any of the elements mentioned in topics 1 to 4.

Thus, dietary supplements are not foods in their natural form, but are not limited to common nutritional agents.

Nutraceuticals, on the other hand, are defined as sophisticated dietary supplements based in concentrated presentations of one or more pure bioactive substances, originally isolated from plant foods, although mineral and animal bioactive molecules are also included. These formulations are prepared in different pharmaceutical dosage forms and are used in dosages many times superior to those detectable in their original sources to improve health in varied aspects (Mechanick et al., 2003).

Most nutraceutical and dietary supplements formulations may be purchased without medical prescription in several countries, and in the latest years, pharmaceutical and health food companies have come up with new formulations claiming to have varied pharmacological effects of interest to prevent diseases (although some of them are still demanding more evidence from clinical studies, as will be discussed in this chapter). Different groups suggest that nutraceuticals present drug-like actions, and therefore, their formulations should be marketed, for instance, as over-the-counter medication. Considering this, a question arises: the rules of Lipinski et al. (1997), widely accepted to characterize a molecule or compound as not "drug-like", states that when a substance falls into one or more of the following properties:

1. More than five hydrogen-bond donors, considering OH and NH moieties;
2. More than ten hydrogen-bond acceptors, considering N and O atoms;
3. Molecular weight beyond 500 g/Mol;
4. Octanol/water partition coefficient log P higher than 5.

Therefore, as it is not reasonable to assume that the chemical properties of all nutraceuticals are within these reference levels, it becomes technically difficult to generalize that nutraceutical formulations could be regulated as over-the-counter drugs. Also, most of the phytomolecules used as nutraceuticals have not shown cytotoxic effects in several *in vivo* and *in vitro* models, being widely recognized as safe for human and animal use (Zhao et al., 2012).

Strong recommendations for consumption of nutraceuticals have become progressively popular to improve health, and to prevent and treat diseases. Nutraceuticals and dietary plant-based supplements, among other properties such as antioxidant and antiproliferative, can stimulate immune response and result in fewer infections or control of infectious diseases, particularly in the elderly and in malnourished, critically ill individuals (Pham-Huy et al., 2008; Lee et al., 2009).

Notwithstanding the incompleteness of an evidence-based use of nutraceuticals, many questions remain unanswered regarding their global effects in humans and animals. Therefore, the aim of this chapter is to provide recent evidence on chemical and pharmacological features of the main phytonutrients explored in nutraceutical formulations, focusing their antimicrobial, anti-oxidant and anti-inflammatory potentials. Also, some insights on drug-phytonutrients interactions will be discussed. With more direction on flavonoids, carotenoids, phytosterols, lauric acid and glucosinolates, we shall present recent evidence of the mentioned pharmacological activities and the possible benefits on the treatment of infectious diseases and cancers with important burden on human health worldwide. However, we do not intend here to exhaust the subject, but to propose discussions to open doors for more advances in this exciting research field.

BACKGROUND

Flavonoids

Flavonoids are a diverse family of phytonutrients derived from phenylpropanoid and malonyl-coenzyme A pathways, characterized by two aromatic cycles (rings A and B) linked to a heterocycle (C ring) (Figure 1).

This phenylpropanoid core with 15 carbon atoms is usually modified by reactions such as alkylation, glycosylation, hydroxylation, methylation, methoxylation and

Figure 1. Structures of the major groups of flavonoids
Authors' personal archive.

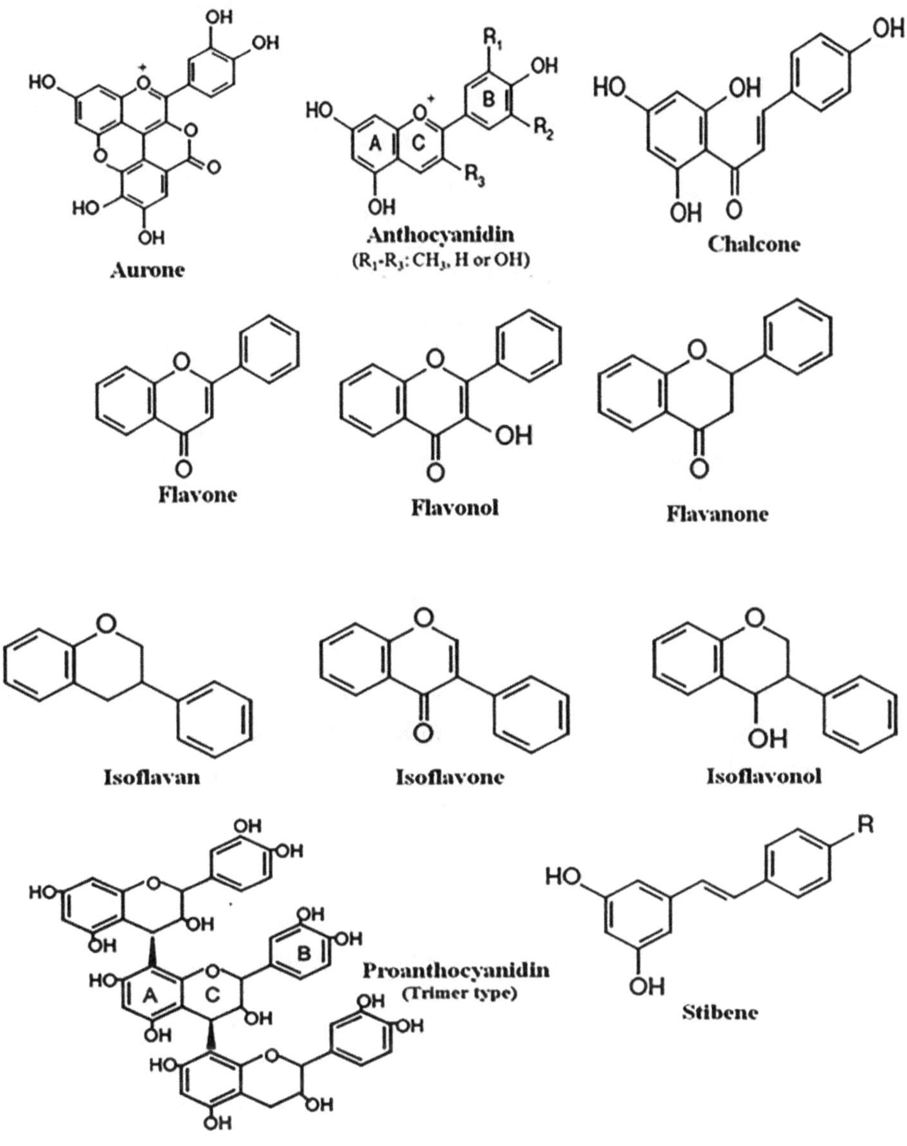

oxidation, generating the major subgroups aurones, anthocyanins, chalcones, flavones, flavonols, flavanones, isoflavans, isoflavones, isoflavonols, stibenes, and proanthocyanidins. Currently, more than 10.000 flavonoid structures had been elucidated, and several pharmacological potentials have been assigned to them, such

Figure 2. Structure of the flavonoids discussed in this chapter
Authors' personal archive.

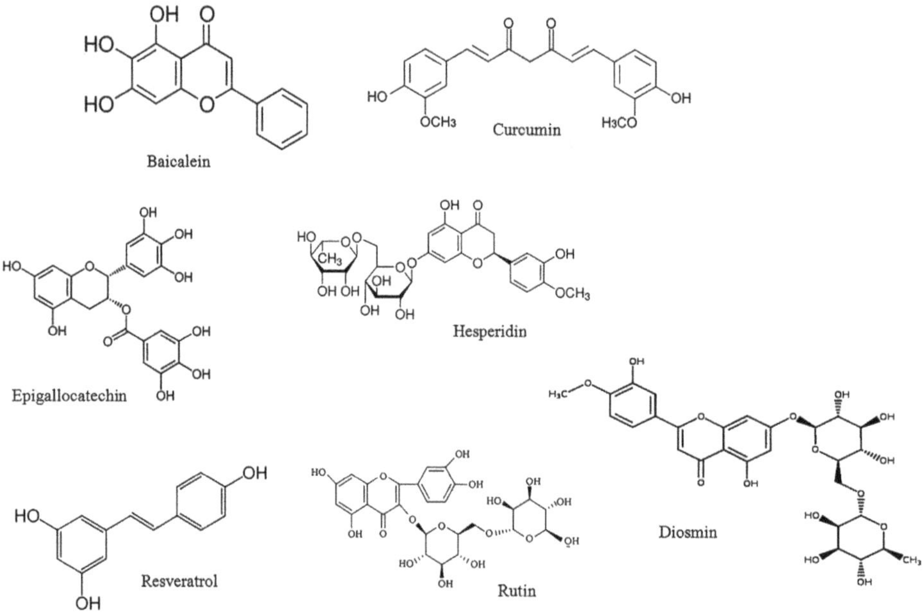

as antiproliferative, wound healing, anti-diabetic, cardioprotective, vasotonic, neuroprotective, antioxidant, antibacterial, antifungal, antiviral, and metabolism booster (Gutteridge, 1994; Haslam, 1996). Following, important flavonoids widely used as nutraceuticals will be discussed (Figure 2).

Baicalein

Baicalein ($C_{15}H_{10}O_5$) is found in citric fruits and mostly in *Scutellaria baicalensis*, a chinese herbal remedy known as skullcap or Huang Qin. Due to its good lipophilicity, baicalein can be transported into cells by passive diffusion. Most of the compound passes through glicuronization and and sulphation during absorption, and becomes too polar to pass through the lipid barriers. being transported in other ways inhibit CYP2C9 enzyme. Baicalein is able to (Stobiecki, 2000; Chen et al., 2006).

Chen et al. (2006) investigated the antimicrobial activity and the possible mechanism of action of baicalein on Methicillin-resistant *Staphylococcus aureus* (MRSA). Changes on membrane penetrability, protein synthesis, DNA topoisomerase activities and restriction map were assessed. The minimum inhibitory concentration reached 0.04 mg/mL, and after 16 h, the total soluble content of proteins decreased 44.62%. The flavonoid inhibited the activities of DNA topoisomerase I and II in a concentration of 0.025 mg/mL. Later, Moghaddam et al. (2014) examined the *in vitro* antiviral activity of baicalin, the main metabolite of baicalein, in different steps of dengue virus replication. Baicalin inhibited virus replication at IC50 = 13.5 ± 0.08 μg/mL with SI = 21.5 following virus internalization by Vero cells. Baicalin exhibited activity against DENV-2 extracellular particles and showed anti-adsorption effect.

Liu et al. (2015) assessed the protective effects of baicalein using an *in vivo* model of polymicrobial sepsis-induced liver injury. Polymicrobial sepsis was induced in C57BL/6 mice, which were treated with intraperitonial 100 mg/kg baicalein after 1, 6 and 12 h of the infection. Baicalein inhibited the mitogen-activated protein kinases (MAPKs) activation and suppressed the transcriptional activity of nuclear factor-kappa B (NF-κB). Resulting effects comprised improved survival of septic mice, ameliorated liver injury, and reduced both neutrophil infiltration and hepatic inflammatory cytokines expression and release.

Li et al. (2013) synthesized baicalein-8 benzyl amino acid derivatives and evaluated their cytotoxicity *in vitro* against HepG2 cells. Substitutions on positions C6 and C8 were considered, and amino acids were subjected to methylation and aminoacylation reactions. Through carboxyl group protection and aminoacylation of amino acid and benzyl protection of baicalein, derivatives of baicalein-6-O-amino acid esters were obtained. A total of 13 novel derivatives were synthesized and chemically characterized. Four derivatives showed a significant increase in cytotoxicity when compared to baicalein. Some baicalein-5-O-amino acid derivatives were also synthesized, but they lost cytotoxic activity. This suggested that 5-OH is an important structural feature for the cytotoxic activity of baicalein and its derivatives.

Luo et al. (2014) studied the *in vitro* antiproliferative effect of 30 novel synthesized baicalein derivatives. Three human cancer cell lines were used: HepG2 (human liver carcinoma), A549 (human alveolar basal epithelial adenocarcinoma) and BCG-823 (gastric carcinoma), and baicalein was used as a comparative control. The compounds were tested over a range of concentrations from 0.1 to 100 M for 48 h, and IC50 values were estimated. Apoptosis mechanism was identified for 8 compounds, which moiety of 7-benzyloxy group exhibited more potent anti-proliferative activity against the tumor cell lines when compared to baicalein. One of the molecules was found to be 14-fold, 16-fold, and 6-fold more potent than baicalein against HepG2, A549 and BCG-823 cancer cell lines, respectively.

Zeng et al. (2015) assessed the anti-allergic and anti-inflammatory activities of baicalein and chrysin, by analysing the interactions between hyaluronidase using experimental methods and molecular docking. With the increase of baicalein or chrysin concentration, the activity of the enzyme decreased significantly and the 50% relative activity (IC50) of baicalein and chrysin were estimated to be 52 ± 7and 267 ± 33 mol/L, respectively. Considering thermodynamic parameters and molecular modeling, authors suggested that each molecule could bind to hyaluronidase spontaneously through electrostatic forces, hydrophobic interactions and hydrogen bonding.

Curcumin

Curcumin ($C_{21}H_{20}O_6$) was firstly isolated from turmeric. The flavonoid is usually a bright orange to yellow powder, with melting point at around 183 ºC, sensible to light and of low bioavailability in humans, but is rapidly metabolized in the liver. Low levels of this substance can be detected in plasma and tissues, and due to its low water solubility and poor absorption, it is quickly excreted. Curcumin inhibits epigenetic enzymes such as histone deacetilases, and has been associated with protection against cancer and cardiovascular diseases. Although the route of biosynthesis of Curcumin is not fully understood, there are two proposed mechanisms that may help to explain its synthesis: the first mentions the extension reaction of cinnamic acid with five malonil-CoA molecules, and the second involves two cinnamate molecules joined by malonil-CoA (Kuzuyama et al., 2005; Rocks et al., 2012).

Rudrappa and Bais (2008) analyzed the effects of curcumin on the virulence of a *Pseudomonas aeruginosa* strain through *in vitro* assays for virulence factors production and tests in pathogenicity models using *Arabidopsis thaliana* and *Caenorhabditis elegans*. Curcumin inhibited the expression of virulence factors such as biofilm, pyocyanin, elastase, protease, and acyl homoserine lactone production, resulting in reduced pathogenicity of the strain. Transcriptomic analysis of the treated strain showed downregulation of quorum sensing genes. Kaur et al. (2010) also described a mechanism for the antimicrobial activity of curcumin in *Bacillus subtilis* and *Escherichia coli*, which relies on growth inhibition by blocking the assembly of the cytoskeletal FtsZ protein, involved in prokaryotic cell division and present in several bacterial species.

The possible synergism of mitomycin C and curcumin was studied by Zhou et al. (2011) in order to suppress human breast cancer *in vitro* and *in vivo*. Experiments were performed through assessing cell cycle phases of MCF-7 cells with flow cytometry. Tumor growth and cell cycle-associated protein expression were also monitored. It was seen that curcumin inhibited MCF-7 breast cancer cell viability in a concentration-dependent manner, and IC_{50} value was of 40 µmol/L.

Chhunchha et al. (2011) investigated the mechanisms involved in the antioxidant activity of curcumin, exploring peroxiredoxin 6 pathway, an anti-ROS pleiotropic oxidative stress-response protein, via specificity of protein 1 activity, against proapoptotic stimuli. Molecular analyses indicated that curcumin enhanced specificity protein 1 and peroxiredoxin 6 mRNA and protein expression in a concentration-dependent manner and downregulated ROS-mediated apoptosis by blunting ROS expression and lipid peroxidation. Curcumin could not activate peroxiredoxin 6 expression in the presence of specificity protein 1 inhibitors, suggesting that curcumin increased expression of peroxiredoxin 6 in a dependent way of specificity protein 1 activity.

Rocks et al. (2012) studied the effects of curcumin complexes with cyclodextrin alone or in combination with gemcitabine on the growth of orthotopically implanted lung tumors *in vivo*. Tumors were monitored on 7, 10, 14, 18 and 21 days after cell injection. Tumors development was almost completely abolished when mice were treated by the association with gemcitabine. The association of curcumin–cyclodextrin-gemcitabine resulted in a two-fold reduction of proliferation index in mouse lung tumours when compared to mice treated with the vehicle alone or non-soluble curcumin.

Diosmin

Diosmin ($C_{28}H_{32}O_{15}$) is a flavone originally isolated from *Teucrium gnaphalodes,* and is quite abundant in citric fruits, with concentrations ranging from 17.8 to 245 mg/100 g. This flavonoid is hydrophobic and has a melting point of around 274 °C, being obtained via dehydrogenation of hesperidin,. Its half life is of around 11 hours, being mostly eliminated (80%) in stool. Diosmin has anti-inflammatory, venotonic vasoprotective effects, being the latest ones associated to the extension of norepinephrin activity in veins, increasing the venous tonus and the intensity and frequency of contractions in the lymphatic vessels (Bae et al., 2000).

Studies of antimicrobial activity of diosmin are, curiously, rare. Bae et al. (1999) described the anti-Helicobacter pylori activity of varied flavonoids, and in their study, the minimum inhibitory concentration of diosmin was higher than 100 µg/mL. Later, Bae et al (2000) assessed the antiviral activity of several flavonoids, and the inhibitory effects of diosmin in cell lines infected wih rotavirus was reached with 10 µg/mL.

Regarding its antioxidant activity, Akroum et al. (2010) described effective free radical scavenging activity of diosmin in the DPPH assay, reaching 50.35% activity at 10 µg/mL. Also, the effect of diosmin in oxidative stress in streptozotocin-nicotinamide induced diabetic rats was studied by Srinivasan and Pari (2012) through assessing lipid peroxidation and ameliorative properties. Diabetic animals had increased plasma glucose concentration with significant decrease in plasma insulin levels. The activity of superoxide dismutase, catalase, glutathione peroxidase and glutathione-S-transferase were reduced. The levels of vitamins C, E and reduced glutathione decreased while lipid peroxidation markers increased in liver and kidney tissues of diabetic control rats, when compared to healthy control rats. The oral treatment with diosmin showed ameliorative effects on the analyzed biochemical parameters.

Barreca et al. (2013) demonstrated that diosmin binding to human serum albumine can contribute to protect it against degradation. Fluorescence experiments indicated that the binding site of the flavonoid involved modifications around Trp214 at the subdomain IIA. A decrease in α-helix structure following flavonoid binding was also detected. *In silico* analyzes suggested that the primary binding site of diosmin was located in a microenvironment able to stabilize the binding of the ligand in non-planar conformations, known as Sudlow's site I.

Using animal model of Wistar rats, Tahir et al. (2013) described the effect of diosmin on attenuation of hepatic toxicity induced by 2-acetylaminofluorene and, the chemopreventive efficacy of the flavonoid against hepatocarcinogenesis induced and increased by diethylnitrosamine and 2-acetylaminofluorene, respectively. The protective effect of diosmin was demonstrated by reductions of visible hepatic nodules, restoration of early tumor markers such as Ki67 and ODC, and reductions of serum cytotoxicity enzyme markers AST and ALT, oxidative stress biomarkers, cell necrosis markers like TNF-α and inflammatory enzymatic markers COX-2 and iNOS.

Epigallocatechin

This polyphenol of molecular formula $C_{22}H_{18}O_{11}$, is available at higher levels in the leaves of *Camelia sinensis* (around 7400mg/100 g as green tea, and around 4300 mg/100 g as white tea). It can also be found in lower concentrations in the skin of apples, plums, onions, walnuts and hazelnuts. This flavonoid is characterized as a white to pink powder, with melting point around 218 °C. Different from other flavonoids, it is soluble in water, and also in ethanol and DMSO (Assis et al., 2015).

Lipson et al. (2015) recently used epigallocatechin against rotavirus. After 3 days in culture, pure epigallocatechin concentrations of 80, 160, and 320 µg/mL reduced the virus infectivity titer levels to 50, 20, and 15% of the control, respectively. No cytotoxicity was detected in the concentrations used.

To increase the antimicrobial activity and stability of epigallocatechin, Sun et al. (2011) complexed the flavonoid with Cu^{+2} into polyvinyl alcohol nanofibers. MICs of the complex against different bacteria and yeasts ranged from 8 to 600 ug/mL, and high values of MIC are related to *S. cerevisiae* and *C. albicans*. The bactericidal activity of the complex against *E. coli* and *P. nitroreducens* was not significantly weaker than that against Bacillus cereus and *B. subtilis*. The activity against *S. aureus* was lower than that against the other bacteria (including Gram-negative).

Nevertheless, epigallocatechin was not effective in eliminating *Streptococcus mutans* from dentin caries-like lesions. Assis et al. (2015) evaluated the efficacy of epigallocatechin at 0.5%, 1%, and 2% concentrations in an in vitro model of dentin caries-like lesions. When compared, chlorhexidine digluconate, an antimicrobial molecule widely used against caries, the antimicrobial efficacy of epigallocatechin was significantly lower against the tested *S. mutans* strain.

Harpole et al. (2015) investigated the effects of epigallocatechin against SK-OV-3 ovarian cancer cell line model, aiming to explore antioxidant exposure to slow the progression of the disease. A statistically significant increase in nitric oxide following the administration of epigallocatechin alone and in combination with thymoquinone was detected at 24, 48 and 72 hours, being approximately three times higher than the control.

Considering that high doses of epigallocatechin can induce toxicity in the liver, kidneys, and intestine, Cai et al. (2015) investigated the proliferation and apoptosis of H9C2 cardiomyocytes treated with high doses of epigallocatechin. Using the CCK8 and TUNEL assays, and western blotting detection of alterations of Sirtuin 1 (SIRT1), it was seen that different from other organs, epigallocatechin inhibited H9C2 cardiomyocytes proliferation and induced apoptosis in a time-dependent and dose-dependent way. The downregulation of SIRT1 protein expression is possibly involved in this mechanism.

Hesperidin

The name "hesperidin" is derived from the term "hesperidium", which means "fruits produced in citric trees". Hesperidin ($C_{28}H_{34}O_{15}$) is able to inhibit LDL oxidation and thus, prevent atherosclerotic plaque growth. It is also able to inhibit the intestinal absorption of cholesterol and increase its hepatic catabolism. It is usually the most abundant molecule among the flavonoids present in lemon or orange. Hesperidin is hydrophobic, of pale yellow color and with melting point ranging from 262 to 258 ºC (Wilcox et al., 2001).

Abuelsaad et al. (2013) performed susceptibility tests through agar-diffusion against *Aeromonas hydrophila.* Hesperidin was tested in the concentrations of 100, 50, 25, and 12.5 mg/ml. The concentration of 100 mg/ml was the most effective in reducing bacterial growth. Using borth microdilution, authors investigated minimal inhibitory concentrations (MIC) and minimal bactericidal concentration (MBC). Hesperidin MBC was of 12.500 µg/mL and MIC was of 3.125 µg/mL. Similarly, Abass et al. (2014) assessed the antimicrobial activity of crude extracts of orange peels, rich in hesperidin, against *Bacillus subtilis, Staphylococcus aureus, Streptococcus pyogenes, Escherichia coli* and *Salmonella typhi* by agar diffusion. The extract was effective mostly against *B. subtilis* (45 µg/mL), and E. coli (75 µg/mL), and less effective against *S. typhy* and *S. aureus* (175 µg/mL)

In one of the first studies with commercial formulations of phytomolecules of nutraceutical importance, using animal (rats) model, Damon et al. (1987) administered hesperidine tablets (Daflon® 500 mg) by gastric intubation for a period of 26 weeks. There were no deaths, no alteration of weight and standard functional tests had no modifications.

Bigoniya & Singh (2014) investigated the anti-ulcer potential of hesperidin through evidences of histological analyzes of its antioxidant activity in mucosal tissue of the stomach. Ulcers were induced with indomethacin (oral doses of 150,

300 and 450 mg/kg) and hypothermic restrain stress. At the doses of 300 and 450 mg/kg, hesperidin induced pH increase, with histological evidences of cytoprotection. Glutathione, super oxide dismutase and catalase, important antioxidant enzyme systems, and mucin levels (for tissue protection) increased significantly at 450 mg/kg. Thus, the antioxidant, mucoprotective and cytoprotective effects of hesperidin are strongly associated to its anti-ulcer properties.

Using a murine model, Man et al. (2015) demonstrated that topical applications of hesperidin improved epidermal functions in aged skin. Hesperidin did not stimulate epidermal proliferation, but decreased the pH in aged skin. Slight increase in transepidermal water loss rates (however ranging within normal loss rates of a healthy skin) was detected in treated skin, and accelerated barrier recovery was detected at 2 and 4 hours after the treatment. The expression of filaggrin, involucrin, and loricrin genes, all trivial for skin integrity, was increased in adult keratinocytes cultures treated with hesperidin. Topical hesperidin increased the levels gene expression of HMG-CoA and FAS in aged skin.

Resveratrol

Resveratrol ($C_{14}H_{12}O_3$) is a stilbene (3,5,4′-trihydroxystilbene) produced by several unrelated plant species like blackberry, ginger, blueberries and grapes, in response to injury, ultraviolet irradiation, microbial infections and other stressing conditions. Takaoka (1939) isolated this flavonoid for the first time from the roots of *Veratrum grandiflorum*. This flavonoid is also present in processed products based on grape and wine, appearing in other foods at lower concentrations. It is poorly soluble in water and is described as a yellowish-white powder, with melting point ranging from 261 to 263 °C. The molecule exists as cis- (Z) and trans- (E) diastereomers. The (E) diastereomer is the form in which resveratrol is found in nature. When exposed to ultraviolet irradiation, resveratrol can undergo isomerisation to the (Z) form.When administered orally, less than 5% of the flavonoid can be found in blood plasma. Among its biological activities, important anti-inflammatory mechanisms comprise the modulation of NF-κB and inhibition of action and expression of cyclooxygenases (COX). It has been described that resveratrol can also induce apoptosis, indicating its antiproliferative potential (Chen et al., 2012; Kumar & Pandey, 2013; Fremont, 2014).

Hwang & Lim (2015) investigated the mechanisms of the antimicrobial potential of resveratrol over E. coli species. It was seen that the production of reactive oxygen species (ROS) increased in the strains, although cell growth was not recovered by ROS quenching. Thus, ROS formation and cell death were not directly correlated to resveratrol treatment. DNA fragmentation increased in cells, and cell elongation was also observed. FtsZ, an essential cell-division protein involved in cell elongation in prokaryotes, had its gene expression and its formation strongly inhibited in *E. coli* strains.

A recent mechanism of the antifungal activity of resveratrol against *C. albicans* yeasts was proposed by Lee & Lee (2015). Interestingly, resveratrol can induce apoptosis in clinical isolates of *C. albicans*, as shown by the loss of mitochondrial membrane potential, an important event in resveratrol-induced apoptosis. Resveratrol also activated metacaspase and promoted cytochrome c release, confirming the apoptosis-induced mechanism.

Resveratrol is effective in scavenging free radicals to prevent LDL oxidation (Chang et al., 2011), and as an effective *in vivo* inhibitor of cyclooxygenase activity, resveratrol can significantly reduce oedema, osteoarthritis, airway inflammation, and can also prevent allograft rejection (Elmali et al., 2005Wu et al., 2005 a and b). In this context, the elegant study of Park et al. (2012) provided data on a new pathway in which resveratrol directly inactivates phosphodiesterase enzymes, indicating that the metabolic effects of this flavonoid are result of competitive inhibition of cAMP-degrading phosphodiesterases, leading to elevated cAMP levels and to a signaling cascade that activates situin 1.

The antiproliferative activity of resveratrol is also widely recognized. Reis-Sobreiro et al. (2009) analyzed the antimyeloma and antileukemia potentials of resveratrol. The flavonoid induced apoptosis in multiple myeloma and leukemia T-cell through coclustering of Fas/ CD95 death receptor and lipid rafts. Resveratrol-induced disruption of mitochondrial transmembrane potential was inhibited by a FADD dominant negative mutant by downstream signaling of Fas/CD95 blockage. This mechanism also inhibited apoptosis induced by resveratrol. Cells deficient in Fas/CD95 did not undergo resveratrol-induced apoptosis.

Frampton et al. (2010) assessed the antiproliferative effects of resveratrol on cholangiocarcinoma cells, in combination to chemotherapeutic drugs. Cholangiocarcinoma cell lines were treated with resveratrol and following, with 5-fluorouracil, gemcitabine, or mitomycin C. The combined treatment with resveratrol decreased cell proliferation and increased apoptosis in all in vitro assays, and more extensively than any of the chemotherapeutic drugs alone.

Scherzberg et al. (2015) studied the antiproliferative effect of the a methylated resveratrol analog Z-TMS [(Z)-3,5,4'-Trimethoxystilbene] over varied cancer cell lines, and compared the analog molecule results to pure resveratrol. Flow cytometric analysis revealed a G2/M cell cycle phases arrest after Z-TMS treatment, whereas resveratrol caused S phase arrest. Furthermore, Z-TMS impaired tubulin and microtubule polymerization, and no beneficial effects on lipid accumulation were observed for this molecule. The lacking beneficial metabolic effects of Z-TMS were assigned to a possible loss of activity on genes that may have the expression regulated by resveratrol.

Rutin

Rutin ($C_{27}H_{30}O_{16}$) has been described to be an effective angiogenesis inhibitor that is also able to block vascular endothelial growth factor (VEGF), what can potentially contribute to the control of some types of cancer. This flavonoid is present in fig, apples and wheat, and is usually presented as a solid yellow to white powder of melting point around 242 °C, being more soluble in methanol than in water. Other pharmacological properties described for rutin comprise anti-inflammatory activity and platelet aggregation inhibition, decreasing capillary permeability and improving microcirculation. These potentials contribute to prevent clots formation and thus, prevention of infarcts and strokes (Haslan, 1996; Ugusman et al., 2014).

Interestingly, the antimicrobial activity of rutin is still controversial somehow. Singh et al. (2008) identified rutin as the major flavonoid in *Pteris vittata* (Brake Fern). Hydromethanolic extracts of *P. vittata* (70, 80, and 90%) were tested against Gram-negative bacteria, and the 70% extract was the most effective against *Pseudomonas aeruginosa* and *Klebsiella pneumoniae*. Orhan et al. (2010) reported antimicrobial activity of rutin against MRSA, *E. coli, P. mirabilis, K. pneumoniae, P. aeruginosa* and *A. baumannii*. However, no activity was observed for rutin against Gram-negative bacteria in the study of Alves et al. (2013).

Ananth et al. (2015) developed thioglycolic acid-capped cadmium telluride quantum dots (TGA-CdTe QDs) and conjugated them to rutin, aiming to enahnce its antimicrobial activity. These complexes were tested against *E. coli*. Adsorption of conjugated QDs on cell wall and its penetration through porins were described as the main possible mechanisms of action of the antimicrobial activity of the complex. QDs also induced stable oxidative stress by ROS production, what contributes to increase the membrane permeability.

Rutin is mostly recognized for its potent antioxidant and anti-inflamatory activities, control of high blood pressure, protection of UV–radiation and mainly, its ability to decrease capillary fragility (Ugusman et al., 2014). Also, effects on bone resorption have been studied. Using a cell culture of bone marrow cells isolated from 4-5-week-old C57BL/6J mice, Kyung et al. (2008) described the effect of rutin on osteoclast formation. Rutin inhibited osteoclast formation induced by receptor activator of NF-κ B ligand (RANKL) at an early stage by reducing levels of ROS and TNF-α, which are elevated via RANKL. Rutin also lowers NF-κ B activation in response to RANKL.

Rutin contains disaccharide moieties and is generally better distributted on the body than other flavonoids. Choi et al. (2013) investigated the mechanisms of rutin and its direct targets involved in reduction of COX-2 expression in JB6 P+ cell lines by benzo[a]pyrene-7,8-diol-9,10-epoxide (B[a]PDE), its active metabolite. AP-1 and NF-kB activities (at DNA level) were mediated by the activation of MAPK-signaling pathways when induced by B[a]PDE, involving ERK, JNK, and p38 proteins. Thus, the transactivation of AP-1 and NF-kB was inhibited, an important mechanism of downregulation that affects the immune system. Rutin suppressed phosphorylation of ERK and upstream kinases such as MEK and Raf induced by B[a]PDE. Akt phosphorylation induced by B[a]PDE was suppressed in JB6 P^+ cells as well. Although rutin reduced B[a]PDE-induced Raf/MEK/ERK and Akt activation, it had no effect on the phosphorylation of the epidermal growth factor receptor (EGFR). Even $EGFR^{-/-}$ mouse embryonic fibroblast cells had COX-2 expression diminished after exposed to B[a]PDE. EGFR appeared to be directly targeted by rutin, and the suppressive effect on COX-2 expression is likely to be mediated by Raf/MEK/ERK and Akt signaling.

Xu et al. (2014) studied the effects of rutin in the clinical evolution of Alzheimer's disease (AD) in a murine model, and proposed the use of this molecule in AD treatments. Orally administered rutin attenuated memory deficits in AD-induced mice, and decreased the levels of oligomeric extracellular β-amyloid (Aβ) plaques. Super oxide dismutase (SOD) activity and glutathione (GSH)/glutathione disulfide (GSSG) ratio were increased, demonstrating its antioxidant activity in the central nervous system. Rutin also reduced GSSG and malondialdehyde (MDA) levels, downregulated microgliosis and astrocytosis, and decreased interleukin (IL)-1β and IL-6 levels in the brain, indicating its anti-inflammatory neuroactivity. The pretreatment with rutin reduced the activity of hepatic transaminases and improved the histological signs of acute liver damage in intoxicated mice. Rutin was effective in the suppression of nitrotyrosine formation, but had weak effects in attenuation of the inflammation in the liver, as indicated by measurements of nuclear factor-kappa B (NF-κB), tumor necrosis factor-α (TNF-α) and cyclooxygenase (COX-2). The expression of inducible nitric oxide synthase (iNOS) was potently suppressed by rutin. Thus, protection against nitrosative stress and hepatocellular damage can be effectively achieved by rutin, in spite of the weak antioxidant and anti-inflammatory activities.

Carotenoids: Lycopene and β-Carotene

Carotenoids are widespread natural pigments (mostly yellow, orange, red, salmon and other variants), and almost all are from the family of terpenoids (tetraterpenes). They can be found in plants, bacteria, fungi, yeasts, algae, and non-mammalian animals. More than 700 different carotenoids have been isolated from natural sources, including some molecules with hydrophilic profile, and more than 600 molecules are fully characterized.

Carotenoids photoprotection and the antioxidant potential for preventing cancer, scavenging of reactive species and diseases of the eye remain important active fields of investigation. Also, carotenoids may boost the immune system by increasing the

Figure 3. Structure of β-carotene and lycopene
Authors' personal archive.

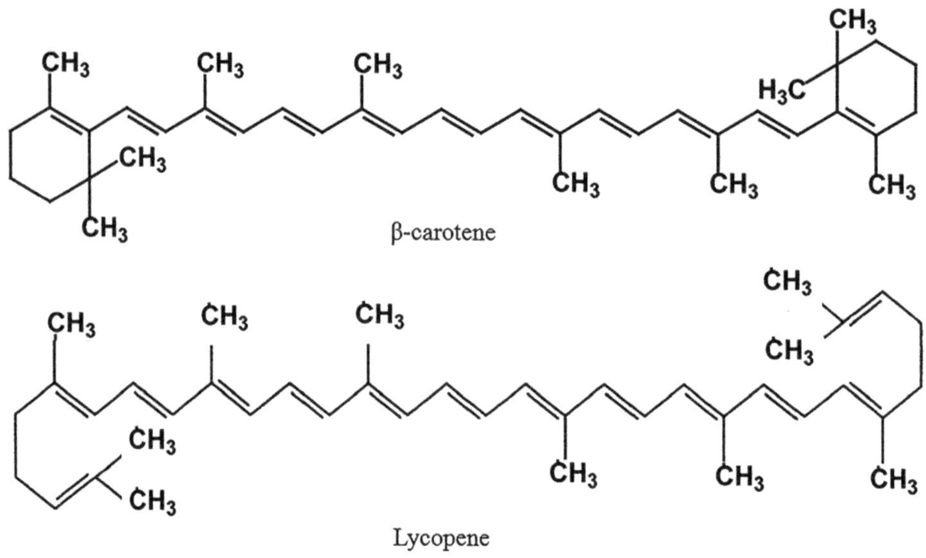

number of white blood cells. On the other hand, rare studies have demonstrated antimicrobial potentials for this chemical group. Until the time of preparation of this chapter, the exact mechanisms of these biological potentials of carotenoids remain unknown.

In humans, the role that carotenoids play in protecting those tissues that are most heavily exposed to light is the most explored. Oral photoprotection formulations, for instance, are already commercially available. β-carotene, α-carotene, lutein, zeaxanthin and β-cryptoxanthin are major carotenoids detected in human blood and tissues; nevertheless, β-carotene and lycopene are the most studied carotenoids, and the most used for nutraceutical purposes. Thus, certain aspects of these molecules will be more explored here (Figure 3).

Lycopene is a red pigment found in plant food like tomatoes, guava and watermelon. This molecule consists in a long acyclic chain of chemical formula $C_{40}H_{56}$. It is usually presented as a dark red hydrophobic solid with melting point ranging between 172 and 173 °C. Lycopene can be found in foods such as tomatoes in an average of around 3.31 mg/100 g, and papaya, in an average of around 3.39 mg/100 g. (Hark & Deen, 2005).

Lycopene levels in vegetables are usually analyzed through spectrophotometric techniques, however, it can be measured indirectly through chromaticity values obtained via colorimetric analysis. This last technique, nevertheless, is recommended for plants with high production of Lycopene.

The synthesis of lycopene and its decomposition are quite pronounced during the ripening of fruit, and at temperatures above 30 °C, the synthesis is inhibited, but it can be reversed as the vegetable return of to lower temperatures. External factors such as pH, temperature and oxidation, can influence the stability of carotenoids.

β-carotene is commonly found in many vegetables, fruits and plants such as carrots. The molecule also has molecular formula $C_{40}H_{56}$. When the cyclisation of lycopene occurs at both ends of the molecule, β-carotene is then formed. It is presented as an orange or red-to-purple solid with a density ranging from 0.935 to 0.947 g/cm^3 and has melting point ranging from 180 to 182 °C. The molecule is hydrophobic and very slightly soluble in methanol.

β-carotene is a precursor of liposoluble retinol. A significant part of the formation of retinol metabolism occurs in the gastrointestinal mucosa, being its absorption pH sensitive. β-carotene is also able to enhance the induction of CYP2E1, important in the metabolism of several drugs. Its average concentration in carrots usually reaches around 7 mg/100 g.

Because the bioavailability of β-carotene is very variable among people, Borel et al. (2015) investigated the possible effects of variations in genes involved in β-carotene absorption and postprandial metabolism on this variability on the bioavailability of the carotenoid. Single-nucleotide polymorphisms (SNPs) were genotyped with the use of whole-genome microarrays. A total of 33 healthy and nonobese adult men were enrolled. After an overnight fast, patients consumed a test meal containing 100 g tomato paste with 0.4 mg β-carotene. Postprandial plasma chylomicron β-carotene concentration was then measured at 8 h intervals, and 54 genes representing 2172 SNPs were investigated. The postprandial chylomicron β-carotene response was highly variable and positively correlated to the fasting plasma β-carotene concentration. A total of 25 SNPs in 12 genes affected the long-term blood β-carotene status and thus, explained (69%) of β-carotene bioavailability variance.

Horváth et al. (2015) proposed that carotenoids might modulate transient receptor potential ankyrin 1 and vanilloid 1 (TRPA1 and TRPV1) activation predominantly on peptidergic sensory nerves, considering that carotenoids are incorporated into membranes. β-carotene, lutein and lycopene were used in a murine model of cutaneous neurogenic inflammation, induced by mustard oil and capsaicin. Administration of 100 mg/kg subcutane lutein or β-carotene (three times during 24 h) resulted in significant swelling reduction, and Lutein decreased neutrophil accumulation induced by TRPA1 activation, although mustard oil-evoked intestinal contraction was not influenced. Curiuously, lycopene had no effect in none of the tested parameters. None of the three carotenoids could overcome capsaicin-evoked inflammation.

Woodside et al. (2015) investigated the possible benefits of anti-inflammatory and antioxidant properties on the risk of diseases that predominate in older people. Authors suggested that carotenoid intake and status are associated with reduced risks of cardiovascular diseases, although β-carotene supplementation increases the risk of lung cancer and does not reduce the risk of cardiovascular diseases. Increased lycopene intake may reduce prostate cancer progression.

Photoprotective effects of these carotenoids are still in debate. Stahl & Sies (2012) reviewed the topic and provided evidence that a carotenoid-rich diet or carotenoid supplementation might have photoprotective benefits through scavenging of ROS. Considering that carotenoids are part of a complex blend nutrients in food, other components can contribute to this effect. As expected, photoprotection through dietary intake of β-carotene or lycopene is lower than the achieved by topical sunscreens. the combination of both strategies, however, increases skin protection against UV irradiation and contributes to preserve skin health and appearance.

Ascenso et al. (2014) proposed that lycopene modulation of gap-junctional communications, involved in cell growth and molecular signalling of proliferation and apoptosis through proteic channels such as connexin 43, are important in cell cycle dynamics and for carotenoids behaviour as cellular anti-oxidants *in vivo*. Fernández-García (2014) assessed the antioxidant effect of lycopene alone or combined to α-tocopherol or naringenin on human dermal fibroblasts (hdf) exposed to ultraviolet-A light. UVA irradiation led to reduced cell viability in a dose dependent manner, and similar effects were observed when cells were exposed to lycopene. However, this reduction was suppressed in the presence of naringenin. α-tocopherol had no effect in this parameter. Lycopene combined to naringenin was able to inhibit ROS formation and increased the stability of the carotenoid. Thus, combinations of dietary antioxidants might be more effective than the sole use of lycopene.

Nevertheless, the work of Sokoloski et al. (2015) reported that lycopene regular intake in pills or tomato paste, although safe and with no side effects, did not provide systemic photoprotection against ultraviolet-B light. A total of 20 subjects using lycopene pills or tomato paste received only ultraviolet B irradiation and the variation of color was compared to normal skin after 24 h. Evaluations were made at baseline and after 4, 8, and 10 weeks. Conversely, no difference was detected in the mean of minimal erythematous dose at baseline between groups.

Phytosterols

In the latest years, several pharmacological potentials of phytosterols have been described, including cardiovascular protection, antiproliferative and antimicrobial effects and lipid metabolism improvement. However, they still lack of evidence generated in clinical studies. Currently, most of their biological activities have been demonstrated *in vitro*, one of the reasons that explains the controversial status of most of the existing investigations. Also, nutraceutical formulations developed with these molecules are scarce, but several types of food are enriched with these compounds, such as dairy products. Phytosterols are of abundant occurrence in plant and marine species, and are hydrophobic white crystalline solids. Phytosterols present from twenty-seven to twenty nine carbon atoms resembling the cholesterol molecule. These can be distinguished by the arrangement of the nucleus, the structure and composition of the side chain and by polar moieties of the molecule (Robbers et al., 1997; Brafau et al., 2008).

The biosynthesis of these compounds usually begins with Coenzyme A generating mevalonate. A set of similar reactions pathways is observed in phytosterols when compared to the synthesis of terpenes. Due to structural characteristics very similar to those of cholesterol, phytosterols are able to perform common cellular functions of cholesterol by interfering in membrane fluidity and water permeability. They can also act as phytormones precursors (Robbers et al., 1997; Thomas et al., 2006).

Phytosterols may be found in foods with high levels of lipids such as sesame seeds, walnuts and peanuts, as well as being present in some vegetables, grains and fruits. These compounds make up part of the unsaponifiable fraction of vegetable oils. In soy and corn, phytosterols might be detected in up to 330 and 970 mg/100g of total oils, respectively (Thomas et al., 2006) (Figure 4).

Monu et al. (2008) investigated the potential antimicrobial activity of a commercial formulation of phytosterols (ss-sitosterol, campesterol, sitostanol, and campestanol) in milk and their effect on yogurt starter cultures. No antimicrobial

Figure 4. Structures of major phytosterols
Authors' personal archive.

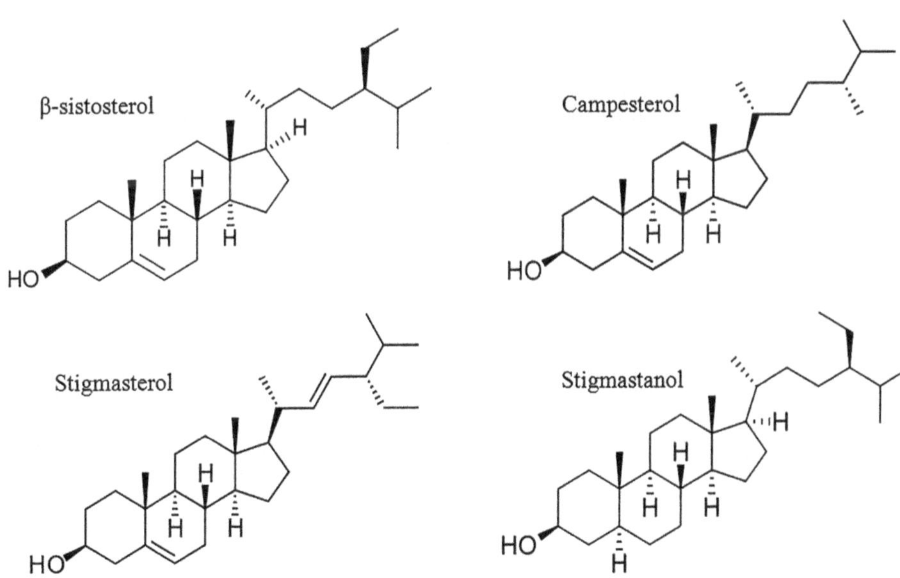

effect was detected on plate count or on psychrotroph population in pasteurized milk stored at 4 °C. A microbial challenge test of the formulation using *Pseudomonas spp.*, *Saccaromyces cerevisiae* and *Aspergillus ochraceous*, in cold milk, confirmed that the blend of phytosterols had no antimicrobial activity. The formulation also had no effect on the growth of *Lactobacillus bulgaricus* and *Streptococcus thermophilus* during yogurt production. When combined to dispersing agents, the formulation presented some antimicrobial effects.

Mahmood et al. (2013) studied the effects antimicrobial activities of β-sitosterol complexed to Cu (II), Co (II), and Fe (III), important trace elements in the human organism. All the complexes presented antimicrobial potential against highly pathogenic bacterial and fungal species. More recently, a group headed by the same author described the complexation of β-sitosterol with Palladium (Pd) (Mahmood et al., 2015). This complex showed significant antibacterial and antifungal activity, being superior to the previous ones.

Ramprasath & Awad (2015) recently reviewed the biological potentials of phytosterols. Although the mechanisms of action remain to be elucidated, improvements in blood lipid profile have been described as the main pathway to its cardioprotective effects. However, the levels of phytosterols in natural diets might range from less than 60 mg to more than 500 mg/2000 Kcal, and in an optmistic perspective, they might reduce only 3-14% LDL levels, what suggests the urgent need of phytosterols-based nutraceutical formulations (Racette et al., 2015). Reductions in growth of various cancer cells have been demonstrated, and mechanisms such as inbihition of cell growth and multiplication, reduction of angiogenesis and impairment of tissues invasion and metastasis, have been proposed to explain its antiproliferative activity (Ramprasath & Awad, 2015).

Ravikumar et al. (2009) isolated both α-spinasterol and spinasterol from a petroleum ether extract fraction of *Polyalthia cerasoides* seeds, and tested them against Caco-2 cell line. These molecules exhibited antiproliferative potential at different concentrations, and IC50 was of 57.7±6.81 nM/mL for spinasterol and 60.0±7.10 nM/mL for α-spinasterol. Carange et al. (2011) analyzed the protective potential of 24-epibrassinolide, a natural brassinosteroid (a type of phytosterol with potential of inducing stress tolerance of vegetables) in an *in vitro* model of Parkinson's disease. Neuronal PC12 cells were treated with 1-methyl-4-phenylpyridinium, which induced oxidative stress and consequent apoptosis in dopaminergic neurons. The treatment with the phytosterol reduced the levels of intracellular ROS and modulated the activity of antioxidant enzymes such as superoxide dismutase, catalase, and glutathione peroxidase. 24-epibrassinolide also inhibited apoptosis by reducing DNA fragmentation as well as the Bax/Bcl-2 protein ratio.

On the other hand, Cilla et al. (2015) tested the antiproliferative effect of β-cryptoxanthin and phytosterols (β-sitosterol, campesterol and stigmasterol) against human colon cancer Caco-2 cells. The molecules showed no antiproliferative activity against Caco-2 cells, nor alone nor in combination. Caco-2 cells were treated with β-cryptoxanthin and/or phytosterols alone or in combination, at concentrations commonly detectable in human serum levels. Decreased cell viability was detected due to apoptosis, which was followed by dephosphorylation of BAD enzyme, mitochondrial depolarization and caspase 3-dependent PARP receptor cleavage. Also, intracellular Ca^{+2} influx and increased ROS/RNS levels were detected.

Lauric Acid

Lauric acid, also known as dodecanoic acid, is a fatty acid of structural formula $CH_3(CH_2)_{10}CO_2H$. Lauric acid is available mainly in coconut oil (from 43 to 53% of total fatty acids), palm kernel oil (40 to 52%) and in smaller fractions in other food, such as 5.8% of the total milk fat, 2.2% of total cow's milk and 4.5% of the fat present in goat's milk. The biosynthesis of this acid occurs through a reverse β-oxidation. Generally, it is presented as a hydrophobic white solid, with slight soap-like odor and lacking uniformity. It has an approximate density of 0.88 g/cm^3, and melting point ranging between 44 and 46 ºC.

Lauric acid can activate the release of interleukin 2 and stimulate the bone marrow to produce white blood cells. The anti-inflammatory potential of lauric acid is belived to be associated to local inhibition of prostaglandin E_2 (PGE_2) and Interleukin 6 synthesis, pro-inflammatory mediators in arthritis, rheumatism and muscle inflammation. Upon arriving in the intestine, it is metabolized by lipases to monolaurin, which is absorbed and has the ability to solubilize virus capsules, causing its destruction, what indicates its antiviral properties. Lauric acid induces the opening of cell membranes allowing glucose and insulin levels to normalize. It is also able to balance HDL levels and to reduce LDL oxidation (Figure 5).

Rouse et al. (2005) combined lauric acid monoesters to lactic, mandelic, malic, or benzoic acid, and evaluated them against MRSA in a murine model of nasopharyngeal colonization. Administration of the molecules 128774-49E or 128774-53A

Figure 5. Lauric acid molecule
Authors' personal archive.

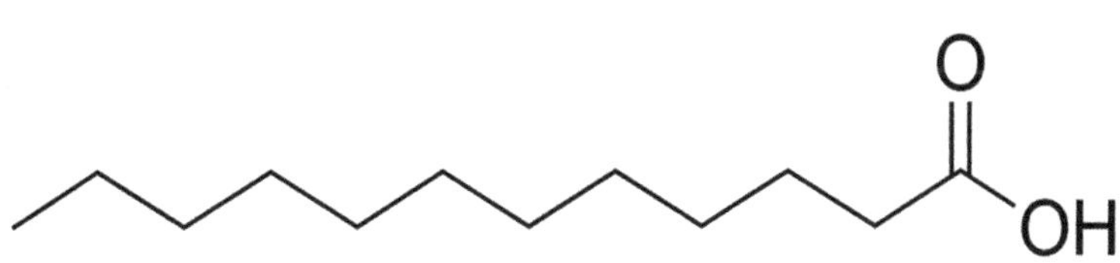

Lauric acid

was associated to reduction of MRSA carriage in 71% and 83% of animals, respectively. Administration of the compound 128774-53A resulted in 50% more reduction of MRSA carriage than mupirocin. Also, in vitro experiments were performed to assess the antimicrobial activity of 13 lauric acid monoester formulations and mupirocin against 30 methicillin-susceptible *S. aureus* (MSSA) isolates and 30 (MRSA) isolates. MSSA and MRSA MIC90 values were 0.25 μg/mL for mupirocin and ≤4 μl/ml for all LAM formulations tested.

Skrivanová et al. (2005) determined the susceptibility of *Clostridium perfringens* strains to C(2)-C(18) fatty acids. Among the tested molecules, lauric acid showed the highest antimicrobial activity, followed by myristic, capric, oleic and caprylic acid. Cultures of *C. perfringens* strains treated with capric and lauric acid at pH 5.0-5.3, the number of viable cells was very reduced; however, only lauric acid reduced the number of viable cells of the strains below 10(2) ml(-1) at pH > 6. The proposed mechanism of action for lauric acid was separation of inner and outer membranes, and cytoplasma disorganization, suggesting its use for controling of clostridial infections.

Nakatsuji et al. (2009) demonstrated that lauric acid can be used to treat acne. This compound showed antimicrobial activity against clinical isolates *of Propionibacterium acnes, Staphylococcus aureus* and *Staphylococcus epidermidis*, both *in vitro* and *in vivo* (using a murine model). Lauric acid yielded minimal inhibitory concentration (MIC) values against more than 15 times lower than those of benzoyl peroxide (a molecule highly used in topical formulations) in the tested species. *P. acnes* was the most sensitive bacteria to lauric acid among the tested species. No cytotoxicity was detected in human sebocytes exposed to lauric acid. *In vivo*, intradermal and epicutaneous applications of lauric acid decreased the count of *P. acnes* isolated from mouse ears.

The antinflammatory potential of lauric acid has been explored in the latest years. The classical study of Henry et al. (2002) described high inhibitory activity of lauric acid over cyclooxygenase enzymes COX-I and COX-II at 100 μg/mL. Further, Fauser et al. (2013) compared lauric acid (C12:0) and butyrate (C4:0) regarding their potentials to induce apoptosis, modify glutathione levels, generate ROS and modify phases of the cell cycle in Caco-2 and IEC-6 cancer cell lines. Lauric acid was more potent to induce apoptosis in Caco-2 and IEC-6 cells when compared to butyrate. In Caco-2 cells, lauric acid was more efficient to reduce GSH availability and in generation of ROS when compared to butyrate. Also, butyrate protected IEC-6 cells from ROS-induced damage, but lauric acid induced high levels of ROS when compared to butyrate.

Glucosinolates

Glucosinolates are generally found in plants with spicy flavor such as leaves and roots of the turnip and mustard seeds, and in vegetables like broccoli and cauliflower. This effect is mostly perceived when these plants are chewed. Most of glucosinlates are water soluble, and when plants suffer mechanical damage, 60 to 80% of total glucosinolates are converted into sulfurano-nitrile compounds. When cooking, the enzyme miriosinase is denatured and glucosinolates can be absorbed with no chemical alteration, being converted into sulforaphane only in the intestines after exposed to bacterial tioglucosidases. Most of the glucosinolates are excreted in the form of N-acetyl-cysteine. among others (Nastruzzi et al., 2000) (Figure 6).

Leoni et al. (1997) investigated the antiproliferative effects of glucosinolates and their isothiocyanate-derived products on K562 (erythroleukemic human) cells. Strong inhibitory activity on K562 cells growth was detected for sinigrin, progoitrin, epi-progoitrin, glucotropaeolin and glucocheirolin. Later, researches conducted by this group (Nastruzzi et al., 2000) described the effects of isothiocyanates and several glucosinolates-derived nitriles (epi-progoitrin, glucocheirolin, glucoraphenin, glucotropaeolin and sinalbin) in an *in vitro* model of colorectal cancer using K562 cells. Isothiocyanates were more potent to inhibit cancer cell growth than the glucosinolates-derived nitriles epi-progoitrin, glucotropaeolin, glucoraphenin, and glucocheirolin.

Lampe and Peterson (2002) reviewed the effects of genetic polymorphisms on the chemoprotective properties of cruciferous vegetables against different types of

Figure 6. General structure of glucosinolates
Authors' personal archive.

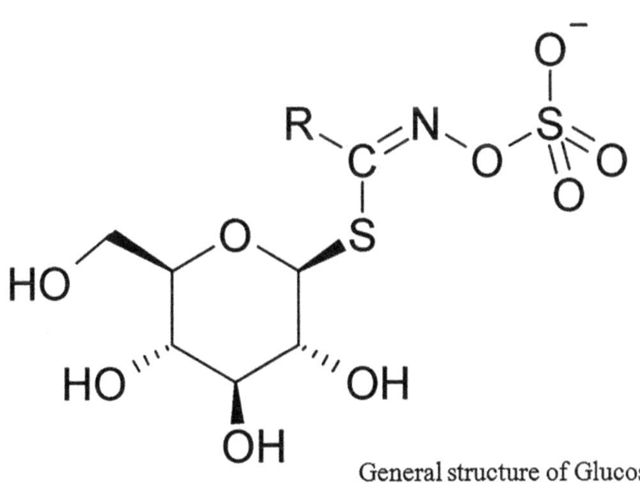

General structure of Glucosinolates

cancer. This pharmacological activity of cruciferous vegetables is generally assigned to the high content of glucosinolates and its metabolites detectable in them. They can modulate important biotransformation enzymatic systems such as the monooxygenases from cytochrome P450, influencing, for instance, scavenging and immune regulation. Beyond the (somehow) expected failure of chemoprotective activity due to genetic and biochemical alterations that influence receptors and transcription factors that interact with these compounds, functional variations due to genetic and biochemical instabilities in enzymes like glutathione S-transferase (mainly M1 and T1 isotypes), which metabolize isothiocyanates, can increase cancer risk due to the intake of cruciferous vegetables.

More recently, Calmes et al. (2015) investigated the mechanism by which glucosinolate-derived isothiocyanates could cause fungal cell death using *Alternaria brassicicola*, a *Brassica* species pathogens. Exposure of the strain to isothiocyanates led to a decreased rate of oxygen consumption, intracellular accumulation of ROS and depolarization of the mitochondrial-membrane, impairing its function in fungal cells. The expression of different oxidative-response genes was increased in the fungus when exposed to isothiocyanates-derived ROS, what may explain the protection of the fungus against isothiocyanates, as mutant strains deficient in the specific transcription factors were hypersensitive to the tested isothiocyanates.

Interactions of Phytomolecules of Nutraceutical Interest and Antimicrobial Drugs

As mentioned, most of the phytonutrients discussed present varied spectrum of antimicrobial activity. Varied practices of traditional medicine in countries such as, Brazil, China, India and several African countries include the use of plant extracts for several illnesses, including infectious diseases. In many cases, patients and health professionals employ a drug-therapy regimen in which the patient used natural products rich in phytonutrients and other phytomolecules of (generally) recognized biological activity combined to medication. However, these interactions are poorly investigated and represent a serious problem in drug therapy due to poorly predictable interactions (Saavedra et al., 2010; Dias-Souza et al., 2013). We will present here in brief some discussion in this topic.

When these combinations include antimicrobial drugs, the risk of favoring microbial resistance is high, given that the efficacy of synthetic antimicrobial drugs can be severely impaired, due to antagonistic interactions. However, it can also be enhanced, as a result of synergic interactions. Saavedra et al. (2010) evaluated the antimicrobial activity of several phytonutrients against *E. coli, P. aeruginosa, L. monocytogenes* and *S. aureus*, and the possible synergism of combinations of streptomycin and these molecules. Phenolic compounds (caffeic acid, chlorogenic acid, ferulic acid, gallic acid, tyrosol, chalcone - phloridzin; flavan-3-ol - (-) epicatechin; seco-iridoid -oleuropein glucoside) and glucosinolate hydrolysis products (allylisothiocyanate, benzylisothiocyanate and 2-phenylethylisothiocyanate) were tested in combination to ciprofloxacin, gentamicin and streptomycin in a disc diffusion assay. All of the tested isothiocyanates had superior antimicrobial activity when compared to phenolic molecules, being *P. aeruginosa* the most sensitive microorganism. Synergy was demonstrated between streptomycin and gallic acid, ferulic acid, chlorogenic acid, allylisothiocyanate and 2-phenylethylisothiocyanate against Gram-negative bacteria.

Sato et al. (2006) provided evidence of the synergic effect of the combination of vancomycin and isoflavones isolated from *Erythrina poeppigiana* against (MRSA). Isolupalbigenin and erythrinin B exhibited the highest anti-MRSA activity. Later, Gould et al. (2009) described the synergic effect of the combination of pomegranate rind extract and cupric sulphate against methicillin-sensitive and resistant *S. aureus,* and Panton-Valentine Leukocidin positive community acquired MSSA. The authors observed reduction in bacterial growth for 80% of the isolates.

Because of the strong resistance of bacteria to the currently available antimicrobial drugs, natural products and specific molecules have been investigated as alternatives to synthetic drugs, and our group has been exploring chemical, microbiological and pharmacological aspects of some natural products that might be interesting candidates for using in antimicrobial therapy (Dias-Souza et al., 2013; Marçal et al., 2014; Figueiredo et al., 2015; Pereira et al., 2015). Concerning drug interactions with natural products, our group is currently investigating possible synergic or antagonist effects of the combination of antimicrobial and antioxidant natural products with synthetic antimicrobial drugs (Dias-Souza et al., 2013; Santos et al., 2015; Santos et al., 2016).

Annacardium occidentale (cashew) is a plant used in Brazil and India for treating infectious diseases and for wound healing, and the fruit is widely explored for juice pulp commercialization. The antimicrobial activity of *A. occidentale* stem bark hydroethanolic extract was demonstrated by our group by the first time against *S. aureus* and *S. epidermidis* by the first time (Dias-Souza et al., 2013), and using an adapted disc diffusion method, strong antagonism was detected when the extract was combined to antimicrobial drugs against *S. aureus* strains (Dias-Souza et al., 2013).

When analyzing specific phytomolecules, we demonstrated that some flavonoids and carotenoids can impair the antimicrobial activity of some drugs, but can also enhance this pharmacological activity. We developed an adaptation to the method used with *A. occidentale* extract and tested phytonutrients against clinical isolates of *S. aureus, E. coli* and *P. aeruginosa*. Interestingly, none of the phytonutrients presented antimicrobial activity against any of *S. aureus* and *E. coli* strains. Nevertheless, most of the tested combinations generated antagonistic effects for these species, being more pronounced for *S. aureus* strains. In investigating *E. coli* strains, the antimicrobial activity of cefalexin and amoxicillin was strongly reduced, whereas most of the drugs tested for *S. aureus* lost their pharmacological activity completely. Conversely, the antimicrobial activity of the drugs tested against *P. aeruginosa* strains was strongly favored, and synergism was evidenced (Santos et al., 2015; Santos et al., 2016).

Like most of the scarce studies on antimicrobials-phytomolecules interactions studies, the mechanisms by which these interactions work remain to be elucidated. We hypothesized that some sort of membrane injury might be involved, considering that, until the preparation of this chapter, the tested phytonutrients does not present any evidence that they may overcome the resistance mechanisms for the tested drugs. An important aspect of investigating such interactions is the necessity of exploration of isolated molecules with pharmacological activity, after the interference of a crude extract on specific drugs is well described.

The research performed by our group and others are being directed for, in a near future, begin investigations with animal models, such that the *in vitro* findings can be confirmed. With *in vivo* data from animal models, it will be possible to plan the use of some associations for clinical studies, in order to reach a combined formulation to be used as a medication.

CONCLUSION

The phytonutrients discussed have many chemical and pharmacological aspects concerning their antimicrobial, antiproliferative and antioxidant activities described, but several points remain to be elucidated, especially the ones related to mechanisms of action. The safety of these molecules for human consumption is largely recognized; however, the combined use with medications may induce unpredictable effects. The evidences of the wide spectrum of antimicrobial and antiproliferative activities of the discussed molecules open doors for more investigations in order to reach the point in which the development of pharmaceutical dosage forms will extrapolate nutraceutical purposes and will be no more a promising alternative to clinical treatments, but effective tools of large scale production against several diseases.

ACKNOWLEDGMENT

The authors are thankful to the researchers and students of the Integrated Pharmacology and Drug Interactions Research Group (GPqFAR). RMDS is recipient of a Master of Science fellowship from CNPq, and MVDS is supported by grants from FAPEMIG.

REFERENCES

Abass, E. H., Zair, S. K., Mohammud, T. K., & Nagem, S. A. (2014). Recovery of pure Hesperidin from Iraqi Sweet Oranges Peel and study the effect in some bacteria. *Baghdad Science Journal, 11*(2), 455–460.

Abuelsaad, A. S., Mohamed, I., Allam, G., & Al-Solumani, A. A. (2013). Antimicrobial and immunomodulating activities of hesperidin and ellagic acid against diarrheic *Aeromonas hydrophila* in a murine model. *Life Sciences, 93*(20), 714–722. doi:10.1016/j.lfs.2013.09.019 PMID:24090709

Akroum, S., Bendjeddou, D., Satta, D., & Lalaoui, K. (2010). Antibacterial, antioxidant and acute toxicity tests on flavonoids extracted from some medicinal plants. *International Journal of Green Pharmacy, 4*(3), 165–169. doi:10.4103/0973-8258.69174

Alves, M. J., Ferreira, I. C., Froufe, H. J., Abreu, R. M., Martins, A., & Pintado, M. (2013). Antimicrobial activity of phenolic compounds identified in wild mushrooms, SAR analysis and docking studies. *Journal of Applied Microbiology, 115*(2), 346–357. doi:10.1111/jam.12196 PMID:23510516

Anand, P., Kunnumakkara, A. B., Newman, R. A., & Aggarwal, B. B. (2007). Bioavailability of Curcumin: Problems and Promises. *Molecular Pharmaceutics, 4*(6), 807–818. doi:10.1021/mp700113r PMID:17999464

Ascenso, A., Ribeiro, H., Marques, H. C., Oliveira, H., Santos, C., & Simões, S. (2014). Chemoprevention of photocarcinogenesis by lycopene. *Experimental Dermatology, 23*(12), 874–878. doi:10.1111/exd.12491 PMID:25040310

Awad, M. (1993). *Fisiologia Pós-colheita de frutos.* São Paulo, SP, Brasil: Nobel.

Bae, E. A., Han, M. J., & Kim, D. H. (1999). *In vitro* anti-Helicobacter pylori activity of some flavonoids and their metabolites. *Planta Medica, 65*(05), 442–443. doi:10.1055/s-2006-960805 PMID:10454900

Bae, E. A., Han, M. J., & Kim, D. H. (2000). *In vitro* inhibitory effect of some flavonoids on rotavirus infectivity. *Biological & Pharmaceutical Bulletin, 23*(9), 1122–1124. doi:10.1248/bpb.23.1122 PMID:10993220

Barreca, D., Laganà, G., Bruno, G., Magazù, S., & Bellocco, E. (2013). Diosmin binding to human serum albumin and its preventive action against degradation due to oxidative injuries. *Biochimie, 95*(11), 2042–2049. doi:10.1016/j.biochi.2013.07.014 PMID:23886889

Bartolotta, S., Garcia, C. C., Candurra, N. A., & Damonte, E. B. (2001). Effect of fatty acids on adenavirus replication: Inhibition of virus production by lauric acid. *Archives of Virology*, *146*(4), 777–790. doi:10.1007/s007050170146 PMID:11402863

Bernard, E., Britz-McKibbin, P., & Gernigon, N. (2007). Resveratrol photoisomerization: An integrative-guide survey experiment. *Journal of Chemical Education*, *84*(7), 1159. doi:10.1021/ed084p1159

Bigoniya, P., & Singh, K. (2014). Ulcer protective potential of standardized hesperidin, a citrus flavonoid isolated from *Citrus sinensis*. *Revista Brasileira de Farmacognosia*, *24*(3), 330–340. doi:10.1016/j.bjp.2014.07.011

Bishayee, K., & Khuda-Bukhsh, A. R. (2013). 5-Lipoxygenase Antagonist therapy: A new approach towards targeted cancer chemotherapy. *Acta Biochimica et Biophysica Sinica*, *45*(9), 709–719. doi:10.1093/abbs/gmt064 PMID:23752617

Brafau, G., Canela, A. M., & Rafecas, M. (2008). Phytosterols: Physiologic and metabolic aspects related to cholesterol-lowering properties. *Nutrition Research (New York, N.Y.)*, *28*(4), 217–225. doi:10.1016/j.nutres.2008.02.003 PMID:19083411

Budavari, S. (1996). *The Merck Index*. Merck and Co.

Cai, Y., Zhao, L., Qin, Y., & He, Y. (2015). High dose of epigallocatechin-3-gallate inhibits proliferation and induces apoptosis of H9C2 cardiomyocytes through down-regulation of SIRT1. *Die Pharmazie*, *70*(1), 12–16. PMID:25975092

Calomme, M., Pieters, L., Vlietnick, A., & Berghe, D. V. (1996). Inibition of bacterial mutagenesis by Citurs flavonoids. *Planta Medica*, *62*(03), 222–226. doi:10.1055/s-2006-957864 PMID:8693033

Carange, J., Longpré, F., Daoust, B., & Martinoli, M. G. (2011). 24-Epibrassinolide, a Phytosterol from the Brassinosteroid Family, Protects Dopaminergic Cells against MPP+-Induced Oxidative Stress and Apoptosis. *Journal of Toxicology*, *2011*, 13. doi:10.1155/2011/392859 PMID:21776258

Cardoso, F. S. P., Moro, A. V., & Correia, C. R. D. (2008, September). *Reação de Heck de estirenos com sais de diazônio: Síntese do Resveratrol e seus análogos*. Paper presented at XVI Congress Internal Scientific Initiation of Unicamp, Campinas, SP.

Carvalho, W., Fonseca, M. E. N., Silva, H. R., Boiteux, L. S., & Giordano, L. B. (2005). Estimativa indireta de teores de licopeno em frutos genótipos de tomateiro via análise colorimétrica. *Horticultura Brasileira*, *23*(3), 819–825. doi:10.1590/S0102-05362005000300026

Chang, H. C., Chen, T. G., Tai, Y. T., Chen, T. L., Chiu, W. T., & Chen, R. M. (2010). Resveratrol attenuates oxidized LDL-evoked Lox-1 signaling and consequently protects against apoptotic insults to cerebrovascular endothelial cells. *Journal of Cerebral Blood Flow and Metabolism*, *31*(3), 842–854. doi:10.1038/jcbfm.2010.180 PMID:20940732

Chen, F., Qian, L.-H., Deng, B., Liu, Z.-M., Zhao, Y., & Le, Y.-Y. (2013). Resveratrol Protects Vascular Endothelial Cells from High Glucose–Induced Apoptosis through Inhibition of NADPH Oxidase Activation–Driven Oxidative Stress. *CNS Neuroscience & Therapeutics*, *19*(9), 675–681. doi:10.1111/cns.12131 PMID:23731528

Chen, Y. X., Zhou, T., & Xie, K. P. (2013). Antibacterial Mechanism of Baicalein on Methicillin-resistant *Staphyloccocus aureus*. *Acta Veterinaria et Zootechnica Sinica*, *44*(12), 2000–2006.

Chhunchha, B., Fatma, N., Bhargavan, B., Kubo, E., Kumar, A., & Singh, D. P. (2011). Specificity protein, Sp1-mediated increased expression of Prdx6 as a curcumin-induced antioxidant defense in lens epithelial cells against oxidative stress. *Cell Death & Disease*, *2*(11), e234. doi:10.1038/cddis.2011.121 PMID:22113199

Choi, K., Jung, M. G., Lee, Y., Yoon, J. C., Kwon, S. H., Kang, H., & Yoon, H. et al. (2009). Epigallocatechin-3-Gallate, a Histone Acetyltransferase Inhibitor, Inhibits EBV-Induced B Lymphocyte Transformation via Suppression of RelA Acetylation. *Cancer Research*, *69*(2), 583–592. doi:10.1158/0008-5472.CAN-08-2442 PMID:19147572

Chun, Y. J., Kim, M. Y., & Guengerich, F. P. (1999). Resveratrol Is a Selective Human Cytochrome P450 1A1 Inhibitor. *Biochemical and Biophysical Research Communications*, *262*(1), 20–24. doi:10.1006/bbrc.1999.1152 PMID:10448061

Cilla, A., Attanzio, A., Barberá, R., Tesoriere, L., & Livrea, M. A. (2015). Antiproliferative effect of main dietary phytosterols and ß-cryptoxanthin alone or combined in human colon cancer Caco-2 cells through cytosolic Ca+2 and oxidative stress-induced apoptosis. *Journal of Functional Foods*, *12*, 282–293. doi:10.1016/j.jff.2014.12.001

Damon, M., Flandre, O., Michel, F., Perdrix, L., Labrid, C., & Crastes de Paulet, A. (1987). Effect of chronic treatment with a purified flavonoid fraction on inflammatory granuloma in the rat. Study of prostaglandin E2 and F2 alpha and thromboxane B2 release and histological changes. *Arzneimittel-Forschung*, *37*(10), 1149–1153. PMID:3481266

Das, S., Taygi, A. K., & Kaur, H. (2000). Cancer modulation by glucosinolates: A review. *Current Science*, *79*(12), 1665–1671.

de Assis, J. S., Lima, R. A., Marques-Lima, J. P., Azevedo-Rodrigues, L. K., & Santiago, S. L. (2015). Effect of epigallocatechin-3-gallate application for remaining carious dentin disinfection. *Journal of Conservative Dentistry*, *18*(1), 51–55. doi:10.4103/0972-0707.148896 PMID:25657528

Deschamps, J. D., Kenyoh, V. A., & Holman, T. R. (2006). Baicalein is a potent in vitro inhibitor against both reticulocyte 15-human and platelet 12-human lipoxygenases. *Bioorganic & Medicinal Chemistry*, *14*(12), 4294–4301. doi:10.1016/j.bmc.2006.01.057 PMID:16500106

Dewick. (2007). Medicinal Natural Products – A biosynthetic Approach. Chippenham, UK: Jhon Wiley & Sons.

Dias-Souza, M. V., Andrade, S., Aguiar, A. P., & Monteiro, A. S. (2013). Evaluation of Antimicrobial and Anti-biofilm activities of Anacardium occidentale stem bark extract. *Journal of Natural Products*, *26*, 198–205.

Dias-Souza, M. V., Caldoncelli, J. L., & Monteiro, A. S. (2013). *Annacardium occidentale* Stem Bark Extract can Decrease the Efficacy of Antimicrobial Drugs. *Revista Ciências Médicas e Biológicas*, *12*, 161–165.

Dos Santos, R. M., Pimenta-Freire, G., Figueiredo, F. J. B., Dias-Souza, M.V. (2016). Interference of flavonoids and carotenoids on the antimicrobial activity of some drugs against clinical isolates of Pseudomonas aeruginosa. International Food Research Journal, 23, 1268-1273.

Dos Santos, R. M., Pimenta-Freire, G., & Dias-Souza, M. V. (2016). Interference of flavonoids and carotenoids on the antimicrobial activity of some drugs against clinical isolates of *Pseudomonas aeruginosa. International Food Research Journal.*

Elmali, N., Esenkaya, I., Harma, A., Ertem, K., Turkoz, Y., & Mizrak, B. (2005). Effect of resveratrol in experimental osteoarthritis in rabbits. *Inflammation Research*, *54*(4), 158–162. doi:10.1007/s00011-004-1341-6 PMID:15883738

Fauser, J. K., Matthews, G. M., Cummins, A. G., & Howarth, G. S. (2013). Induction of apoptosis by the medium-chain length fatty acid lauric acid in colon cancer cells due to induction of oxidative stress. *Chemotherapy*, *59*(3), 214–224. doi:10.1159/000356067 PMID:24356281

Figueiredo, F. J. B., Dias-Souza, M. V., Nascimento, E., & Lima, L. R. P. (2015). Physicochemical Characterization and Flavonoid Contents of Artisanal Brazilian Green Propolis. *International Journal of Pharmacy and Pharmaceutical Sciences*, *7*, 64–68.

Fremont, L. (2014). Efeitos biológicos de resveratrol. *Ciências da Vida*, *66*, 663–673.

Garg, A., Garg, S., Zaneveld, L. J. D., & Singla, A. K. (2001). Chemistry and pharmacology of the citrus bioflavonoid hesperidin. *Phytotherapy Research*, *15*(8), 655–669. doi:10.1002/ptr.1074 PMID:11746857

Gould, S. W., Fielder, M. D., Kelly, A. F., & Naughton, D. P. (2009). Anti-microbial activities of pomegranate rind extracts: Enhancement by cupric sulphate against clinical isolates of *S. aureus*, MRSA and PVL positive CA-MSSA. *BMC Complementary and Alternative Medicine*, *9*(23). PMID:19635137

Gu, X., Creasy, L., Kester, A., & Zeece, M. (1999). Capillary Electrophoretic Determination of Resveratrol in Wines. *Journal of Agricultural and Food Chemistry*, *47*(8), 3223–3227. doi:10.1021/jf981211e PMID:10552635

Gunstone, F. D., & Padley, F. B. (1997). *Lipid technology and applications*. New York, NY: Marcel Dekker Inc.

Hark, L., & Deen, D. (2005). *Saúde e Nutrição. S.l.* DK Civilização.

Harpole, J. L., Tucci, M., & Benghuzzi, H. (2015). Pathophysiological Effects of Thymoquinone and Epigallocatechin-3-Gallate on SK-OV-3 Ovarian Cancer Like Cell Line. *Biomedical Sciences Instrumentation*, *51*, 31–39. PMID:25996696

Havsteen, B. (1983). Flavonoids, class of natural of high pharmacological potency. *Biochemical Pharmacology*, *32*(7), 1141–1148. doi:10.1016/0006-2952(83)90262-9 PMID:6342623

Henry, G. E., Momin, R. A., Nair, M. G., & Dewitt, D. L. (2002). Antioxidant and cyclooxygenase activities of fatty acids found in food. *Journal of Agricultural and Food Chemistry*, *50*(8), 2231–2234. doi:10.1021/jf0114381 PMID:11929276

Horváth, G., Kemény, Á., Barthó, L., Molnár, P., Deli, J., Szente, L., & Helyes, Z. et al. (2015). Effects of some natural carotenoids on TRPA1- and TRPV1-induced neurogenic inflammatory processes *in vivo* in the mouse skin. *Journal of Molecular Neuroscience*, *56*(1), 113–121. doi:10.1007/s12031-014-0472-7 PMID:25645682

Hui, K. M., Wang, X. H., & Xue, H. (2000). Interaction of Flavones from the Roots of *Scutellaria baicalensis* with the Benzodiazepine Site. *Planta Medica*, *66*(1), 91–93. doi:10.1055/s-0029-1243121 PMID:10705749

Hurst, W. J., Glinski, J. A., Miller, K. B., Apgar, J., Davey, M. H., & Stuart, D. A. (2008). Survey of the trans-Resveratrol and trans-Piceid Content of Cocoa-Containing and Chocolate Products. *Journal of Agricultural and Food Chemistry*, *56*(18), 8374–8378. doi:10.1021/jf801297w PMID:18759443

Hwang, D., & Lim, Y. H. (2015, May5). Resveratrol antibacterial activity against Escherichia coli is mediated by Z-ring formation inhibition via suppression of FtsZ expression. *Scientific Reports*, *5*, 10029. doi:10.1038/srep10029 PMID:25942564

Kaur, S., Modi, N. H., Panda, D., & Roy, N. (2010). Probing the binding site of curcumin in *Escherichia coli* and *Bacillus subtilis* FtsZ--a structural insight to unveil antibacterial activity of curcumin. *European Journal of Medicinal Chemistry*, *45*(9), 4209–4214. doi:10.1016/j.ejmech.2010.06.015 PMID:20615583

Kita, T., Ima, S., Sawada, H., Kumagai, H., & Seto, H. (2008). The Biosynthetic Pathway of Curcuminoid in Turmeric (Curcuma longa) as Revealed by 13C-Labeled Precursors. *Bioscience, Biotechnology, and Biochemistry*, *72*(7), 1789–1798. doi:10.1271/bbb.80075 PMID:18603793

Krewson, C. F., & Naghski, J. (2006). Some physical properties of rutin. *Journal of the American Pharmaceutical Association*, *41*(11), 582–587. doi:10.1002/jps.3030411106 PMID:12999623

Kumar, S., & Pandey, A. K. (2013). Chemistry and Biological Activities of Flavonoids: An Overview. *TheScientificWorldJournal*, *29*, 162750. PMID:24470791

Kuzuyama, T., Noel, J. P., & Richard, S. B. (2005). Structural basis for the promiscuous biosynthetic prenylation of aromatic natural products. *Nature*, *435*(7044), 983–987. doi:10.1038/nature03668 PMID:15959519

Laczkowski, M. S., & Laczkowski, I. M. (2013, October). *Microencapsulaçcão de curcumina com maltodextrin, avaliação daestabilidade e aplicação em alimentos.* Paper presented at VIII Meeting of Scientific Production and Technology, Paraná, Brasil.

Lagouge, M., Argmann, C., Gerhart-Hines, Z., Mezaine, H., Lerin, C., Daussin, F., & Auwerx, J. et al. (2006). Resveratrol Improves Mitochondrial Function and Protects against Metabolic Disease by Activating SIRT1 and PGC-1a. *Cell*, *127*(6), 1109–1122. doi:10.1016/j.cell.2006.11.013 PMID:17112576

Lee, W. J., Shim, J., & Zhu, B. T. (2005). Mechanisms for the Inhibition of DNA Methyltransferases by Tea Catechins and Bioflavonoids. *Molecular Pharmacology*, *68*(4), 1019–1030. doi:10.1124/mol.104.008367 PMID:16037419

Li, L., Liu, W. Y., Feng, F., Wu, C. Y., & Xie, N. (2013). Synthesis and *in vitro* cytotoxicity evaluation of baicalein amino acid derivatives. *Chinese Journal of Natural Medicine*, *11*(3), 284–288. doi:10.1016/S1875-5364(13)60030-8 PMID:23725843

Lipinski, C. A., Lombardo, F., Dominy, B. W., & Feeney, P. J. (1997). Experimental and computational approaches to estimate solubility and permeability in drug discovery and development settings. *Advanced Drug Delivery Reviews*, *23*(1-3), 3–25. doi:10.1016/S0169-409X(96)00423-1 PMID:11259830

Lipson, S. M., Ozen, F. S., Louis, S., & Karthikeyan, L. (2015). Comparison of a-glucosyl hesperidin of citrus fruits and epigallocatechin gallate of green tea on the Loss of Rotavirus Infectivity in Cell Culture. *Frontiers in Microbiology*, *6*, e359. doi:10.3389/fmicb.2015.00359

Liu, A., Wang, W., Fang, H., Yang, Y., Jiang, X., Liu, S., & Dirsch, O. et al. (2015). Baicalein protects against polymicrobial sepsis-induced liver injury via inhibition of inflammation and apoptosis in mice. *European Journal of Pharmacology*, *748*, 45–53. doi:10.1016/j.ejphar.2014.12.014 PMID:25533331

Luo, R., Wang, J., Zhao, L., Lu, N., You, Q., Guo, Q., & Li, Z. (2014). Synthesis and biological evaluation of baicalein derivatives as potent antitumor agents. *Bioorganic & Medicinal Chemistry Letters*, *24*(5), 1334–1338. doi:10.1016/j.bmcl.2014.01.053 PMID:24507925

Mahmood, T., Bibi, Y., Ishaq, H., Mahmood, I., Wahab, A., & Sherwani, S. (2013). Complexation and Antimicrobial activities of ß sitosterol with trace metals.(Cu (II), Co (II), and Fe (III)). *European Academic Research*, *1*(5), 677–685.

Mahmood, T., Bibi, Y., Zafar, R., Wahab, A., Mahmood, I., Arshad, N., & Sherwani, S. K. (2015). Report: Complexation of ß-sitosterol with tris (dibenzylideneacetone) dipalladium and its anti-microbial activity. *Pakistan Journal of Pharmaceutical Sciences*, *28*(2), 631–634. PMID:25730794

Man, G., Mauro, T. M., Zhai, Y., Kim, P. L., Cheung, C., Hupe, M., & Man, M. Q. et al. (2015). Topical hesperidin enhances epidermal function in an aged murine model. *The Journal of Investigative Dermatology*, *135*(4), 1184–1187. doi:10.1038/jid.2014.486 PMID:25402552

Manolova, Y., Deneva, V., Antonov, L., Drakalsa, E., Momekova, D., & Lambov, N. (2014). The effect of the water on the curcumin tautomerism: A quantitative approach. *Spectrochimica Acta. Part A: Molecular and Biomolecular Spectroscopy*, *132*, 815–820. doi:10.1016/j.saa.2014.05.096 PMID:24973669

Manzan, A. C. C. M., Toniolo, F. S., Bredow, E., & Povh, N. P. (2003, November). Extration of essential oil and pigments from *Curcuma longa L.* by steam distillation and extraction with volatile solvents. *Journal of Agricultural and Food Chemistry*, *51*(23), 6802–6807. doi:10.1021/jf030161x PMID:14582978

Marambuad, P., Zhao, H., & Davies, P. (2005). Resveratrol Promotes Clearance of Alzheimer's Disease Amyloid-β Peptides. *The Journal of Biological Chemistry, 280*(45), 37377–37382. doi:10.1074/jbc.M508246200 PMID:16162502

Marçal, P. H. F., Dias-Souza, M. V., Villela, E. G., Luz, L. M., Pereira, M. K., Vale, C. H. B., & Rabelo, F. L. A. (2014). Qualidade Físico-Química, Microbiológica e Microscópica de Polpas de Frutas Congeladas Comercializadas no Município de Governador Valadares, MG. Nova. *Revista Científica, 2*, 1–10.

Markham, K. R. (1982). *Techniques of flavonoid identification*. New York, NY: Academic Press.

Mechanick, J. I., Brett, E. M., Chausmer, A. B., Dickey, R. A., & Wallach, S. (2003). American Association of Clinical Endocrinologists medical guidelines for the clinical use of dietary supplements and nutraceuticals. *Endocrine Practice, 9*(5), 417–470. doi:10.4158/EP.9.5.417 PMID:14583426

Midio, A. F. M. (2000). *Toxicologia de Alimentos*. São Paulo, SP: Livraria Varella.

Mithen, R. F., Dekker, M., Verkerk, R., Rabot, S., & Jhonson, T. (2000). The nutritional significance, biosynthesis and bioavailability of glucosinolates in human foods. *Journal of the Science of Food and Agriculture, 80*(7), 967–984. doi:10.1002/(SICI)1097-0010(20000515)80:7<967::AID-JSFA597>3.0.CO;2-V

Monforte, M. T., Trovato, A., Kirjavainen, S., Forestieri, A. M., Galati, E. M., & Lo Curto, R. B. (1995). Biological effects of hesperidin, a citrus flavonoid. (note II): Hypolipidemic activity on experimental hypercholesterolemia in rat. *Pharmacology, 50*(9), 595–599. PMID:7495469

Monu, E., Blank, G., Holley, R., & Zawistowski, J. (2008). Phytosterol effects on milk and yogurt microflora. *Journal of Food Science, 73*(3), 121–126. doi:10.1111/j.1750-3841.2008.00668.x PMID:18387114

Nakatsuji, T., Kao, M. C., Fang, J.-Y., Zouboulis, C. C., Zhang, L., Gallo, R. L., & Huang, C.-M. (2009). Antimicrobial Property of Lauric Acid Against *Propionibacterium acnes*: Its Therapeutic Potential for Inflammatory Acne Vulgaris. *The Journal of Investigative Dermatology, 129*(10), 2480–2488. doi:10.1038/jid.2009.93 PMID:19387482

Orhan, D. D., Ozçelik, B., Ozgen, S., & Ergun, F. (2010). Antibacterial, antifungal, and antiviral activities of some flavonoids. *Microbiological Research, 165*(6), 496–504. doi:10.1016/j.micres.2009.09.002 PMID:19840899

Park, S. J., Ahmad, F., Philp, A., Baar, K., Williams, T., Luo, H., & Chung, J. H. et al. (2012). Resveratrol ameliorates aging-related metabolic phenotypes by inhibiting cAMP phosphodiesterases. *Cell*, *148*(3), 421–433. doi:10.1016/j.cell.2012.01.017 PMID:22304913

Quintin, J., & Lewin, G. (2004). Semisynthesis of linarin, acacetin and 6-iodoapiagenin derivatives from diosmin. *Journal of Natural Products*, *67*(9), 1624–1627. doi:10.1021/np040079b PMID:15387678

Racette, S. B., Lin, X., Ma, L., & Ostlund, R. E. (2015). Natural Dietary Phytosterols. *Journal of AOAC International*, *98*(3), 679–684. PMID:26086252

Ramprasath, V. R., & Awad, A. B. (2015). Role of Phytosterols in Cancer Prevention and Treatment. *Journal of AOAC International*, *98*(3), 735–738. PMID:26086253

Ravikumar, Y. S., Mahadevan, K. M., Manjunatha, H., & Satyanarayana, N. D. (2010). Antiproliferative, apoptotic and antimutagenic activity of isolated compounds from Polyalthia cerasoides seeds. *Phytomedicine*, *17*(7), 513–518. doi:10.1016/j.phymed.2009.09.005 PMID:19879119

Reis-Sobreiro, M., Gajate, C., & Mollinedo, F. (2009). Involvement of mitochondria and recruitment of Fas/CD95 signaling in lipid rafts in resveratrol-mediated antimyeloma and antileukemia actions. *Oncogene*, *28*(36), 3221–3234. doi:10.1038/onc.2009.183 PMID:19561642

Robbers, E. J. (1997). *Farmacognosia e Farmacobiotecnologia*. São Paulo, SP, Brasil: Premier.

Rocks, N., Bekaert, S., Coia, I., Paulissen, G., Gueders, M., Evrard, B., & Cataldo, D. et al. (2012). Curcumin-cyclodextrin complexes potentiate gemcitabine effects in an orthotopic mouse model of lung cancer. *British Journal of Cancer*, *107*(7), 1083–1092. doi:10.1038/bjc.2012.379 PMID:22929882

Rouse, M. S., Rotger, M., Piper, K. E., Steckelberg, J. M., Scholz, M., Andrews, J., & Patel, R. (2005). *In Vitro* and *In Vivo* Evaluations of the Activities of Lauric Acid Monoester Formulations against *Staphylococcus aureus*. *Antimicrobial Agents and Chemotherapy*, *49*(8), 3187–3191. doi:10.1128/AAC.49.8.3187-3191.2005 PMID:16048923

Rudrappa, T., & Bais, H. P. (2008). Curcumin, a known phenolic from *Curcuma longa*, attenuates the virulence of *Pseudomonas aeruginosa* PAO1 in whole plant and animal pathogenicity models. *Journal of Agricultural and Food Chemistry*, *56*(6), 1955–1962. doi:10.1021/jf072591j PMID:18284200

Saavedra, M. J., Borges, A., Dias, C., Aires, A., Bennett, R. N., Rosa, E. S., & Simões, M. (2010). Antimicrobial activity of phenolics and glucosinolate hydrolysis products and their synergy with streptomycin against pathogenic bacteria. *Medicinal Chemistry (Shariqah, United Arab Emirates)*, *6*(3), 174–183. doi:10.2174/1573406411006030174 PMID:20632977

Sato, M., Tanaka, H., Tani, N., Nagayama, M., & Yamaguchi, R. (2006). Different antibacterial actions of isoflavones isolated from *Erythrina poeppigiana* against methicillin-resistant *Staphylococcus aureus*. *Letters in Applied Microbiology*, *43*(3), 243–248. doi:10.1111/j.1472-765X.2006.01963.x PMID:16910926

Scherzberg, M. C., Kiehl, A., Zivkovic, A., Stark, H., Stein, J., Fürst, R., & Ulrich-Rückert, S. et al. (2015). Structural modification of resveratrol leads to increased anti-tumor activity, but causes profound changes in the mode of action. *Toxicology and Applied Pharmacology*, *287*(1), 67–76. PMID:26044878

Si, D., Wang, Y., Zhou, Y., Guo, Y., Wang, J., Zhou, H., & Fawcett, J. P. et al. (2009). Mechanism of CYP2C9 inhibition by flavones and flavonols. *Drug Metabolism and Fawcett*, *37*(3), 629–634. doi:10.1124/dmd.108.023416 PMID:19074529

Singh, M., Govindarajan, R., Rawat, A. K. S., & Khare, P. B. (2008). Antimicrobial Flavonoid Rutin from *Pteris vittata L.* Against Pathogenic Gastrointestinal Microflora. *American Fern Journal*, *98*(2), 98–103. doi:10.1640/0002-8444(2008)98[98:AFRFPV]2.0.CO;2

Skrivanová, E., Marounek, M., Dlouhá, G., & Kanka, J. (2005). Susceptibility of *Clostridium perfringens* to C-C fatty acids. *Letters in Applied Microbiology*, *41*(1), 77–81. doi:10.1111/j.1472-765X.2005.01709.x PMID:15960756

Srinivasan, S., & Pari, L. (2012). Ameliorative effect of diosmin, a citrus flavonoid against streptozotocin-nicotinamide generated oxidative stress induced diabetic rats. *Chemico-Biological Interactions*, *195*(1), 43–51. doi:10.1016/j.cbi.2011.10.003 PMID:22056647

Stobiecki, M. (2000). Application of mass spectrometry for identification and structural studies of flavonoid glycosides. *Phytochemistry*, *54*(3), 237–256. doi:10.1016/S0031-9422(00)00091-1 PMID:10870178

Sun, L. M., Zhang, C. L., & Li, P. (2011). Characterization, antimicrobial activity, and mechanism of a high-performance (-)-epigallocatechin-3-gallate (EGCG)-CuII/polyvinyl alcohol (PVA) nanofibrous membrane. *Journal of Agricultural and Food Chemistry*, *59*(9), 5087–5092. doi:10.1021/jf200580t PMID:21417240

Tahir, M., Rehman, M. U., Lateef, A., Khan, A. Q., Khan, R., Qamar, W., & Sultana, S. et al. (2013). Diosmin abrogates chemically induced hepatocarcinogenesis via alleviation of oxidative stress, hyperproliferative and inflammatory markers in murine model. *Toxicology Letters*, *220*(3), 205–218. doi:10.1016/j.toxlet.2013.04.004 PMID:23665045

Takaoka, M. (1939). Resveratrol, a new phenolic compound, from *Veratrum grandiflorum*. *Journal of the Chemical Society of Japan*, *60*(1), 1090–1100.

Thomas, S. C., Beveridge, T. H. J., & Drover, J. C. G. (2006). Phytosterol content of sea buckthorn (*Hippophae rhamnoides L.*) seed oil: Extraction and identification. *Food Chemistry*, *101*(4), 1633–1639.

Vanamala, J., Reddivari, L., Yoo, K. S., Pike, L. M., & Patie, B. S. (2006). Variation in the content of bioactive flavonoids in different brands orange and grapefruit juices. *Journal of Food Composition and Analysis*, *19*(2-3), 157–166. doi:10.1016/j.jfca.2005.06.002

Walters, D. R., Walker, R. L., & Walker, K. C. (2003). Lauric Acid exhibits antifungal activity against plant pathogenic fungi. *Journal of Phytopathology*, *151*(4), 228–230. doi:10.1046/j.1439-0434.2003.00713.x

Wang, H., Hui, K. M., Xu, S., Chen, Y., Wong, J. T., & Xue, H. (2002). Two flavones from Scutellaria baicalensis Georgi and their binding affinities to the benzodiazepine site of the GABAA receptor complex. *Die Pharmazie*, *57*(12), 857–858. PMID:12561253

Wilcox, L. J., Borradaile, N. M., de Dreu, L. E., & Huff, M. W. (2001). Secretion of hepatocyte apoB is inhibited by the flavonoids, naringenin and hesperetin, via reduced activity and expression of ACAT2 and MTP. *Journal of Lipid Research*, *42*(5), 725–734. PMID:11352979

Williamson, E., Driver, S., & Baxter, K. (2009). *Interações medicamentosas de Stockley*. Porto Alegre, Rio Grande do Sul, Brasil: Artmed.

Woodside, J. V., McGrath, A. J., Lyner, N., & McKinley, M. C. (2015). Carotenoids and health in older people. *Maturitas*, *80*(1), 63–68. doi:10.1016/j.maturitas.2014.10.012 PMID:25466302

Wu, S. L., Pan, C. E., Yu, L., & Meng, K. W. (2005). Immunosuppression by combined use of cyclosporine and resveratrol in a rat liver transplantation model. *Transplantation Procedures*, *37*(5), 2354–2359. doi:10.1016/j.transproceed.2005.03.112 PMID:15964415

Wu, S. L., Yu, L., Meng, K. W., Ma, Z. H., & Pan, C. E. (2005). Resveratrol prolongs allograft survival after liver transplantation in rats. *World Journal of Gastroenterology, 11*(30), 4745–4749. doi:10.3748/wjg.v11.i30.4745 PMID:16094722

Yankah, V. V. (2006). Lipids phytosterols and human healtl. In *AKOH, Casimir C. Handbook of functional lipids* (pp. 403–418). New York, NY: CRC.

Yu, C., Shin, Y. G., Chow, A., Li, Y., Kosmeder, J. W., Lee, Y. S., & Van Breemen, R. B. et al. (2002). Human, rat and mouse metabolism of resveratrol. *Pharmaceutical Research, 19*(12), 1907–1914. doi:10.1023/A:1021414129280 PMID:12523673

Zatta, L., Nepel, A., Barison, A., & Wypych, F. (2012). Montmorilonita modificada como catalisador heterogêneo em reações de esterificação (m)etílica de ácido láurico. *Quimica Nova, 35*(9), 1711–1718. doi:10.1590/S0100-40422012000900002

Zeng, H. J., Hu, G. H., You, J., Yang, R., & Qu, L. B. (2015). Spectroscopic and molecular modeling investigation on theinteractions between hyaluronidase and baicalein and chrysin. *Process Biochemistry, 50*(5), 738–745. doi:10.1016/j.procbio.2015.02.007

Zhang, L., Lin, G., Kovács, B., Jani, M., Krajcsi, P., & Zuo, Z. (2007). Mechanistic study on the intestinal absorption and disposition of baicalein. *European Journal of Pharmaceutical Sciences, 31*(3-4), 221–231. doi:10.1016/j.ejps.2007.04.001 PMID:17507208

Zhou, Q. M., Wang, X. F., Liu, X. J., Zhang, H., Lu, Y. Y., & Su, S. B. (2011). Curcumin enhanced antiproliferative effect of mitomycin C in human breast cancer MCF-7 cells *in vitro* and *in vivo*. *Acta Pharmacologica Sinica, 32*(11), 1402–1410. doi:10.1038/aps.2011.97 PMID:21986579

Chapter 4
Millets as an Integral Part of Nutritional Diet in India

T. K. Hrideek
Kerala Forest Research Institute, India

K. U. K. Nampoothiri
Central Plantation Crops Research Institute, India

ABSTRACT

Millets are small grained cereals belonging to the family Gramineae and they include major millets and minor millets. Millets are quite important from the point of food and nutritional security at regional and house hold level. In India's dry lands, they play a significant role in meeting food and fodder requirements of farming communities. Millets are found to have high nutritive value comparable and even superior to major cereals with respect to protein, energy, vitamins and minerals. They are also rich sources of phytochemicals and micronutrients. Since millet is gluten-free, it is an excellent option for the people who are suffering from atherosclerosis, diabetics and heart disease. In the face of increasing population and stagnant wheat and rice production, millets can be a promising alternative in solving the problem of food insecurity and malnutrition, because of their sustainability in adverse agro-climatic conditions. These crops have substantive potential in broadening the genetic diversity of the food basket and ensuring improved food and nutrition security.

DOI: 10.4018/978-1-5225-0607-2.ch004

INTRODUCTION

Millets are small grained cereals belonging to Gramineae family which include major millets like sorghum and pearl millet (which are tall growing and fairly drought tolerant) and minor millets with short slender culm and small grains possessing remarkable drought tolerance (ICRISAT and FAO, 1996). The term "millet' is often used loosely to refer to several types of small seeded annual grasses. Millets share a set of characteristics which make them unique amongst cereals. They belong to five genera, namely *Panicum*, *Setaria*, *Echinochola*, *Pennisetum, Paspalum*, and *Eleusine*. The genus *Pennisetum* includes about 140 species, some of which are domesticated and some grow in the wild. Most of the genera are widely distributed throughout the tropics and subtropics of the world (De Wet et al, 1984). Millets can be a valuable source of forage because of their rapid growth, high nutritive value and ability to survive stressful conditions such as drought. According to Hulse *et al*. (1980), the most important cultivated millet species are pearl millet *(Pennisetum typhoides),* also known as bulrush millet; proso millet (*Panicum miliaceum)*, also known as common millet; foxtail millet (*Setaria italica*); Japanese barnyard millet *(Echinochloa crus- galli*var *or E. colona*); finger millet (*Eleusine coracana*), also known as birds foot millet or African millet and kodo millet (*Paspalum scorbiculatum*). Other millets include little millet (*Panicum sumatrense*), tef millet (*Eargrostis tef*) and fonio millet *Digitaria exilis* and *D. iburua*) (Dogget, 1989). The vernacular names of millets in India are given in Table 1.

India is also the home for the species *Echinochola colona (Sawa)* under barnyard millet. Many indigenous communities in Asia preferred millets as their grain crop for shifting cultivation. The long history of minor millet cultivation and their spread to different regions of the world, which are notable for extremely harsh farming conditions, had generated considerable genetic variability in these crops. Kodo millet is very hardy and possesses the highest drought resistance with potential to offer a good yield in a growing period between 80-135 days. Barnyard millet could be said to be the second hardiest millet with the ability to give a modest yield in 50-100 days. Finger millet is more widely grown in Africa and Asia, differentiated in to five races and shows wide variability in appearance, adaptability, maturity period, yield and quality. Foxtail millet may be ranked fourth in yielding ability. The yield potential of little and proso millets are relatively lower with proso millet being hardier. Brief details of millet crops are given in Table 2.

Table 1. Vernacular names of millets

English	Alternate Names	Botanical	Hindi	Kannada	Tamil	Telugu	Malayalam	Marathi
Sorghum	Great Millet/ Milo/Chari	*Sorghum vulgare*	Jowar	Jola	Cholam	Jonnalu	Cholam	Jwari
Pearl Millet	Spiked Millet/ Bullrush	*Pennisetum typhoideum*	Bajra	Sajje	Kambu	Gantilu/ Sazzalu	Kambu	Bajri
Finger Millet	Rajika	*Eleusine coracana*	Mandua/ madua	Ragi	Kelvargu/ kezhvaragu	Ragulu	Muthari	Nachni
Barnyard Millet	Japanese Millet/ Sawank	*Echinochola frumantacea*	Jhangora/ Shama	Samai	Kuthiravaali	Odalu/ Bonta/ Chamula	–	Shamul
Foxtail Millet	Moha Millet/ Italian Millet	*Setarai italica*	Kangni	Navane/ PriyanguThene	Tenai	Korra/ Korralu	Thina	Rala
Kodo Millet	Pakodi/ Manakodra	*Paspalum scrobiculatum*	Kodra	Harka	Varagu	Arikelu	Varagu	Harik
Proso Millet	French Millet/ Common Millet	*Panicum miliaceum*	Barri	Baragu	Panivaragu	Varigulu/ Varagalu	Panivaragu	Vari
Little Millet	Goudli/ Gondola	*Panicum miliare*	Kutki	Same	Samai	Sama	Chama	Sava

HISTORY

NABARD (2007) summarized the history of millets as follows: From African highlands finger millet was taken to India about 3000 years ago and to Europe at the beginning of the Christian era. Later, the crop was widely distributed both in many African countries as well as in the Indian subcontinent. They have been a part of the human food system from time immemorial. Many types of millets have been found in Harrapa and Mohenjadaro archaeological sites. Africans were known to use millets in their myriad culinary courses. The leader of the Shang Dynasty in the 2nd millennium BC was known as Hou Chi, 'The ruler of Millet'. Indian vedic scriptures like Sathapatha Brahmana have ample references to millets. Kalidasa, in his legendary literary masterpiece 'Shakuntala', has sage Kanva pouring foxtail millet while bidding farewell to Shakuntala in Dushanta's court.

The oldest historical roots of millet are found in China, where it was considered a sacred crop. One of the earliest recorded writings dates from 2800 BC giving directions for growing and storing of the grain. During prehistoric times, people of Northern India were also cultivating millet. Millet's travel continued throughout the Middle East and Northern Africa where it became a staple food. It further became a

Table 2. Details of small millet crops

Crops	Particulars	
Barnyard Millet: *Echinochola colona* (L.) Link.	Origin	India
	Existential	Minuscule food, cattle fodder, cattle and poultry feed.
	Ecology	Adapted to temperate climate and grows well in tropics as well as on soils with fragile ecology
	Temperature	Tolerant to wide temperature range
	Altitude	Up to 2700 metres
	Rainfall	200-400 mm.
	Distribution	
	Global	Tansaniaand Malawi republic of Africa, India, Nepal, Japan, Korea and China.
	India	Andhra Pradesh, Gujarat, Madhya Pradesh, Maharashtra,Tamilnadu and Uttarakhand
Common(Proso) Millet: *Panicum milliaceum* L.	Origin	Central and Eastern Asia
	Existential	Minuscule food with medicinal properties being rich in Choline with traces of manganese, copper and zinc and minerals like calcium, phosphorous and iron. Used for hog feed, cattle fodder, bedding and starch for textiles.
	Soils	Marginal shallow lands with low humus
	Temperature	Tolerant to very wide temperature range
	Altitude	Up to 2700 metres
	Rainfall	200-400 mm.
	Pollination	Partly cross-pollinated
	Distribution	
	Global	Neolithic Europe, Volga region of Russia, Khazakhistan, Bangladesh, Srilanka, Nepal and China, North and West America, Kenya, Zimbabwe Ethiopia and India.
	India	Andhra Pradesh, Bihar, Gujarat, Karnataka, Maharashtra, Rajasthan and Tamilnadu
Foxtail Millet: *Setaria italica* Beauv.	Origin	Eastern Asia.
	Existential	Minuscule food rich in minerals, popped culinary and cattle fodder
	Ecology	Adapted to hot and dry climate. Grown in temperate regions to tropics
	Soils	Marginal shallow lands with no humus. Grown mostly as companion crop with cotton/pulses/oilseeds
	Temperature	Tolerant to very wide temperature range
	Rainfall	200-400 mm
	Distribution	
	Global	Eurasia, Ethiopia, Zimbabwe, Japan, China, Nepal and India
	India	Andhra Pradesh, Gujarat, Maharashtra, Rajasthan and Tamilnadu

continued on following page

Table 2. Continued

Crops	Particulars	
Kodo Millet: *Paspalum scrobiculatum* L.	Origin	India
	Existential	Minuscule food, cattle and cattle fodder
	Ecology	Koda millet can grow even where no other cereal grows. Adapted to very hot and dry climate.
	Soils	Marginal soil with no humus, hilly slopes/edges
	Distribution	
	Global	Uganda
	India	Andhra Pradesh, Gujarat, Karnataka,Maharashtra, Chhattisgarh, Madhya Pradesh and Tamilnadu
Little Millet: *Panicum sumatrense* Roth Ex. Roem & Schult	Origin	Arid Western and North America.
	Existential	Minuscule food, cattle fodder
	Ecology	A very hot and dry season crop grown on marginal lands and hilly slopes.
	Temperature	Tolerant to very wide temperature range.
	Rainfall	200-400 mm
	Altitude	Up to 2100 metres
	Distribution	
	Global	South East Asia, China and India
	India	Andhra Pradesh, Bihar, Gujarat, Karnataka, Maharashtra, Madhya Pradesh, Odisha and Tamilnadu
Finger Millet: *Eleusine coracana*	Origin	Ethiopian region of Africa
	Existential	Across the states in India. A famine crop in Ethiopia, staple food in the regions of perturbed ecology across the globe. Used for beverages, baby food, cattle fodder and for thatching
	Ecology	A warm season crop grown from sea level to 3000 metres (above msl.), C4 plant
	Soils	Grows well on well drained soils with steady supply of moisture
	Rainfall	500-2000 mm
	Temperature	Optimum 15-27^{0}C
	Distribution	
	Global	South East Asia, Africa, China and India
	India	Andhra Pradesh, Bihar, Gujarat, Karnataka, Maharashtra, Madhya Pradesh, Odisha and Tamilnadu

typical food of the Sumerian diet in about 2500 BC. Millet was even mentioned in the Hebrew bible. The idyllic Hanging Gardens of Babylon were said to have included millet among their treasured plants. Through trading with Eritrea and Somalia circa 3000 BC, the early Egyptians learned from the Africans how to cultivate millet, which would grow well in the dry Sahara, where wheat and barley were unable to thrive. Millets made their way from China to the Black Sea region of Europe by 5000 BC. Romans and Gauls made porridge from it and in the middle ages millet was more extensively eaten than wheat. The interesting fact is that millet is also pointed out in the Bible as used to prepare bread during those days.

Genetic Resources

Even the limited millet genetic resources are getting eroded in a fast pace mainly due to neglect, among other reasons, resulting in replacement with more remunerative commercial or non-food crops (Balaravi e*t al*., 2010). Despite national efforts to collect minor millet germplasm from farmers, research to improve these crops has been negligible. Liberalization of the Indian seed sector in the 1990s favoured dry land cereals and legumes, with little impact on research and formal distribution channels for minor millets. Neglected and underutilized crop genetic resources are very vital for sustainable agriculture (Bhag Mal, 2007) and minor millets belong to this important group of crops (Dutta *et al*., 2007). Plant genetic resources play a critical role in enhancing adaptation and resilience of agricultural production systems (Jarvis *et al*., 2007). Currently, states of Andhra Pradesh, Karnataka, and Tamil Nadu lead in crop improvement research on minor millets. but the range of improved varieties is narrow. Private companies show little interest in developing

Table 3. Some released varieties of millets in India

SL No.	Crop	Name of the Variety
1	Finger Millet	GPU 45, Chillika OEB 10, TANU 946, VL 315 & GPU 48, VL 149, PR 202, GPU 26 and CO 11 PES 176, PES 110, Pant Mandua 3, PRM 1, PRM 2,(Ranichouri) CO 10,CO 11,Paiyur 1, CO 12, TRY 1, CO 13 Indira Ragi -1(BR-7), Dapoli Safed-1
2	Foxtail millet	Meera (SR 16), Sri Lakshmi, Prathap kangni 1(SR 1), SR 51, PRK 1 & TANU 196 Pant Setaria - 4, PRK-1
3	Kodo millet	Jawahar kodo 48 (JK 48) & KK 2 GPUK 3 and JK 48 Indira Kodo-1(BK-1) CO 3, APK1,Vamban 1
4	Barnyard millet	VL Madira 181and VL 172 CO1
5	Little millet	Tarini (OLM 203), Kolab (OLM 36) & OLM 20 TNAU 63 CO 2, Paiyur1, CO 3, Paiyur2
6	Proso millet	GPUP 8 & GPUP 21 PRC - 1 BR 7 and K 1 CO 2,CO 3,CO 4

new varieties, due to their lack of commercial importance and the limited scope for developing new hybrids. Minor millet with a higher yield potential have been recommended for cultivation in India are given in Table 3 and some of these varieties are mentioned in the publication by ICAR(2013)

Kolli Hills of Tamil Nadu, Koraput of Odisha and Dharvad in Karnataka have a genetically diverse pool of minor millet varieties being grown by the tribal farming communities for their own consumption without formal trade. Lack of attention of researchers, policy makers, donors, farmers and consumers is increasingly threatening the genetic diversity of minor millets. This is an irreversible loss to the humanity, particularly the poor who heavily depend on these crops for their food and nutritional security and income generation (Prabhakaran *et al.* 2012).

Figure 1. Phenotypic variation in fingers of Eleusine coracana from Odisha region of India

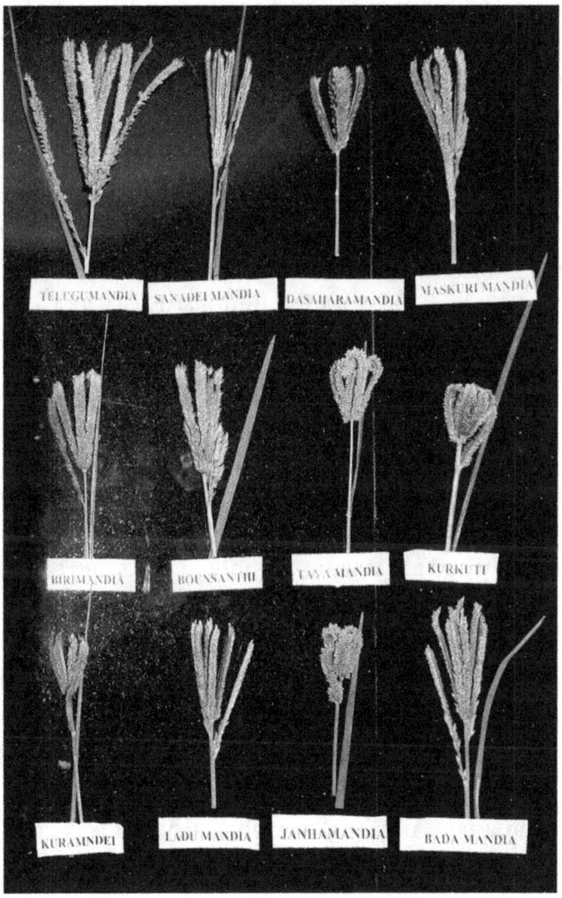

Very recently minor millets, especially finger millet has received better attention by research and development agencies in terms of agronomy and improved varieties. About 86 improved varieties of finger millet have been released during 1935-2008 with seed production system available for a few of these varieties. These crops are virtually free from insect-pests in the field, though they are affected by a few major diseases. Plant protection measures, which are seldom used by farmers, can contribute to productivity increase by minimizing the disease-induced yield losses. The Variation in Finger shape of *Eleusine coracana* is shown in Figure 1.

With regard to the conservation of the genetic resources of minor millets, the largest *ex situ* collection at international level is maintained by the Consultative Group on International Agricultural Research (CGIAR). These collections hold 46,231 accessions and 16.7% of them has been duplicated and deposited with the Global Crop Diversity Trust for safe storage at the Svalbard Gene Bank in Norway. The largest CGIAR collection is being held at ICRISAT (10,193 accessions). India holds the largest national collection at the National Bureau of Plant Genetic Resources (21,226 accessions) in New Delhi. A working collection of 13,296 accessions is being maintained by the All India Coordinated Small Millet Improvement Project at the University of Agricultural Sciences, Bangalore (Karnataka). Minor millet germplasm collections are also maintained at the N.I.Vavilov Research Institute of Plant Industry (VIR) in Russia and at CIRAD, France. Very scarce information is available with regard to *in situ*/on-farm conservation of minor millets. On-farm conservation is a dynamic process, because varieties managed by the farmers continue to evolve in response to natural and human selection leading to crop populations with better adaptive potential for the future (Brush, 2000).

ADVANTAGES OF MILLETS

Millets are versatile in that they perform well in regions with erratic rainfall or in low-quality arable land. They are highly nutritious, the grains have a good storage capacity, mature quickly and are less susceptible to pests and diseases. The extraordinary hardiness of many of these species and their ability to cope with adverse growing and climatic conditions offer great promise in the context of climate change. Though millets occupy relatively a lower position among food crops in Indian agriculture, they are quite important from the point of food security at regional and house hold level. Small millets can be grown even in poor soil and climatic conditions. They have short growing season and can be very well fitted into multiple cropping systems both under irrigated as well as dry farming conditions. They can provide nutritious grain and fodder in a short span of time. Small millets have a capacity for wide adaptation. They can withstand a certain degree of soil acidity

Table 4. Food value of millets compared to rice (%)

Name of Millet	Moisture	Protein	Carbohydrate	Fat	Fibre	Mineral	Calcium	Phosphorous	Calorific Value (100g)
Finger millet	13.0	8.0	72.0	1.3	3.0	2.70	0.3	0.3	332
Common millet	11.1	13.71	72.26	1.76	0.10	1.07	0.01	0.2	341
Foxtail millet	11.9	9.7	72.4	3.5	1.0	1.5	0.04	0.3	353
Little millet	11.1	13.4	72.3	1.8	0.10	1.1	0.02	0.3	360
Kodo millet	11.6	10.6	59.2	4.2	10.2	4.4	0.04	0.3	346
Tef	11.2	9.1	74.3	2.2	-	-	-	-	-
Japanese Barnyard millet	11.9	6.2	65.5	2.2	9.8	4.4	-	-	-
Hungry rice	6.0	8.7	81.0	1.1	1.1	2.1	-	-	-
Polished rice	13.2	7.5	76.7	1.0	0.3	1.6	0.01	0.17	348

Source: FAO 2001.

and alkalinity, stress due to moisture and temperature and variation in soils from heavy to sandy infertile ones. It is important to enhance production and productivity of these crops to ensure food and nutritional security (Stanly *et al.*, 2013).The small seeds have a long shelf life and can be stored for a long period without insect damage, which makes them good reserves for famine-prone areas. Millets provide the cheapest source of calories in people's diet, but unfortunately the support for production and consumption of rice and wheat through public distribution system has resulted in neglect of various millets by a significant number of small rain fed farmers engaged in its cultivation. This has led to reduction in conservation, cultivation and consumption of these crops (Yenag *et al.*, 2011).

Nutritional Value of Millets

Nutritional quality of food is a key element in maintaining overall human health. An increasingly important determinant in food choice is the growing consumer concern about nutrition and health (Nehir and Simsek, 2012). Therefore, for solving the problem of deeprooted food insecurity and malnutrition, dietary quality should be taken into consideration (Singh and Raghuvanshi, 2012). In addition to their cultivating advantages, millets are found to have high nutritive value comparable to that of major cereals such as wheat and rice (Parameswaran and Sadasivam 1994). It has also been reported that millet proteins are good sources of essential amino acids-

Table 5. Amino acid profiles of millet grains

Amino Acids (g/100g)	Foxtail Millet (Defatted Flour) (a)	Proso Millet (Dehulled Grain) (b)	Pearl Millet (True Prolamine) (c)	Finger Millet (Native Grain) (d)
Essential Amino Acids				
Isoleucine	4.59	4.1	5.1	4.3
Leucine	13.6	12.2	14.1	10.8
Lysine	1.59	1.5	0.5	2.2
Methionine	3.06	2.2	1	2.9
Phenylalanine	6.27	5.5	7.6	6
Threonine	3.68	3	3.3	4.3
Valine	5.81	5.4	4.2	6.3
Histidine	2.11	2.1	1.7	2.3
Tryptophan	NA	0.8	1.2	NA
Non-Essential Amino Acids				
Alanine	9.3	10.9	8.1	6.1
Arginine	3	3.2	0.9	3.4
Aspartic acid	7.71	6.2	6.2	5.7
Cystine	0.45	NA	0.8	NA
Glutamic acid	22	21.3	22.8	23.2
Glycine	2.91	2.1	0.7	3.3
Serine	4.56	6.3	5.4	5.3
Tyrosine	2.44	4	2.7	3.6
Pronile	5.54	7.3	8.2	9.9
*PER (b)	0.8	1.1	1.6	2

References: (a) Bagdia *et al.*. (2011); (b) Devi *et al.* (2011).
*Protein efficiency ratio (PER). NA: Not available.

except lysine and threonine -but are relatively high in methionine. Millets are also rich sources of phytochemicals and micronutrients (Mal *et al.*, 2010; Singh *et al.*, 2012). The various types of millets and their food values are given in Tables 4 and 5.

However, millet seeds have a seed coat which gives a darker color, chewy texture and musky odour. These characteristics reduce the applicability of millet in the food industry. Millets are highly nutritious, non-glutinous and non-acid forming foods. Hence they are soothing and easy to digest. They are considered to be the least allergenic and most digestible grains available. Compared to rice (especially polished rice), millets release lesser percentage of glucose. Finger millet is the richest in calcium, about 10 times that of rice or wheat. Considering the nutrient richness of these grains they are now considered as 'nutri-cereals' and not as 'coarse cereals'.

Though millets are generally regarded as "coarse" grains, their potential for augmenting the grain supplies, as also to considerably bridge the protein gap is being increasingly realized. Millet, besides being a rich source of carbohydrates, is very easy to digest; it contains a high amount of lecithin and is excellent for strengthening the nervous system. Millets are rich in B vitamins, especially niacin, pyridoxine and folic acid, as well as the minerals calcium, iron, potassium, magnesium and zinc.

Finger millet carbohydrates comprise of free sugars (1-2%), starch (75-80%) and non-starchy polysaccharides consisting of cellulose and hemicellulose. It is a very good source of dietary fibre, micronutrients and polyphenols. Fermented finger millet extract suppresses growth of *Salmonella* sp. and *Escherichia coli*. It is reported to have many nutraceutical and functional properties. The extremely good storage property of finger millet and its processed foods could be attributed to its polyphenol content (Mathangi, *et al.*, 2012).

The seed husk of millet is an excellent source of phytochemicals (polyphenols up to 3%) and dietary fibre (Palanisamy, Bruntha Devi *et al.*, 2011). Certain parts of the seed contain anti-nutritive compounds such as phytates (0.48%), polyphenols, tannins (0.61%), tripsin inhibitory factors and hydrochloric acid which require processing for the promotion of millets for nutritional and organoleptic acceptance (Jingju, 2007; Shobana, 2007; Bagdia *et al..*, 2011).

In general, cereal proteins including millets are limited in lysine and tryptophan content and vary with cultivars. However, most cereals contain the essential amino acids as well as vitamins and minerals (Devi *et al..*, 2011; FAO, 2009). Millets generally contain significant amounts of essential amino acids particularly the sulphur containing amino acids (methionine and cysteine); they are also higher in fat content than maize, rice and sorghum (Obilana and Manyasa, 2002; Mal *et al.*, 2010). Though millets are not the important part of daily diet of American and European people, now these countries have recognized its importance as an ingredient in multigrain and gluten-free cereal products. However, in many Asian and African countries millet is the staple food of the people in millet producing areas and they prepare various traditional foods and beverages, breads as well as infant and snack foods from it (Chandrasekara and Shahidi, 2011). Whilst a number of traditional foods are made in the domestic household, the lack of large-scale industrial utilization discourages the farmers from raising millet crops (Subramanian and Viswanathan, 2003). Therefore, many countries including India, China, USA etc. have now started research to develop process technology for nutritional improvement, to fully take advantage of the health benefits and to promote them as food on a larger scale. 21st century challenges like climate change, water scarcity, increasing world population, rising food prices and other socio economic impacts are expected to generate a great threat to agriculture and food security worldwide, especially for the poorest people who live in arid and sub-arid regions (Saleh *et al.*, 2013). Millets have relatively poor digestibility and low bio-availability of minerals due to the presence of inherent anti-nutritional factors. The difficulties in millet grain processing present a challenge but nutritional as well as health benefits and consumer demand for health foods provide opportunities in processing, development of suitable technology for newer products and process mechanization.

Millet grains are nutritionally comparable and even superior to major cereals with respect to protein, energy, vitamins and minerals (Sehgal and Kawatra, 2003). Millets are a rich source of minerals, nutraceuticals and higher dietary fibers when compared to rice or wheat and contains 9-14% protein and 70-80% carbohydrates (Hadimani and Malleshi, 1993). These are rich sources of phytochemicals and micronutrients (Singh *et al.*, 2012b). The quality of protein is mainly a function of its essential amino acids. Finger millet contains 44.7% essential amino acids of the total amino acids (FAO, 1991; Mbithi *et al.*, 2000). The characterization of the proteins of millet grains shows that prolamin fraction constitutes the major storage protein of the grain and lysine is the most limiting amino acid followed by cystine but millets are relatively high in methionine (Monteiro *et al.*, 1987; Sudharshana *et al.*, 1987; Kumar and Parmeswaran, 1999). The true digestibility and biological value of these millets range between 95.0 to 99.3 and 48.3 to 56.5 respectively (Geerwani and Eggum, 1989). Among the millets, pearl millet (*Bajra*) has the highest content of macronutrients and iron, zinc, Mg, P, folic acid and riboflavin. It is significantly rich in resistant starch and soluble and insoluble dietary fibres (Antony *et al.* 1996; Ragaee *et al.*, 2006). Finger millet seed coat is an edible material and contains good proportion of dietary fibre, minerals and phytochemicals. The seed coat matter (SCM) forms a by-product of millet milling, malting and decortication industries which can be profitably utilized as composite flour in biscuit preparation (Krishnan *et al.*, 2011). Finger millet is an extraordinary source of calcium. Kodo millet and little millet are also reported to have 37% to 38% of dietary fiber, which is the highest among them (Malleshi and Hadimani 1993; Antony *et al.*, 1996). Kodo millet has the highest free radical (DPPH) quenching activity followed by great millet (sorghum) and finger millet (Hegde and Chandra, 2005). The niacin content in pearl millet is higher than all other cereals. In addition, millets are gluten-free, easy to digest and are a great source of antioxidants and might have anti-carcinogenic properties (Dykes and Rooney, 2006). The lipid content is generally high (3–6%) for pearl millet - higher than that of sorghum and most other common cereals. About 75% of the fatty acids in pearl millet are unsaturated and linoleic acid is particularly high (46.3%). For this reason energy content of millet is greater than sorghum and nearly equal to that of brown rice. Finger and teff millet are good sources of dietary calcium and magnesium and iron content is significant.

Health Benefits of Millets

Millets are still the staple food for millions of poor people in Africa and Asia. Like many other cereals, millets are nutritious and high in carbohydrate energy content, making them useful components for dietary and nutritional balance in foods. Millets offer unique advantage for health being rich in micronutrients, particularly minerals and B vitamins as well as nutraceuticals. Combination of millets with other sources of protein would compensate the deficiency of certain amino acids such as lysine. Successful improvement of these attributes would be a crucial key to expand the spectrum of applications of millet grains (Issoufou Amadou *et al* 2013). If included in the daily diet, millets provide adequate nutrition and offer health benefits especially in the management of disorders like diabetes mellitus, obesity, hyperlipidemia, etc. (Veena, 2003).

Since millet is gluten-free, it is an excellent option for people suffering from celiac diseases often irritated by the gluten content of wheat and other more common cereal grains and also useful for people who are suffering from atherosclerosis and diabetic heart disease (Gélinas *et al.*, 2008). Finger millet diets have been found to lower blood glucose and cholesterol. It has a potent therapeutic role as dietary supplement for the prevention of glycation induced complications, as in diabetes or aging. The grain is also rich in phytochemicals, including phytic acid, which is believed to lower cholesterol, and phytate, which is associated with reduced cancer risk (Coulibaly *et al.*, 2011). These health benefits have been partly attributed to the wide variety of potential chemo preventive substances, called phytochemicals, including antioxidants present in high amounts (Izadi *et al.*, 2012). Chandrasekara and Shahidi (2010) reported that non processed brown finger millet had the highest radical quenching activity than the processed one and postulated that tannins and phytic acid were responsible for the activity. Millet extract from the seed coat were reported to have shown high antibacterial and antifungal activity compared to whole flour extract due to high polyphenol content in seed coat (Viswanath *et al.*, 2009). It maintains cardiovascular health and helps to reduce acidity problems. Epidemiological evidence from research studies has shown that diets rich in plant foods are protective against several degenerative diseases such as cancer, cardiovascular ailments, diabetes, metabolic syndrome and Parkinson's disease (Manach *et al.,* 2005; Scalbert *et al.,* 2005; Chandrasekara and Shahidi 2012). In addition, there is strong epidemiological evidence that whole-grain cereals protect the body against age-related diseases such as diabetes, cardiovascular diseases and some cancers (Fardet *et al.* 2008).

The chemical reaction between the aldehyde group of reducing sugars and the amino group of proteins is a major factor responsible for the complications of diabetes and aging (Monnier 1990). Millet grains are rich in antioxidants and phenolics; it has been established that phytates, phenols, and tannins can contribute to antioxidant activity, important in health, aging, and metabolic syndrome (Bravo 1998). It has also been found that methanolic extracts from finger millet and kodo millet inhibited glycation and cross-linking of collagen (Hegde *et al.,* 2002). Therefore, there is potential usefulness of millets in the protection against aging (Issoufou Amadou *et. al* .2013).

Value Addition

All millets are cooked after dehulling and dehulled grain is milled into flour. Traditional way of hulling Finger millet is given in Figure 2. Italian millet is consumed as stiff porridge called sargatic or as roti. Proso millet flour is also used as a substitute for rice flour in various snack foods. Millet protein lacks gluten, hence it is unsuitable as the sole material for preparation of bakery products. Mudde from millet flour is prepared by steaming the dough and making it into balls. Millet flours are soaked overnight in cold water containing a little butter milk and the slurry after fermentation is used to prepare porridge. Millets and black gram mixed in the ratio of 3:1 are wet ground and fermented overnight which can be steamed to make idli or baked on hot pan to prepare dosa or wet pan cakes. Non-conventional foods like flakes and extruded products can be prepared from millets. Flakes are prepared by soaking pearl millets in water and then steamed under pressure for complete

Figure 2. Traditional method of dehusking finger millet

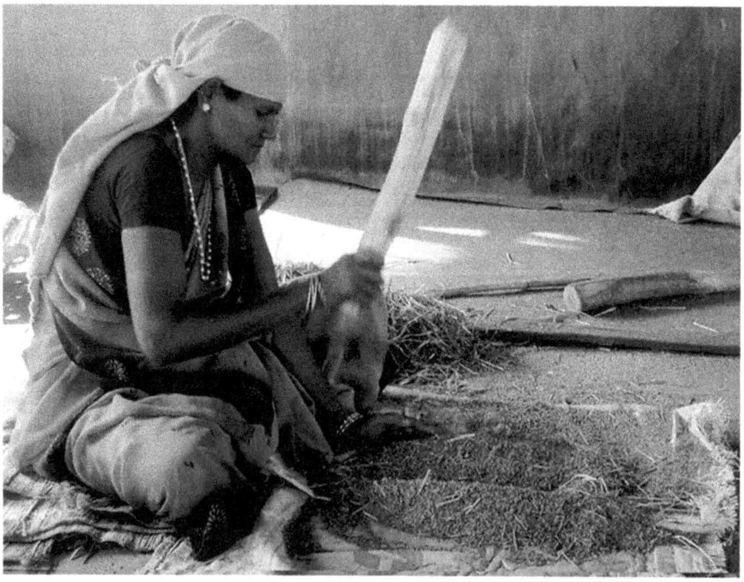

gelatination of the starch and dried to about 18% moisture. Then they are pressed to requisite thickness between heavy duty rollers and dried to prepare flakes which hydrate quickly when added to warm water or milk. Noodle like products can be prepared from millet flours. They form nutritionally balanced food which is used as supplementary or weaning foods.

Typical grain texture and hard seed coat of millets increases their keeping quality but makes them difficult to process as well as cook in convenient form. Absence of appropriate primary processing technologies to prepare ready-to-use or ready-to-cook products and also secondary as well as tertiary processing to prepare ready-to-eat value added products have been the major limiting factors for their diversified food uses (Malleshi, 2014). Par boiling improves the quality and is also used to prepare expanded grains. Millets are rarely used to produce starch for industrial uses. Their starches generally exhibit higher gelatinization temperature, higher water binding capacity and are slow in enzymatic hydrolysis than that of wheat and rice. Millets may also find use for formulating high fibre and diabetic foods.

In collaboration with agricultural universities in Bangalore and Dharwad as well as Bioversity International, M.S. Swaminathan Research Foundation (MSSRF) has been working with tribal farming families in the Indian states of Uttarakhand, Odisha, Tamil Nadu and Karnataka to increase production and to facilitate commercialization of little millet, finger millet and foxtail millet. Traditional milling and grinding using pestle and mortar and manual grinding stones take several hours. To reduce the drudgery of processing, simple mechanical pulverisers and dehulling units were introduced and women trained to operate and maintain them. Using the new machines, processing was reduced to ten minutes and consequently led to a revival of interest amongst the women for cultivating and consuming millets to a greater extent. Attempts were also made, along with rural women to add value and develop popular snack foods such as ragi powder, *murukku*, *laddu* etc. By training the women in maintaining quality, standardization, packaging and production, new millet-based recipes were developed for urban consumers and schools, which led to increased sales of millet based products. The new recipes were cost effective without being labour or time intensive, leaving the women with more time for carrying out other responsibilities. The new recipes were also promoted to combat nutritional deficiencies among school going children, as the snacks are higher in protein and vitamins than equivalent products made of rice or wheat. In another initiative, women who produced and packaged a finger millet-based, hot malt drink testified that it tasted similar to chocolate, with more nutrients. These opened opportunities to provide it for the benefit of both mothers and children creating a higher demand and increased profits. But much desires to be done to take these initiatives to a marketable proposition.

Cultivation: Indian Scenario

India is the largest producer of many kinds of millets and it remains a staple crop for numerous households. In India's dry lands, they play a significant role in meeting food and fodder requirements of farming communities. Millets are invariably grown in the semi-arid and mountainous regions of tropics and subtropics, where monsoon failure and drought are frequent, soil fertility is poor and land terrain is difficult. These regions are also hot spots of poverty and frequent starvation. Traditional agriculture in these regions has found more dependability on minor millets because of their extreme hardiness. Millets are grown in an area of 3.5 million hectares in India, their cultivation extending from sea level in coastal Andhra Pradesh up to an altitude of 8000 feet above sea level in hills of Uttaranchal and North-Eastern states (Table 6). They offer satisfactory yields from shallow and less fertile soils and in steep slopes of hillocks and mountainous terrains. Their yield varies widely from very low to modestly high across regions and years depending on the soil, management and weather. Millets have retained their primacy under these farming conditions to provide livelihood and food security to the poor people. Millets have been farmed at subsistence level with years of experience and traditional wisdom embedded in the varietal choice and farming systems. These systems are invariably structured on location specific multiple or intercropping systems to safeguard livelihood even under unforeseen weather. These farming systems and underlying economic compulsions have discouraged extensive use of fertilizers, herbicides or pesticides in minor millet farming. Farmers in each region have been innovative in developing many local cultivars, which are well adapted to their farming conditions. Millets have hardly received any attention from national or global food policy makers in research funding and improvement of these crops. Hence they continue to be grown largely under traditional practices using traditional cultivars under subsistence farming.

Millets, and particularly small millets, are in a crisis situation in India. The period between 1961 and 2009 saw a dramatic decrease in cultivated area under millets (80% for small millets, 46% for finger millet, 59% for sorghum and 23% for pearl millet); a 76% decrease in total production of small millets; a significant decrease in per capita availability of all millets (despite high productivity gains for some varieties); and a steep fall in overall millet consumption. Almost 50% area under millets has been diverted largely to soybean, maize, cotton, sugarcane and sunflower. A combination of factors like low remuneration compared to other food crops, lack of input subsidies and price incentives, subsidized supply of fine cereals through Public Distribution System (PDS), and change in consumer preference coupled with difficulty in processing, low shelf life of flour and low social status attached to millets, have led to shift from production of millets to other competing crops.

Table 6. Trend in harvested area, production, and consumption of millets in India

Years	Harvested Area (in 0000' M. Ha)	Growth %	Production (in 0000' M. MT)	Growth %	Consumption (in 0000' M. MT)	Growth %
2001	12000	-7.87%	900	0.00%	900	0.00%
2002	9000	-25.00%	700	-22.22%	700	-22.22%
2003	13100	45.56%	900	28.57%	900	28.57%
2004	11000	-16.03%	800	-11.11%	800	-11.11%
2005	10500	-4.55%	900	12.50%	900	12.50%
2006	10300	-1.90%	900	0.00%	900	0.00%
2007	10800	4.85%	1000	11.11%	1000	11.11%
2008	10000	-7.41%	1000	0.00%	1000	0.00%
2009	10400	4.00%	700	-30.00%	700	-30.00%
2010	11150	7.21%	1200	71.43%	1200	71.43%
2011	10800	-3.14%	1500	25.00%	1500	25.00%
2012	8500	-21.30%	1200	-20.00%	1200	-20.00%

Source: Ministry of Agriculture, Govt. of India and United States Department of Agriculture.

Constraints Limiting Productivity of Millets

Millets have traditionally played an important role in farming and food culture in many regions of the world, including Sub-Saharan Africa and South Asia (McDonough *et al.*, 2000) with India being the world's largest producer of these crops. Millets mature quickly, a valuable trait important for rain-fed farming, and require relatively few inputs compared to major cereals. They grow under a range of day lengths and in poor soil, making them an attractive crop for marginal farming environments. In addition to these agronomic advantages, millets can offer other benefits in ecological, nutritional, and socioeconomic areas. Though overall production of millets in India has increased over the past few decades, from 7.7 million tons in 1961 to 10.7 million tons in 2012, the area dedicated to minor millets has fallen; finger millet declined from 2.3 million ha in 1951–1955 to 1.35 million ha in 2006–2010. Other minor millets declined even more precipitously, from 5.29 million ha to 0.97 million ha over the same period. Productivity of finger millet, in terms of yield per ha, doubled from 704 to 1471 kg ha^{-1} largely thanks to improved varieties more than making up for the decrease in area. According to Mal and Padulosi.,2013, the other minor millets recorded more modest gains in productivity, from 410 to 480 kg ha^{-1} and total production is less than a quarter of its 1950 value (2.177 MT in 1951–1955 *vs.* 0.467 MT in 2006–2010). The decline in minor millets in India can be attributed to many factors; agronomic, economic and social. The green revolution of the 1970s saw government promotion of rice and wheat pushing minor millets into even more marginal areas. Unfortunate consequence is that in those areas, millets have come to be regarded as crops of the poor, which they are, and thus to be avoided. Policy-makers have contributed to this by keeping millets largely out of the scope of both official research and development and price support agreements. Continuing neglect hastens the loss of genetic diversity and traditional knowledge on the production, processing and use of millets. Production is inefficient as a result of lack of suitable higher yielding varieties, poor quality seeds and unimproved cultivation practices. Traditional processing methods considerably increase the daily drudgery of women who prepare millets. Coupled with unfavourable environmental policy, there is a lack of attractive recipes for adding value, lack of awareness of the nutritional value of millets, poorly organized integration with markets, and generally unfavourable environmental policy.

The major constraints can be summarized as follows:

1. Millets are grown on poor shallow and marginal soils under rain fed conditions. The soils on which these are gown have mostly low moisture retention capacity. Some of these are still grown in the hilly areas under shifting cultivation which is one of the most primitive ways of cultivation.
2. Shortage of improved seeds as there is no organized programme for production and supply of seeds with high yield potential. Seed is usually farm saved and of poor quality. Poverty and lack of food security also threaten the seed supply sometimes forcing farmers to eat their saved seed.
3. Seeds are often broadcast. This is a major bottle neck in taking inter-cultivation operation and effective weed control. Mixed cropping practices adopted by the farmers are often suited to sustenance agriculture and many of them are not remunerative.
4. Research has paid little attention to improve the genetic potential of the crop and the way it is cultivated and used. Even the known crop management practices are not able to be adopted by the farmers due to their socio-economic constraints ((Balakrishnan *et al.*, 2002, Stefano *et al.*, 2015).
5. Typical grain texture and hard seed coat of millets make them difficult to process as well as cook in convenient form. Absence of appropriate primary processing technologies to prepare ready-to-use or ready-to-cook (RTC) products and also secondary as well as tertiary processing to prepare ready-to-eat value added products make it difficult to exploit their diversified food uses (Malleshi, 2014) The grains are to be hulled, cleaned and often powdered before use. These are cumbersome tasks often carried out by women and in the

absence of affordable small scale processing units, act as a deterrent factor in taking up millet cultivation.

6. There is no ready market for the disposal of surplus produce at a remunerative price. So also extension and development support are unsatisfactory.
7. More recently, farmers have turned to cash crops such as cassava, and even eucalyptus where promotional schemes are available, resulting in a decline in millet cultivation.
8. The yield gap in millets is largely due to existing poor cultivation technology that leaves ample scope for improvement.
9. Lack of awareness on the nutritive value and health benefits of millets.

FUTURE STRATEGY

1. **Strengthening Breeding Programmes:** Added research efforts are required in collection of traditional cultivars and their breeding to provide improved seeds with high yield potential and other desirable traits like drought tolerance. Development of varieties/ hybrids should better be taken up with active participation of farmers (participatory millet breeding) to take full advantage of local resources and indigenous knowledge. Conventional breeding as well as marker-assisted breeding for bio fortification and for incorporating other traits such as better root architecture.
2. **Seed Production:** Efficient seed production measures with public, private, NGO partnership and establishment of seed villages to make quality seeds available in sufficient quantity.
3. **Improved Agro Techniques:** Concurrent work is required to develop specific management practices to realize full potential of the newly evolved varieties. Strategies for zero tillage under rice fallows are required. Validation and refinement of indigenous technology under various farming situations will be rewarding.
4. **Processing Facilities:** Development of small scale processing units for dehusking and powdering of small millets coupled with proper packaging facilities.
5. **Value Addition:** Processing technologies to prepare ready-to-use or ready-to-cook products and also secondary as well as tertiary processing to prepare ready-to-eat value added products.
6. **Government Support:** Support to farmers in terms of subsidy and loan for various farm operations is required, considering the poor financial position of the millet farmers. Better procurement prices and insurance coverage to mitigate hardship of millet farmers in view of the serious yield loss under climate change.

7. **Inclusion of Millets in the PDS System:** This recommendation made by M.S. Swaminanthan and accepted by the Government of India has to be properly implemented.
8. **Post-Harvest Technology:** Research for better post-harvest management, especially for enhancing the shelf life of millets and prevention of wastage.
9. **Validation of Health Benefits:** Consortium-mode research may be pursued for validating the advantages of millets as health and functional foods.
10. **Marketing:** Markets and entrepreneurship development through modern and innovative approaches coupled with storage and marketing facilities at village level.
11. **Public Awareness:** Proper advertisement strategies are necessary to increase awareness on the nutritional advantages and health benefits of millets.

CONCLUSION

In the face of increasing population and stagnant wheat and rice production, millets can be a promising alternative in solving the problem of food insecurity and malnutrition, because of their sustainability in adverse agro-climatic conditions. These crops have substantive potential in broadening the genetic diversity of the food basket and ensuring improved food and nutrition security. Through millet consumption, we will be encouraging farmers in dry land areas to grow crops suited for these regions. This is a step towards introducing diversity in our diets, by using the local biodiversity.

These facts call for added attention to promote their cultivation and consumption. Enhancement of millet cultivation gives an interesting opportunity to bridge the yield gap in food production. According to one estimate, "increasing yields to 50% of the potential yield in all low-performing areas could increase annual production, which is enough to meet the basic caloric requirements of 850 million people". While annual yield increase (as a percentage of current yield) in staples like rice and wheat are below 1%, directing greater research attention to nutritious cereals like millets would be a strategic choice, because it would be more viable and would offer greater benefits in terms of lower water requirement and adaptation to climate change. This creates social impact in terms of greater self-reliance of local population as well as more resilience to food systems. There is further opportunity to provide better adapted and higher yielding materials both for grain and forage, but these will require added research efforts, development of niche markets and improvement in management techniques.

Millets are drought, temperature and pest tolerant and hence are grains for the future in an environment of climate change and global warming. Despite these attributes, these cops are loosing their pride of place both in terms of production and consumption, for a variety of reasons, including unfavourable policy initiatives. Though they have not enjoyed technological breakthroughs like the green revolution for rice and wheat, their productivity has increased. Confined to poor lands, productivity is affected resulting in a wide gap between potential productivity and productivity in farmers' fields. Scientific, technological and behavioural engineering involving convergence of efforts of agricultural scientists, food technologists, home scientists, policy makers, and media is needed to revitalise millets. Nutritional as well as health benefits and consumer demand for health foods provide opportunities in processing, development of suitable technology for newer products and process mechanization. This change in technology and consumer food preference would help in increasing the area under millets, maintaining ecological balance, ensuring food security, preventing malnutrition and increasing the scope for utilization of millet grains on an industrial scale.

REFERENCES

Amadou, , Gounga, & Le. (2013). Millets: Nutritional composition, some health benefits and processing – A Review.Emir. *Journal of Food & Agriculture*, *25*(7), 501–508. doi:10.9755/ejfa.v25i7.12045

Antony, U., Sripriya, G., & Chandra, T. S. (1996). Effect of fermentation on the primary nutrients in finger millet (*Eleusine coracana*). *Journal of Agricultural and Food Chemistry*, *44*(9), 2616–2618. doi:10.1021/jf950787q

Bagdia, A. B. G., Schmidtb, J., Szatmária, M., Schoenlechnerb, R., Berghoferb, E., & Tömösközia, S. (2011). Protein Characterization and Nutrient Composition of Hungarian Proso Millet Varieties and the Effect of Decortication. *Acta Alimentaria*, *40*(1), 128–141. doi:10.1556/AAlim.40.2011.1.15

Bala Ravi, S., Swain, S., Sengotuvel, D., & Parida, N. R. (2010). *Promoting nutritious millets for enhancing income and improved nutrition (p- 37). A case study from Tamil Nadu and Orissa*. Chennai, India: Minor Millets in South Asia.Published by Bioversity International, Rome, Italy and MSSRF.

Balakrishnan, R., Alagukannan, G., Kumar, N. A., Nambi, V. A., Balakrishnan, V., Balasubramanian, K., & Girigan, G. et al. (2002). *Rural and Tribal Women in Agrobiodiversity Conservation; An Indian Case Study, RAP Publication 2002/08*. Chennai, India: MS Swaminathan Research Foundation.

Bravo, L. (1998). Polyphenols: Chemistry, dietary sources, metabolism and nutritional significance. *Nutrition Reviews*, *56*(11), 317–333. doi:10.1111/j.1753-4887.1998.tb01670.x PMID:9838798

Brush, S. B. (Ed.). (2000). Genes in the Field: On-Farm Conservation of Crop Diversity. RC/IPGRI/Lewis Publishers.

Chandrasekara, A., & Shahidi, F. (2010). Content of insoluble bound phenolics in millets and their contribution to antioxidant capacity. *Journal of Agricultural and Food Chemistry*, *58*(11), 6706–6714. doi:10.1021/jf100868b PMID:20465288

Chandrasekara, A., & Shahidi, F. (2011). Determination of antioxidant activity in free and hydrolyzed fractions of millet grains and characterization of their phenolic profiles by HPLC-DAD-ESI-MSn. *Journal of Functional Foods*, *3*(3), 144–158. doi:10.1016/j.jff.2011.03.007

Chandrasekara, A., & Shahidi, F. (2012). Bioaccessibility and antioxidant potential of millet grain phenolics as affected by simulated in vitro digestion and microbial fermentation. *J Funct Foods*, *4*(1), 226–237. doi:10.1016/j.jff.2011.11.001

Coulibaly, A., Kouakou, B., & Chen, J. (2011). Phytic acid in cereal grains: Structure, healthy or harmful ways to reduce phytic acid in cereal grains and their effects on nutritional quality. *Am. J. Plant Nutr. Fert. Technol*, *1*(1), 1–22. doi:10.3923/ajpnft.2011.1.22

De Wet, J. M. J., Prasada Rao, K. E., Brink, D. E., & Mengesha, M. H. (1984). Systematic and Evolution of *Eleusine coracana*. *American Journal of Botany*, *71*(4), 550. doi:10.2307/2443330

Devi, P. B., Vijayabharathi, R., Sathyabama, S., Malleshi, N. G., & Priyadarisini, V. B. (2011). Health benefits of finger millet (*Eleusine coracana* L.) polyphenols and dietary fiber: A review. *J. Food Science and Technology (Campinas.)*. doi:10.1007/s13197-011-0584-9

Dutta, M., Phogat, B. S., & Dhillon, B. S. (2007). Genetic improvement and utilization of major underutilized crops in India. In Breeding of Neglected and nderutilized Crops, Spices and Herbs (pp. 251-298). Science Publishers.

Dykes, L., & Rooney, L. W. (2006). Sorghum and millet phenols and antioxidants. *Journal of Cereal Science*, *44*(3), 236–251. doi:10.1016/j.jcs.2006.06.007

FAO. (1991). Food and Agriculture Organization.Amino Acid Scoring Pattern. In: Protein quality evaluation. FAO/WHO Food and Nutrition Paper, Italy.

FAO. (2001). *Post harvest operations*. Millet: Kajuna.

FAO. (2009). *FAOSTAT. Food and Agriculture Organisation of the United Nations*. Retrieved from http://faostat.fao.org/site/339/default.aspx

Fardet, A., Rock, E., & Remesy, C. (2008). Is the in vitro antioxidant potential of whole-grain cereals and cereal products well reflected in vivo? *International Journal of Food Science & Technology*, *43*(7), 1245–1252.

Geerwani, P., & Eggum, B. O. (1989). Nutrient composition and protein quality of minor millets. *Plant Foods for Human Nutrition (Dordrecht, Netherlands)*, *39*(2), 201–208. doi:10.1007/BF01091900 PMID:2548175

Gélinas, P., McKinnon, C. M., Mena, M. C. & Méndez, E. (2008). *Gluten contamination of cereal*. Academic Press.

Hadimani, N. A., & Malleshi, N. G. (1993). Studies on milling, physico-chemical properties, nutrient composition and dietary fiber content of millets. *Journal of Food Science and Technology*, *30*, 17–20.

Hegde, P. S., & Chandra, T. S. (2005). ESR spectroscopic study reveals higher free radical quenching potential in kodo millet (*Paspalum scrobiculatum*) compared to other millets. *Food Chemistry*, *92*, 177–182. doi:10.1016/j.foodchem.2004.08.002

Hegde, P. S., Chandrakasan, G., & Chandraa, T. S. (2002). Inhibition of collagen glycation and crosslinking in vitro by methanolic extracts of Finger millet (*Eleusine coracana)* and Kodo millet (*Paspalum scrobiculatum*). *The Journal of Nutritional Biochemistry*, *13*(9), 517–521. doi:10.1016/S0955-2863(02)00171-7 PMID:12231421

Hulse, J. H., Liang, E. M., & Pearson, O. E. (1980in press). *Sorghum and the millets: Their composition and nutritive value*. London: Academic Press.

ICAR. (2013). *Handbook of Agriculture*. New Delhi: Indian Council of Agricultural Research.

ICRISAT & FAO. (1996). *The world sorghum and millets economies: Facts, trends and outlook, joint study report by ICRISAT and FAO*. ICRISAT.

Izadi, Z., Nasirpour, A., Izadi, M., & Izadi, T. (2012). Reducing blood cholesterol by a healthy diet. *Int. Food Res. J*, *19*(1), 29–37.

Jarvis, D. I., Padoch, C., & Cooper, H. D. (Eds.). (2007). *Managing Biodiversity in Agricultural ecosystems*. Bioversity International, Rome, Italy.

Jingju, N. L. Z. C., Huiyuan, Y., & Ying, X. (2007). "Optimization of stress medium enhance hydroxyl radical inhibition by water-soluble protein from germinated millet." LWT – *Fd Sci. Technol*, *40*, 1630–1636.

Krishnan, R., Dharmaraj, U., & Malleshi, N. G. (2011). Quality characteristics of biscuits prepared from finger millet seed coat based composite flour. *Food Chemistry*, *129*(2), 499–506. doi:10.1016/j.foodchem.2011.04.107

Kumar, K. K., & Parmeswaran, K. P. (1999). Characterization of storage protein from selected varieties of foxtail millet (*Setaria italica* L. Beauv). *Journal of the Science of Food and Agriculture*, *77*(4), 535–542. doi:10.1002/(SICI)1097-0010(199808)77:4<535::AID-JSFA77>3.0.CO;2-G

Mal, B. (2007). Neglected and underutilized crop genetic resources for sustainable agriculture. *J. Plant Genet. Resour*, *20*(1), 1–14.

Mal, B., & Padulosi, S. (2013). Best Practices, Methods and Tools in Minor Millets Value Chains and Uptaking Processes. Bioversity International.

Mal, B., Padulosi, S., & Ravi, S. B. (2010). Minor millets in South Asia: learnings from IFAD-NUS Project in India and Nepal. *Swaminathan Research Foundation*, *32*(2), 1–185.

Malleshi, N. G. (2014). *Post-harvest processing of millets for value addition*. Retrieved from http://isites.harvard.edu /fs/docs/icb.topic868074

Malleshi, N. G., & Hadimani, N. A. (1993). Nutritional and technological characteristics of small millets and preparation of value added products from them. In Advances in Small Millets (pp. 271-287). Oxford IBH Publishing Co. Pvt. Ltd.

Manach, C., Mazur, A., & Scalbert, A. (2005). Polyphenols and prevention of cardiovascular diseases. *Current Opinion in Lipidology*, *16*(1), 77–84. doi:10.1097/00041433-200502000-00013 PMID:15650567

Mathanghi, S.K. & Sudha, K. (2012). Functional and phytochemical properties of Finger Millet _*Eleusine coracana* L.) for health. *International Journal of Pharmaceutical, Chemical and Biological Sciences,* 2(4), 431-438.

Mbithi-Mwikya, S., Ooghe, W., Van Cam, J., Nagundi, D., & Huyghebaert, A. (2000). Amino acid profile after sprouting, autoclaving and lactic acid fermentation of finger millet (*Elusine coracana*) and kidney beans (*Phaseolus vulgaris* L.). *Journal of Agricultural and Food Chemistry*, *48*(8), 3081–3085. doi:10.1021/jf0002140 PMID:10956072

McDonough, C. M., Rooney, L. W., & Serna-Saldivar, S. O. (2000). The Millets. In Handbook of Cereal Science and Technology (2nd ed.; pp. 177–210). CRC Press.

Monnier, V. M. (1990). Nonenzymatic glycosylation, the Maillard reaction and the aging process. *Journal of Gerontology, 45*(4), 105–111. doi:10.1093/geronj/45.4.B105 PMID:2195101

Monteiro, P. V., Sudharshana, L., & Ramchandra, G. (1987). Japanese barnyard millet (*Echinochloa frumentacea*): Protein content, quality and SDSPAGE of protein fractions. *Journal of the Science of Food and Agriculture, 43*(1), 17–25. doi:10.1002/jsfa.2740430104

NABARD. (2007). *Millets in your meals (ppt – 21)*. NABARD.

Nehir, E. I. S., & Simsek, S. (2012). Food technological applications for optimal nutrition: An Overview of opportunities for the Food Industry. *Comprehensive Reviews in Food Science and Food Safety, 11*(1), 1–11. doi:10.1111/j.1541-4337.2011.00167.x

Obilana, A. B., & Manyasa, E. (2002). Millets. In P. S. Belton & J. R. N. Taylor (Eds.), Pseudo cereals and less common cereals: Grain properties and utilization potential (pp. 177–217). Springer-Verlag.

Padulosi, S., Mal, B., King, O., & Gotor, E. (2015). Minor Millets as a Central Element for Sustainably Enhanced Incomes, Empowerment, and Nutrition in Rural India. *Sustainability, 7*(7), 8904–8933. doi:10.3390/su7078904

Palanisamy Bruntha Devi, R. V., Sathyabama, Malleshi, & Priyadarisini. (2011). Health benefits of finger millet (*Eleusine coracana* L.) polyphenols and dietary fiber: a review. *J Food Sci Technol.*

Parameswaran, K., & Sadasivam, S. (1994). Changes in the carbohydrates and nitrogenous components during germination of proso millet (*Panicum miliaceum*). *Plant Foods for Human Nutrition (Dordrecht, Netherlands), 45*(2), 97–102. doi:10.1007/BF01088466 PMID:8153070

Prabhakaran, T. R., Das, Balaravi, & King. (2012). *Assessing farmers willingness to participate in the on-farm conservation of minor millet using direct compensation payment*. Working Paper 73/2012.

Ragaee, S., Abdel-Aal, E. M., & Noaman, M. (2006). Antioxidant activity and nutrient composition of selected cereals for food use. *Food Chemistry, 98*(1), 32–38. doi:10.1016/j.foodchem.2005.04.039

Saleh, A. S. M., Zhang, Q., Chen, J., & Shen, Q. (2013). Millet Grains: Nutritional Quality, Processing, and Potential Health Benefits. *Comprehensive Reviews in Food Science and Food Safety, 12*(3), 281–295. doi:10.1111/1541-4337.12012

Scalbert, A., Manach, C., Morand, C., Remesy, C., & Jimenez, L. (2005). Dietary polyphenols and the prevention of diseases. *Critical Reviews in Food Science and Nutrition, 45*(4), 287–306. doi:10.1080/1040869059096 PMID:16047496

Sehgal, A., & Kwatra, A. (2003). Processing and utilization of pearl millet for Nutrition Security. In *Proceeding of national seminar on Recent Trend in Millet Processing and Utilization.*

Shobana, S., & Malleshi, N. G. (2007). Preparation and functional properties of decorticated finger millet (*Eleusine coracana*). *Journal of Food Engineering, 79*(2), 529–538. doi:10.1016/j.jfoodeng.2006.01.076

Singh, K. P., Mishram, H. N., & Saham, S. (2012). Changes during accelerated storage in millet–wheat composite flours for bread. *Food and Bioprocess Technology Journal, 5*(5), 2003–2011. doi:10.1007/s11947-011-0769-2

Singh, P., & Raghuvanshi, R. S. (2012). Finger millet for food and nutritional security. *African Journal of Food Science, 6*(4), 77–84.

Stanly, Raj, & Shanmugam. (2013). A study on millets based cultivation and consumption in India. *International Journal of Marketing, Financial Services & Management Research, 2*(4), 49-58.

Subramanian, S., & Viswanathan, R. (2003). Thermal properties of minor millet grains and flours. *Biosystems Engineering, 84*(3), 289–296. doi:10.1016/S1537-5110(02)00222-2

Sudharshana, L., Monteiro, P. V., & Ramchandra, G. (1987). Studies on proteins of kodo millet (*Paspalum scroculatum*). *Journal of the Science of Food and Agriculture, 42*(4), 315–323. doi:10.1002/jsfa.2740420405

Veena, B. (2003). *Nutritional, functional and utilization studies on barnyard millet.* (M. Sc. Thesis). University of Agricultural Sciences Dharwad, Karnataka, India.

Viswanath, V., Urooj, A., & Malleshi, N. G. (2009). Evaluation of antioxidant and antimicrobial properties of finger millet polyphenols (*Eleusine coracana*). *Food Chemistry, 114*(1), 340–346. doi:10.1016/j.foodchem.2008.09.053

Yenagi, N. B., Naik, & Josna. (2011). Knowledge, Attitude and Practice of Farm Women of Millet Growing Areas Towards Millet Consumption. *National symposium on recapturing of nutritious millets for Health and Management of diseases.* NAIP Project.

Chapter 5
Bioactive Compound Analysis of *Coriandrum Sativum* L against Microbial Keratitis

V. Nithya
Alagappa University, India

ABSTRACT

In recent years, multiple drug resistance has been developed due to indiscriminate use of existing drugs in the treatment of infectious diseases. One such herbal drug is Coriandrum Sativum L that possesses potential pharmaceutical activities and used in several ayurvedic formulations. Keratitis caused by bacteria, viruses, fungi and parasites. The main goal of this study is to evaluate the antibacterial, antifungal activity, anti-oxidant activity and anti-inflammatory activity of Coriandrum Sativum L leaves and seeds using various organic solvent of plant extract against keratitis disease. The present study carried out the effect on various organic solvents extract of leaves and seeds of Corindrum sativum not only on the bacterial and fungal populations isolated from the conjunctivitis infected eyes but also to screen the phytochemical, anti-inflammatory and in vitro antioxidant potential of the leaf and seed extracts.

DOI: 10.4018/978-1-5225-0607-2.ch005

INTRODUCTION

Microbial keratitis is a major cause of monocular blindness in developing countries. Corneal scarring listed second only to cataracts as an important cause of blindness and visual impairment in many developing countries in Asia, Africa and the Middle East. India too suffers a major setback in public health due to blindness caused by microbial keratitis (Alexandrakis, Alfonso, & Miller, 2000). Corneal lesions were found to be responsible for 9% of all blindness in India in a recent national survey. The factors that can predispose to infectious keratitis include age, occupation, environmental factors, trauma into the eye, foreign bodies, extended wear of conventional contact lenses (Alfonso, Mandelbaum, Fox, et al., 1986). chronic ocular surface disease, prior ocular surgery, diabetes mellitus, leprosy, rheumatoid arthritis, use of topical corticosteroids. Rapid initiation of treatment is required to halt the progression of disease so that the extent of corneal scarring can be limited and thereby loss of vision (Ahmadi & McKenna 2003; Baker, Smith, & Cowan, 2003).

The antibiotics and steroid-based eye drops for the management of ophthalmic disorder has been found clinically unsafe in recent times and a current demand is to investigate alternative drug. A serious adverse drug reactions (ADRs) occurring due to use of herbal drugs is very rare event. A common argument that favours the use of herbal medicines is that they have a longstanding history of traditional use. Even after being used from ancient times, plant-derived medicines can result in some adverse reaction so needs have been raised for safety evaluation. Microorganisms develop resistance to present day antibiotics that has created immense clinical problem in the treatment of infectious diseases. However, today it is necessary to provide scientific proof as to whether or not it is justified to use a plant or its active principles. It is still a problem to use these medicinal plants for ophthalmic problems.

Coriandrum is the dried fruit of the tall perennial herbaceous plant, *Coriandrum Sativum*, and belonging to the family Apiaceae. This herb is cultivated commercially in Europa, Asia and Africa. The leaves are lanceolate, green or dark green, glabrous on both surfaces with acuminate apex. The fruit are, ovoid. The Coriandrum seeds have a warm, slightly pungent and highly aromatic flavour. Therefore, it is used as a spice in meat products such as Bologna and Frankfurter. Coriandrum oil is used in food, perfumery, and liquor in pharmaceutical industries as a flavour and a carminative. In medicine, it is used as a powerful aromatic, antiseptic, stimulant, carminative, stomachic, expectorant, anti-spasmodic and diuretic. In some parts of the world, especially the Near East and Saudi Arabia, Coriandrum is used mostly in the preparation of "Gahwa" a strong Coriandrum coffee concoction.

The World Health Organization (WHO) noted that the majority of the world's population depends on traditional medicine for primary healthcare. Medicinal and aromatic plants are widely used as medicine and constitute a major source of natural organic compounds. Some medicinal plants have been used for a wide variety of purposes such as food preservation, pharmaceutical, alternative medicine, and natural therapies for many thousands of years (Chopra, Nayar, & Chopra,1965). It is generally considered that compounds produced naturally, rather than synthetically, will be biodegraded more easily and therefore be more environmentally acceptable.

In the present study, the *Coriandrum Sativum* L was extracted by using various solvents of increasing polarity like petroleum ether, benzene, ethyl acetate, acetone, methanol and water. These extracts were characterized to demonstrate photochemical screening of secondary metabolites, antimicrobial property against microbes causing eye infections such as bacteria and fungi. The active antioxidants property and scavenging free radical activity was evaluated using FRAP assay. The anti-inflammatory activity of plant extracts using UV-VIS.

BACKGROUND

Plants have a vast potential for their use as curative medicine. In India, medicinal plants are widely used by all sections of people both directly as folk medicines in different indigenous systems of medicine like Siddha, Ayurveda and Unani and indirectly in the pharmaceutical preparations. India has about 4.5 million plant species and among them, several thousands have been claimed to possess medicinal properties against human diseases (Nadakarni, 1973). Although traditional medicinal healers have used medicinal plants for treatment of ailments for hundreds of years, there has always been a lingering question in scientific circles about their therapeutic efficacy. As a consequence, the pharmacological activity of many medicinal plants has been studied, even though the vast majority of medicinal plants remain to be studied for their phytochemical components and pharmacological effects (Tripathi, 1994).

C. sativum extract protects liver from oxidative stress induced by carbon-tetrachloride (CCl4) and thus helps in evaluation of traditional claim on this plant. Pretreatment of rats with different doses of plant extract (100 and 200 mg/kg) significantly lowered serum glutamate oxaloacetate transaminase (SGOT), serum glutamate pyruvate transaminase (SGPT), and TBARS levels against CCl4 treated rats. Hepatic enzymes like superoxide dismutase (SOD), catalase (CAT), and glutathione peroxidase (GPx) were significantly increased by treatment with plant extract, against CCl4 treated rats. Oral administration of the leaf extract at a dose of 200 mg/kg significantly reduced the toxic effects of CCl4. The activity of leaf extract at this dose was comparable to the standard drug, silymarin (Ohkawa, Ohishi, & Yagi,1979).

Coriandrum essential oil is obtained by steam distillation of the dried fully ripe fruits (seeds). Based on the results of a 28-day oral gavage study in rats, a no-observed effect level (NOEL) for Coriandrum oil is approximately 160 mg/kg/day. In a developmental toxicity study, the maternal no-observed adverse effect level (NOAEL) of Coriandrum oil was 250 mg/kg/day and the developmental NOAEL was 500 mg/kg/day. Coriandrum oil is not clastogenic, but results of mutagenicity studies for the spice and some extracts are mixed. The major component of the essential oil, linalool, is non-mutagenic. Coriandrum oil has broad-spectrum, antimicrobial activity. Coriandrum oil is irritating to rabbits, but not to humans; it is not a sensitizer, although, the whole spice may be. Based on the history of consumption of Coriandrum oil without reported adverse effects, lack of its toxicity in limited studies and lack of toxicity of its major constituent, linalool, the use of Coriandrum oil as an added food ingredient is considered safe at present levels of use. The median lethal dose (LD50) of C. sativum essential oil was determined as 2.257 ml/kg. C. sativum as an oilseed crop grown in Italy was investigated regarding anti-nutritive compounds such as glucosinolates, sinapine, inositol phosphates, and condensed tannins, which can adversely affect the nutritional value of residues from the oilseed processing. All these compounds were found in C. sativum fruits in different amounts.

MAIN FOCUS OF THE CHAPTER

Preparation of *Coriandrum Sativum* L Extract of Leaves and Seeds

The *Coriandrum Sativum* L leaves and seeds will be collected and identified. The leaves were shade dried at room temperature and powdered the dried leaves and seeds. 500gm of *Coriandrum Sativum* L. leaves and seeds powder was taken in a beaker. Extracts will be prepared in the series of 500ml of different solvents based on increasing polarity (Ethyl acetate, Acetone, Methanol, and Water) using Soxhlet extraction method.

Macroscopic and Microscopic Studies

Macroscopic studies were carried out by simple determination, technique like the shape, size, colour, odour, margin and apex. The stem and leaf specimens were fixed in FAA and microtome slides were prepared and stained. Photomicrographs of with different magnifications were taken with microscopic unit.

Determination of Physicochemical Parameters

Total ash value, water and acid, soluble and insoluble ash value, and moisture content will be determined as per Indian pharmacopoeia.

Preliminary Phytochemical Analysis

The preliminary phytochemical analysis of the various organic solvent extract will be carried out using standard methods. The presence and absence of the secondary phytoconstituents such as alkaloids, steroid and /or triterpenoids and their glycosides, tannins, flavonoids and their glycosides, carbohydrates and cardiac glycosides using different phytochemical tests will be noted.

Sample Collection

All patients were examined under a slit-lamp biomicroscope by an ophthalmologist. Corneal scrapings were collected after instillation of 4% lignocaine without preservative under aseptic conditions from each ulcer by an ophthalmologist using a sterile Bard Parker blade. Scrapings were directly inoculated onto the surface of solid media such as sheep blood agar, chocolate agar and Sabouraud Dextrose Agar (SDA) in a row of C- shaped streaks and also deep inoculation in the liquid media such as Brain Heart Infusion (BHI) broth without gentamicin sulphate and thioglycollate medium.

Isolation of Bacteria from Sample

As per the standard protocol, microbial cultures were considered positive only if growth of the same organism was demonstrated on 2 or more solid media or there was confluent growth at the site of inoculation on 1 solid medium and which was subsequently sub-cultured and Gram stained for identification.

Identification of Bacteria

Both morphological and biochemical test for microorganism identifications were carried out. The biochemical tests were performed in order to identify the unknown bacteria. Some of the tests provided immediate results while others had to be incubated for a period of time.

Isolation of Fungi from Sample

Fungi were identified by their colony characteristics on PDA by their microscopic appearance in Lactophenol cotton blue. Fungal cultures from cases with smears negative for fungi were discarded as possible contaminants, although Chin et al., pointed out that negative smears and cultures do not necessarily rule out fungal infection Garg, Gopinathan, Choudhary, & Rao, 2000).

Determination of Antibacterial and Antifungal Activity of Plant Leaves and Seed Extract Using Agar Well Diffusion Method

Antibacterial activities of all the solvent extracts of plant leaves and seed will be determined by agar well diffusion method (Alastruey-Izquierdo et al.,2008). The extracts were dissolved in DMSO (dimethylsulphoxide). The microbial cultures were revived at 37°C for 18h in a broth medium. The 20µl of the culture was spread on Muller Hinton agar plates and wells of 9mm diameter were punched into the agar plates. 100µl of the solvent-free extracts of concentration 0.5mg/100µl and 1mg/100µl were used for determination of ZOI (Zone of Inhibition). After holding the plates at room temperature for 2 hours to allow diffusion of the extract into the media, the plates were incubated at 37ºC for 24h. DMSO and Gentamicin was used as a negative control and as reference antibiotic (positive control) respectively. The test was performed in triplicates and the final results were presented as the mean zone of inhibition (Barik, Yegneswaran, Tayung, & Sahu, 2011).

Determination of Ferric Reducing Antioxidant Potential (FRAP)

The ferric reducing power of the plant extracts was determined by using potassium ferricyanide-ferric chloride method (Oyaizu, 1986). Different dilutions of extracts amounting to 1 ml were added to 2.5ml 0.2M phosphate buffer (pH6.6) and 2.5ml potassium ferriocyanide (1%). The mixtures were incubated at 500C for 20 minutes, after which 2.5ml trichloroacetic acid (10%) was added. 2.5 ml of the mixture was taken and mixed with 2.5ml water and 0.5ml 1% FeCl3. The absorbance at 700 nm was measured after allowing the solution to stand for 30 minutes. A graph of absorbance vs. plant extract concentration was plotted to observe the reducing power.

Antioxidant Activity of Fruit Juices by DPPH Free Radical Scavenging Assay

The scavenging activity of the extract was determined based on 2,2-diphenyl-1-picryl hydrazyl free radical (DPPH) scavenging assay described by Lai et al. (2001). The pepper extract (200 µl) was mixed with 800 µl of 100mM TrisHCl buffer, pH 7.4. The mixture was then added to 1.0ml of 500 µM DPPH (previously prepared in methanol). This was made up to the DPPH final concentration of 250 µM. The control was performed by mixing 200 µl of methanol with 1.0 ml DPPH. The mixture was then shaken vigorously and left to stand for 20 min at room temperature in a dark room. The absorbance was read using a UV-vis spectrophotometer at 517 nm with methanol as the blank. Triplicate measurements were carried out and their activity was calculated based on the percentage of scavenged DPPH.

Anti-Inflammatory Activity of Plant Extract Using UV-VIS Effect on Protein Denaturation

Protein denaturation was performed as described with slight modifications (Park, 2006). Test solution consisting of 1ml of different concentrations of Herbal Preparation (HP-4) ranging from 100-500 µg/ml or standard acetylsalicylic acid 100 and 200 µg/ml was mixed with 1ml of egg albumin solution (1mM) and incubated at 27 ±1°C for 15 minutes. Denaturation was induced by keeping the reaction mixture at 70°C in a water bath for 10 minutes. After cooling the turbidity was measured spectrophotometrically at 660 nm. Percentage inhibition of denaturation was calculated from control where no drug was added. Each experiment was done in triplicate and the average was taken.

SOLUTIONS AND RECOMMENDATIONS

Anatomical Studies

Fresh Coriandrum leaf, stem, and root were collected and used to take hand section to study the internal features. The materials were trimmed and placed in thermocol and hand section were taken with safety blade. The thin section were selected, stained with Toluidine blue, observed and the microscope, the photographs were taken, with help of Olympus microscope. The images were saved and printed shown in Figures 1, 2, and 3. The photographs were taken in 10x and 45x magnification.

Figure 1.

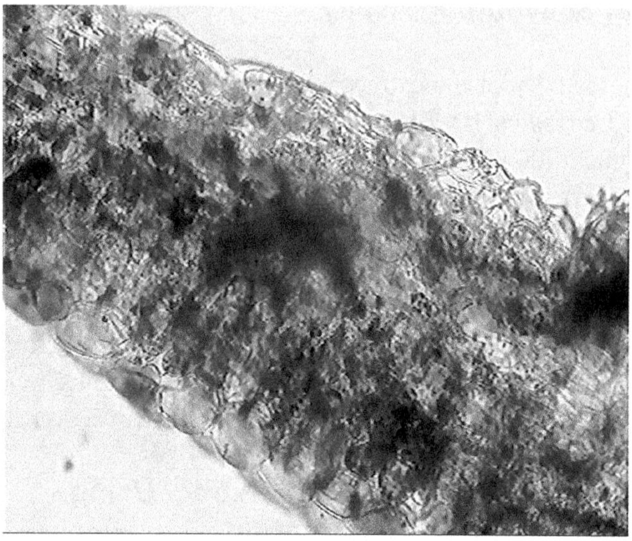

Figure 2. Cross section of Coriandrum stem

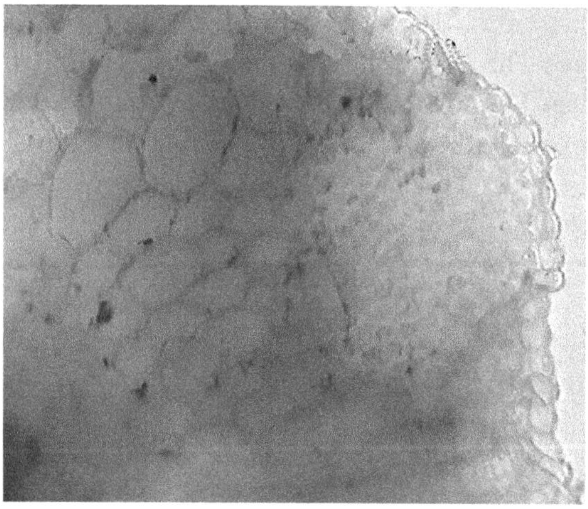

The leaf has upper and lower epidermis. The epidermis is single layered with barrel shaped cells. The radial cells of thick in between the dermises. Meshophile tissue is present palisade parenchyma and sponge parenchyma. The cells of the palisade parenchyma is having chloroplast. The median central vein has both xylem and phloem as the connecting tissue. The stem is more are less circulating outline having single layered epidermis without any intracellular spaces, it is followed by

Figure 3. Cross section of Coriandrum root

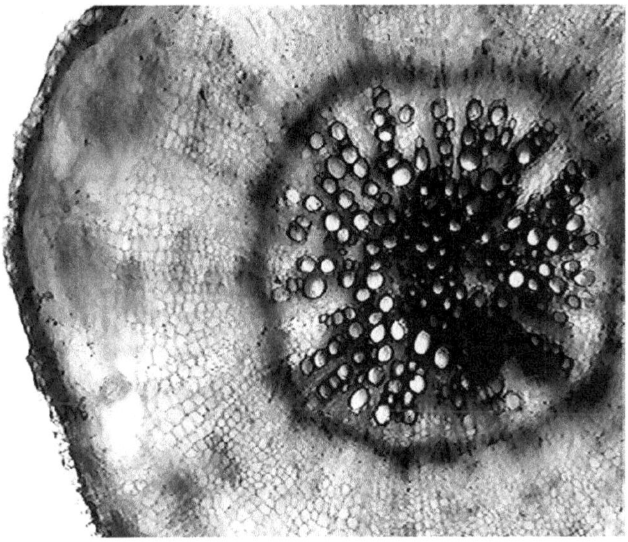

hypodermis having small is isodiametric cell it is four to five layer. The hypodermal layer is followed by large thin walled cortical cells having large intracellular spaces. The vascular bundle are arranged, peripherally. The vascular bundle are central arranged form of a ring plate. The root is circular outline the root epidermis layer followed by five to six hypodermis. The root cortex of made up of parenchyma, which is 20 to 25 layered. The next to root cortex, single layer endodermis is present. The central region root is having exact vascular bundle without any pitch.

Total Ash Value Content

The qualitative analysis of Coriandrum sativum L. powder of moisture content, total ash value, water soluble ash, acid soluble ash, content are shown in Table 1.

Table 1. Coriandrum sativum L. powder of moisture content, total ash value, water soluble ash, acid soluble ash, content

Ash Type and Content	Total gm per Sample
Total ash	1.7
Insoluble ash in hcl	O.23
Soluble ash in distilled water	1.2

The results of physical constance of raw material lie within the limit, which is mentioned in Table 2. This signifies that the quality and purity of raw material was good enough. It is absorbed the moisture content of the material was found to be (2.3 gm). Which signify that the drug is properly dried and stored. The total ash (1.7 gm) particularly important in the evaluation of purity of material. The water soluble ash was found to be (1.2 gm) whereas the acid insoluble ash was found to be (0.23 gm) which is within fairly wide limit. As the ash value of the plant material with in the fair limit which signify is quality, purity and give an idea about the total inorganic compounds.

In the aqueous extract, alkaloids, flavanoids, carbohydrate, tannins, saponins, terpenoids, phenolic compounds are present and quinones and anthocyanin are absent. The carbohydrate saponins, terpenoids are absent in the acetone extract of Coriandrum sativum L and other also present.

In the methanolic extract of Coriandrum sativum L. contains the phytochemical constituent are alkaloids, carbohydrate, flavanoids, tannins, saponin, terpenoids, phenol, and anthocyaanin are present except quinones. The chloroform extract having alkaloids, tannins, terpenoids, and anthocyanin are present (Table 3) from the result the aqueous and methanolic plant extract showed. More phytochemical constuients when compare with other extract.

The results of quantitative estimation of protein, phenol, and flavanoids are tabulated in Tables 3 and 4. The total phenol content was significantly high in aque-

Table 2. Phytochemical studies on Coriandrum sativum L. with various extract

PhytochemicalConstituents	Phytochemical Test	Aqueous	Acetone	Methanol	Chloroform
Alkaloids Test	Wagners	+	+	+	+
Carbohydrate Test	Molischs Test	+	_	+	_
Carbohydrate Test	Fehlings Test	+	_	+	_
NaOH Test	Flavonoids	+	_	+	_
Ferric Chloride Test	Tannins	+	+	+	+
Foam Test	Saponins	+	_	+	_
Quinones Test	Quinones	_	+	_	_
Libermann-Burchard Test	Terpenoids	+	-	+	+
Libermann-Burchard Test	Sterols	+	+	_	_
Libermann-Test	Phenols	+	+	+	_
Naoh Test	Anthocyanin	+	+	+	+

+ Present; - Absent

Table 3. Total phenolic content

Plant Constituents	Aqueous Extract	Methanol Extract
phenols	1.24mg	1.1g

Table 4. Total flavonoid content

Plant Constituents	Aqueous Extract	Methanol Extract
Flavonoides	0.92mg	0.88g

ous extract Coriandrum sativum L.When compared with methanolic extract likewise the total flavanoid content was significantly high in methanolic extract Coriandrum sativum L. followed by aqueous extract.

Antibacterial Activity

The antibacterial activity of selected reference drugs against microorganisms was determined using three different concentrations. The development of drug resistance in human pathogens against commonly used antibiotics has necessitated a search for new antimicrobial substances from other sources including plants and microbes. The results on antimicrobial screening of the crude extracts of the *Coriandrum Sativum* L. plants are shown in Table 5. The antibacterial activity of the crude extract of plant extracts resulted in clear inhibition zones of at least 10mm for all the strains tested. showed high degree of antibacterial activity tested against bacterial species. Different extracts of activity against *Coriandrum Sativum L.* plants showed antibacterial

Table 5. The antibacterial activity of Coriandrum Sativum L

Microorganisms	Zone of Inhibition (mm)			
	Antibiotic Disc	AQE	ME	AE
E. coli	Amp -	22	24	15
Shigella. flexneri	Str 7	15	14	12
Salmonella	Str 5	12	22	17
Vibrio	Str 8	20	22	17
Pseudomonas aeroginosa	Amp -	12	18	16
Proteus	Pen -	15	20	11
Streptococcus pyogens	Pen -	7	16	12
Staphylococcus	Amp -	12	15	13
Klebsiella	Pen -	19	25	20
Bacillus	Amp-	10	16	15

Amp=Ampicillin, Str=Streptomycin, Pen=Penicillin, - =No zone, Aqe=Water Extract, Me=Methonal Extract, Ae =Acetone Extract.

activity against *Proteus* and *Bacillus,salmonella,shigella flexneri, pseudomonas, E.coli, streptocoocus pyogens,staphylococcus aureus,klebsiella,vibrio,*. reported that *Coriandrum Sativum L.* contains large amount of phytoconstitutents and the antibacterial activity may be indicating the presence of some secondary metabolites.

Antifungal Activity

Antifungal activity of the methanol, acetone and aqueous extracts of *Coriandrum sativum L.* were determined against *Candida albicans andAspergillus* were shown in Table 6. Maximum inhibition zones of Coriandrum plant extracts against *C. albicans* were obtained in 20, 40, 60, µl concentraion respectively. It should be noted that, the Coriandrum plant extracts had antifungal activity in 20,40,60 µl concentration. It is shown that there is direct relationship between concentration and inhibition zone against standard antibiotic components of the clotrimazole and amphotericin B. The results are shown in Table 6.

Antioxidant Result

The data for the antioxidant capacity by phosphomolybedenum method and the antioxidant capacity of fraction was measured spectro photometrically through phosphomolybedenum method, which was based in the reduction of Mo (VI) to Mo (V) by the sample analytic and the supssequent formation of green phosphate Mo (V) compounds with a maximum absorbtion at 695 nm. The antioxidant capacity of the extract Coriandrum sativum L. was found to increase in methanolic extract and comparing in aqueous extract (Table 7).

REDUCING POWER ASSAY

Table 8 shows the reducing power of the Coriandrum sativum L extract by both the method. In this assay the yellow colour of the test solution changes to various shades of green and blue, depending on the reducing power of each compound.

Table 6. The antifungal activity of Coriandrum Sativum L

Microorganisms	Zone of Inhibition (mm)			
	Antibiotic Disc	AQE	ME	AE
Aspergillus	Amphotericin. B 7	10	18	14
Candida albicans	Clotrimazole10	12	16	13

Aqe=Aqueous Extract, Me=Methonal Extract=, Ae=Acetone Extract.

Table 7. Antioxidant activity of Coriandrum sativum L, leaves in methonal extract using phospho molybdate assay

Tests	Ascorbic Acid	Methanol Extract
B	0,00	0.00
S1	0.136	0.99
S2	0.137	0.162
S3	0.150	0.179
S4	0.158	0.280
S5	1.161	1.179

Table 8. Antioxidant activity of Coriandrum sativum L, leaves in aqueous extract using determination of reducing power assay

Tests	Ascorbic Acid	Aqueous Extract
B	0.00	0.00
S1	0.136	0.19
S2	0.137	0.21
S3	0.150	0.33
S 4	0.158	0.47
S 5	1.161	0.77

The presence of reducers causes the reduction of the Fe3+/ ferricyanide complex to the ferrous form. Therefore by measuring the formation of perl,s prussion blue at 700 nm, we can monitor the Fe2+ concentration. The reducing properties as generally of reductones, which have been showed to extract antioxidant action by breaking the free radical chain by donating a hydrogen atom. However as anticipated the reduction power of ascorbic acid was relatively more pronounced than that of Coriandrum sativum L. sativum L. was found to increase in methanolic extract and comparing in aqueous extract.

The major thrust is to establish alternative antimicrobial agent in order to treat microbial infections with less or no toxicity and less or negligible side effects. The herbal medicines have shown potential to overcome the limitation associated with conventional drugs. The herbal drug is *Coriandrum Sativum* L that possesses potential pharmaceutical activities and used in several ayurvedic formulations. Coriandrum is a very good disinfectant and has antimicrobial properties which protect the eyes from contagious diseases like conjunctivitis.

The electron donating ability of fruits and vegetables is a suitable parameter to establish the possession of oxidative stress quenching ability and their health studies have shown that are good sources of antioxidants. Though, high correlations have often been observed between phenolics and antioxidant capacity, our esults indicate that flavonoids which are a group in phenolic compounds had highest correlation coefficient with antioxidants capacity.

Phenolics are most abundant in plants and are very common in fruits, vegetables, seeds, stems, and flowers and in tea. In plants, accumulation of phenolics varied from one part to another part and also depended on the age and developmental stage of the concerned plant parts; hence the differences observed in phenolics content in *Coriandrum Sativum* L.leaves and rhizomes extracts. In the present study, we employed DPPH assay to determine the antioxidant potential of *Coriandrum Sativum* L. leaves. The antioxidant capability of the medicinal plants is also often measured by their reducing power.

In our present study, the antioxidant property, of 50% ethanolic extract of *Coriandrum Sativum* L. was found to be changed in SOD, CAT, and LPO levels in rat gastric mucosa. During the ulcer condition there is an increase in gastric mucosal SOD and LPO activities. This indicated that the generation of reactive oxygen species during stress might be the causative factor for the inactivation of gastric peroxidase. Moringa oleifera Lam. exerts its antioxidant defense mechanism probably by metabolising lipid peroxides and scavenging endogenous H2O2. The superoxide anion (O2 -), H2O2 and hydroxyl radical (OH-) are the major reactive oxygen species (ROS) which induce cell degeneration by increasing LPO of cell membrane lipids. The toxic end products of peroxidation induce damage of the structural and functional integrity of cell membrane, break DNA strands and denature cellular proteins. The natural cellular antioxidant enzyme includes SOD, which scavenges superoxide radicals by speeding up their dismutation, CAT, a heame enzyme which removes H2O2. Detoxification of the superoxide anion is not a terminating step in free radical scavenging, since the enzyme catalysed dismutation results in the production of H2O2 which ultimately accumulates in the mitochondria and cytosol.

Phenolic compounds are secondary metabolites in fruits and vegetables. They have been re-ported to exhibit antioxidant activity which allows them to scavenge both active oxygen species and electrophiles, to inhibit nitrosation and to chelate metal ions, to have the potential for autoxidation and the capability to modulate certain cellular enzyme activities. Flavonoids, a class of phenolic compounds has been shown to possess anti-inflammatory, antiviral, anticarcinogenic, antithrom-botic, antiallergic and hepatoprotective. Carotenes have been proved to possess antioxidant activity due to their ability to quench singlet oxygen and inhibit lipid per oxidation. Thus, diets rich in fruits and vegetables are believed to play an important role in preventing diseases but human choices of diet are driven by necessity and economy. Lack of knowledge on the importance of good diet and prevalence of poverty has influenced the composition of diets taken by Nigerians. Coupled with this, the exposure to different kinds of toxic substances such as smoke from generators, sec-ond-hand vehicles and pesticide which are capable of in-ducing oxidative stress through production of free radicals.

FUTURE RESEARCH DIRECTION

Furthermore, the molecular docking studies carry out by using in silico studies used to initiate appropriate anti microbial therapy. The present study is used to create an efficient public health programme for rapid referral and treatment of microbial keratitis in the population at risk.

Molecular Docking Process Based on *In Silico* Approach

Microbial infections are a growing problem in contemporary medicine in keratitis, yet only a few antimicrobial agents are used in clinical practice. Most drug molecules inhibit the specific activity of a specific protein by blocking its active site. Docking methods are used to predict the manner in which a ligand binds to a protein receptor. The protein structure from the causative organism that contains the bound ligands most similar to the docked ligand increases docking accuracy for all methods ("similarity selection"). Identifying the most successful protein conformer ("best selection") and similarity selection substantially reduce the difference between self-docking and average cross-docking accuracy.

CONCLUSION

The research work was carried out on the ten selected medicinalplants which shows that phytochemical constituent's i.e., terpenoids, flavonoids, alkaloids, reducing sugars and tannins are either present or absent in these plants and the results were summarized. In our studies it was investigated that alkaloids and flavonoids are present in *Coriandrum Sativum*.L and tannins, whereas reducing sugars and terpenoids were found to be absent. In previous studies it was reported that flavonoids and terpenoids were present in aqueous extract of the while alkaloids and phlobatannins were found to be absent in it. The recent research studies and previous research studies results were different so it might be due to the change in location and genetic variation due to cross pollination, so their genetic makeup were changed and that is why shows the different results.

It was observed that *Coriandrum Sativum*.Lshowed highest concentration of phytochemicals by qualitative and quantitative. So it can be used as a good source of secondary metabolites. Herbs are enormously important in both traditional and western medicine. Hence it is essential to analyze the phytochemicals present in the plant through a potential technique. Based upon the qualitative and quantitative it can be concluded that this analytical technique is a convenient method to identify the presence of numerous constituents present in the methanolic, aqeoues acetone and chloroform extract. The qualitative concentration of flavonoides and phenols in herbs have high amount of constituents.

The plant extract studied could be an answer to the people seeking for better therapeutic agents from natural sources which is believed to be more efficient with little or no side effects when compared to the commonly used synthetic chemotherapeutic agents. The present study verified the traditional use of *Coriandrum Sativum*. L plants for various human ailments especially for various infectious diseases. Thus this plant could be utilized as an alternative source of useful antimicrobial drugs. Further studies are needed to isolate, characterize and elucidate the structure of the bioactive compounds of this plant for antimicrobial drug formulation.

REFERENCES

Ahmadi, S., & McKenna, K. (2003). Keratitis-ichthyosis-deafness syndrome and carotenaemia. *Clinical and Experimental Dermatology*, *28*(4), 394–396. doi:10.1046/j.1365-2230.2003.01316.x PMID:12823302

Alastruey-Izquierdo, A., Cuenca-Estrella, M., Monzon, A., Mellado, E., & Rodriguez-Tudela, J. L. (2008). Antifungal susceptibility profile of clinical Fusarium spp. isolates identified by molecular methods. *The Journal of Antimicrobial Chemotherapy*, *61*(4), 805–809. doi:10.1093/jac/dkn022 PMID:18263569

Alexandrakis, G., Alfonso, E. C., & Miller, D. (2000). Shifting trends in bacterial keratitis in south Florida and emerging resistance to fluoroquinolones. *Ophthalmology*, *107*(8), 1497–1502. doi:10.1016/S0161-6420(00)00179-2 PMID:10919897

Alfonso, E. C., Mandelbaum, S., Fox, M. J., & Forster, R. K. (1986). Ulcerative keratitis associated with contact lens wear. *American Journal of Ophthalmology*, *101*(4), 429–433. doi:10.1016/0002-9394(86)90641-0 PMID:3963102

Baker, G. C., Smith, J. J., & Cowan, D. A. (2003). Review and re-analysis of domain specific 16s primers. *Journal of Microbiological Methods*, *55*(3), 541–555. doi:10.1016/j.mimet.2003.08.009 PMID:14607398

Barik, B. P., Yegneswaran, P. P., Tayung, K., & Sahu, H. K. (2011). Molecular Identification and in-vitro Antifungal Susceptibility of Fusarium sp. isolated from Corneal Scrape. *Journal of Life Science*, *3*(2), 127–130.

Chopra, R. N., Nayar, S. L., & Chopra, I. C. (1965). Glossary of Indian Medicinal Plants with active principles Part-I (a-k). National Institute of Science Communication.

Garg, P., Gopinathan, U., Choudhary, K., & Rao, G. N. (2000). Keratomycosis: Clinical and microbiologic experience with dematiaceous fungi. *Ophthalmology*, *107*(3), 574–580. doi:10.1016/S0161-6420(99)00079-2 PMID:10711898

Lai, L. S., Chou, S. T., & Chao, W. W. (2001). Studies on the antioxidative activities of hsian-tsao (Mesona procumbens Hemsl) leaf gum. *Journal of Agricultural and Food Chemistry*, *49*(2), 963–968. doi:10.1021/jf001146k PMID:11262057

Nadakarni, A. K. (1973). *Indian Meteria Medica*. Mumbai. *Popular Prakashan*, *1*(1), 72.

Ohkawa, H., Ohishi, N., & Yagi, K. (1979). Assay for lipid peroxidase in animal tissues by thiobarbituric acid reaction. *Analytical Biochemistry*, *95*(2), 351–358. doi:10.1016/0003-2697(79)90738-3 PMID:36810

Oyaizu, M. (1986). Studies on products of browning reactions: Antioxidative activities of products of browning reaction prepared from glucosamine. *Japanese Journal of Nutrition*, *44*(6), 307–315. doi:10.5264/eiyogakuzashi.44.307

Park, E. K., Ryu, M. H., Kim, Y. H., Lee, Y. A., Lee, S. H., Woo, D. H., & Kim, K. S. et al. (2006). Anti-inflammatory effect of an ethanolic extract from Clematis mandshurica Rupr. *Journal of Ethnopharmacology*, *108*(1), 142–147. doi:10.1016/j.jep.2006.04.025 PMID:16787723

Tripathi, K. D. (1994). Essentials of Medical Pharmacology. Jaypee Brothers Medical Publishers.

KEY TERMS AND DEFINITIONS

Antibacterial: Anything that destroys bacteria or suppresses their growth or their ability to reproduce.

Antifungal: A medication that limits or prevents the growth of yeasts and other fungal organisms.

Anti-Inflammatory: Acting to reduce certain signs of inflammation, as swelling, tenderness, fever, and pain.

Antioxidant: A substance that reduces damage due to oxygen, such as that caused by free radicals.

Free Radicals: An especially reactive atom or group of atoms that has one or more unpaired electrons.

Keratitis: An inflammation of the cornea, the transparent membrane that covers the colored part of the eye (iris) and pupil of the eye.

Phytochemicals: Chemical compounds that occur naturally in plants.

Chapter 6
Breeding for Improving Human Nutrition and Grain Quality through Biofortification of Traditional Land Races and Improved Cultivars in Rice (*Oryza sativa* L.)

P. Savitha
Tamil Nadu Agricultural University, India

R. Usha Kumari
Tamil Nadu Agricultural University, India

ABSTRACT

Rice (Oryza sativa L.) which belongs to the family poaceae, is the life and the prince among cereals as this unique grain helps to sustain two thirds of the world's population. India have traditionally been used or rice cultivation due to availability of water and conductive soil (Nadesa panic). Rice was grown in 155.30 million hectares and around 600 million tonnes of rice harvested each year globally. About 114 countries produce rice with China and India supporting 50 per cent of total production. India stands first in area under cultivation (41.85 mha) and ranks second in production, where as China ranks first in production with just half of the area. India's production is 89.13 million tonnes with a productivity of 2130 kg/ha. Among the rice producing states of India, Tamil Nadu ranks sixth in production (6.53 mil-

DOI: 10.4018/978-1-5225-0607-2.ch006

lion tonnes) and second in productivity of 3918 kg/ha with an area of 20.16 lakh ha (Season and Crop Report, 2012). Local farmers in such farming systems retain the traditional varieties based on their knowledge of the quality of the rice varieties and their adaptation to varying agro-ecological situations created by diverse seasons and land situations (Tapasi das & Ashesh Kumar Das, 2014). Among the major micronutrient deficiencies common in rice consuming countries, iron and zinc deficiencies ("hidden hunger"), affect over three billion people worldwide, mostly in developing countries (Welch & Graham, 2004).

NUTRITIONAL REQUIREMENT

Iron deficiency anemia is by far the most common micronutrient deficiency in the world affecting more than two billion people. Zinc deficiency is more extensive in developing countries where more than 60 per cent of the population is at risk. Zinc deficiency in grown up children and adolescent males causes retarded growth and dwarfism, retarded sexual development, impaired sense of taste and poor appetite and mental lethargy (Walker & Black, 2007). Coloured rice (black and red) are rich in minerals (iron and zinc) polyphenols and have antioxidant properties. Though the red of the grain colour is confined to the bran layer, a tinge of red remains even after a high degree of milling. The colour of the bran ranges from light to dark red. The zinc and iron content of red rices is 2-3 times higher than that of white rices.

Ayurveda considered red rice (rakta shali) the best among the shali varieties of rice. Red rices were highly valued as they had the power to redress the imbalance in the tridosha (the cornerstone of ayurvedic medicine is the concept of doshas. 'Laicha' rice of Chattisgarh and 'Navara' rice of Kerala are the medicinal rice varieties that had been evidently treating diseases like chronic gastritis and peptic ulcer for a long time. The 'Bhat moori' of Tamil Nadu which cures anemia and enhances blood circulation in women after child birth, contains folic acid which helps in the assimilation of dietary iron. Parmai-sal of West Bengal has special nutritive properties for strength, Kabiraj-sal of Orissa is fed to convalescing patients to quicken the recovery (Rajukkannu et al, 2009). Among the cereals, rice is a major crop of this region with considerable variability in duration, adapting to various agro-climatic and cultural situations and seasons, seed coat colour, shape, size, pigmentation of plant parts, plant height, tillering, lodging, grain, cooking quality and aroma (Latha et al, 2013). Considering that the highest antioxidant activity due to the presence of polyphenols in red rices than in white rices, red rices offer great hope for health conscious consumers.

TRADITIONAL RICE VARIETIES

Traditional landraces like Navara, Kavuni, Veeradangan and Kathanellu is highly nutritive and are rich in minerals like potassium, calcium, magnesium, micronutrients like iron and zinc. Though there is no scientific data on the medicinal properties, they are being used in ayurveda in treating diseases like arthritis, cervical spondylitis, muscle wasting, skin diseases and neurological problems (Deepa et al, 2008). Other medicinal landraces from different parts of the country which are not popularized are equally potent in the nutritive values. “Harvest Plus”, a research progarmme implemented with the International Research Institutes of the CGIAR, targets a multitude of crops that are a regular part of the staple food based diet of the poor and to breed crop varieties with rich in iron and zinc content. The main emphasis of rice varietal improvement in all countries and in international research institutions has been on increasing the production per unit area followed by imparting resistance against malnutrition and on grain quality. To take a more sophisticated and comparative approach to the understanding and management of biodiversity is underscored by the controversy that has surrounded a number of major international attempts at biodiversity preservation (Stewart Lockie & David Carpenter 2011).

BACKGROUND

The main objective of the present research work is to study the gene action of yield contributing and the nutritive characters of the traditional landraces of rice collected from Tamil Nadu and Kerala. The experimental material consists of six high yielding ruling rice varieties *viz.,* IR 72, ADT 43, ADT 45, ASD 16, TPS 4 and ADT 39, were utilized as female parent. Four nutritive and medicinal landraces in rice consumed by the people in different parts of Tamil Nadu and Kerala *viz.*, Veeradangan, Kavuni, Kathanellu and Navara were collected and used as male parents. The details of the parental genotypes are presented in Table 1.

Five generations (P_1, P_2, F_1, F_2 and F_3) in six cross combinations were raised.

MEAN PERFORMANCE OF PARENTS FOR GRAIN QUALITY AND NUTRITIONAL TRAITS

Mean performance of parents for grain quality and nutritional traits are presented in Table 2. The high hulling percentage (89.11) was exhibited by IR 72 followed by ADT 39 (89.10) and TPS 4 (86.30). However, Veeradangan registered the lowest

Table 1. Details of parents

Sl. No.	Genotype	Pedigree/Source	Duration (Days)
Female Parents			
1.	IR 72	IR 19661-9-2-3 x IR 15795-199-3-3 x IR 9129-209-2-2-2-1.	95-100
2.	ADT 39	IR 8 x IR 20	120-125
3.	ADT 45	IR 50 x ADT 37	105-115
4.	ADT 43	IR 60 x W. Ponni	110-115
5.	ASD 16	ADT 31 x CO 39	115-120
6.	TPS 4	TS 29 x ASD 16	110-115
Male Parents			
7.	Veeradangan	Orunooranvayal, Kanyakumari,Tamil Nadu	100-110
8.	Kavuni	Chettinadu,Tamil Nadu	125-135
9.	Navara	Palaghat, Kerala	90-100
10.	Kathanellu	Orunooranvayal, Kanyakumari, Tamil Nadu	105-115

hulling percentage of 78.30. ADT 43 recorded the lowest milling per centage of 64.09 whereas, IR 72 recorded the highest milling percentage of 77.83 followed by TPS 4 (76.30), ADT 39 (74.71) and Navara (73.54). Among the ten parents studied, Navara had the highest head rice recovery (68.13 per cent) and ADT 39 recorded the minimum of 51.38 with the grand mean of 58.63 per cent. The parents, Kavuni (63.15), ASD 16 (62.16), TPS 4 (61.82) and Kathanellu (61.82) recorded significantly higher head rice recovery. IR 72 showed the highest kernel length (6.82 mm) followed by ADT 45 (5.71 mm) and the lowest kernel length was noticed in TPS 4 (4.96 mm). Kathanellu recorded the maximum kernel breadth of 2.81 mm and the minimum was in IR 72 (2.01 mm). Significant kernel breadth were recorded in Veeradangan (2.63 mm), TPS 4 (2.62 mm) and Kavuni (2.41 mm). IR 72 recorded the highest kernel L/B ratio (3.39) and the lowest was noticed in Kathanellu (1.83). The parents, ADT 45 (2.76), ASD 16 (2.66) and ADT 43 (2.50) recorded significant kernel L/B ratio. Kernel length after cooking was highest in ADT 39 (8.53 mm) followed by ADT 45 (8.52 mm) and lowest in Kavuni and Kathanellu (6.20 mm). Kernel breadth after cooking was highest in Kathanellu (3.00 mm) and lowest in Kavuni (2.49 mm). Significant values were recorded in IR 72 (2.89 mm), ADT 39 (2.90 mm), Navara (2.90 mm) and Kathanellu (3.00 mm). Linear elongation ratio was highest in ADT 39 (1.64 mm) followed by ADT 45 (1.49 mm) and lowest in IR 72 (1.10 mm). Significant values were recorded by three parents *viz.,* ADT 39 (1.64 mm), ADT 45 (1.49 mm) and TPS 4 (1.52 mm). Mean performance of parents for grain quality and nutritional traits are presented in Table 2 and Figures 1 and 2.

Table 2. Mean performance of grain quality and nutritional traits in parents

Parents	HP (%)	MP (%)	HRR (%)	KL (mm)	KB (mm)	KLBR	KLAC (mm)	KBAC (mm)	LER	VER	ASV	AC (%)	Ca (mg/100 g)	Mg (mg/100 g)	Fe (mg/100 g)	Zn (mg/100 g)
Female Parents																
IR 72	89.11*	77.83*	53.19	6.82*	2.01	3.39*	7.50	2.89*	1.10	5.29*	4.66*	21.10	6.61	68.02	0.57	1.36
ADT 39	89.10*	74.71*	51.38	5.19	2.31	2.25	8.53*	2.90*	1.64*	4.79*	3.66	20.11	6.28	46.14	0.52	1.63
ADT 45	81.90	66.07	54.67	5.71*	2.07	2.76*	8.52*	2.51	1.49*	4.21	3.66	22.32	7.12	48.12	0.51	0.91
ADT 43	82.69	64.09	53.51	5.63	2.25	2.50*	6.59	2.70	1.17	4.32	4.33	21.79	6.03	64.33	0.63	1.26
ASD 16	83.90	72.30	62.16*	5.38	2.02	2.66*	6.70	2.60	1.24	4.10	3.33	20.11	6.22	68.04	0.60	1.33
TPS 4	86.30*	76.30*	61.82*	4.96	2.62*	1.89	7.57	2.80	1.52*	4.39	4.66*	20.52	6.28	56.11	0.56	1.34
Male Parents																
Veeradangan	78.30	68.50	56.51	5.52	2.63*	2.09	6.41	2.71	1.16	4.59	3.66	25.09*	8.26*	120.27*	1.61*	2.73*
Kavuni	79.90	70.10	63.15*	5.10	2.41*	2.11	6.20	2.49	1.21	3.40	4.33	27.19*	12.30*	118.04*	1.32*	2.79*
Navara	82.35	73.54*	68.13*	5.54	2.36	2.35	6.30	2.90*	1.20	4.90*	3.66	20.12	7.10	92.93*	0.96*	1.68
Kathanellu	83.14	72.39	61.82*	5.16	2.81*	1.83	6.20	3.00*	1.13	5.39*	3.33	24.59*	9.20*	131.59*	0.77	2.14*
Grand mean	83.59	71.56	58.63	5.50	2.34	2.38	7.50	2.75	1.29	4.54	3.93	22.29	7.54	81.36	0.80	1.71
SE	0.72	0.64	0.67	0.09	0.03	0.02	0.12	0.03	0.01	0.06	0.32	0.39	0.16	1.29	0.04	0.15
CD (5%)	2.17	1.91	2.01	0.27	0.11	0.08	0.38	0.12	0.05	0.19	0.97	1.18	0.31	3.85	0.13	0.48

Figure 1. Mean performance of parents for grain quality

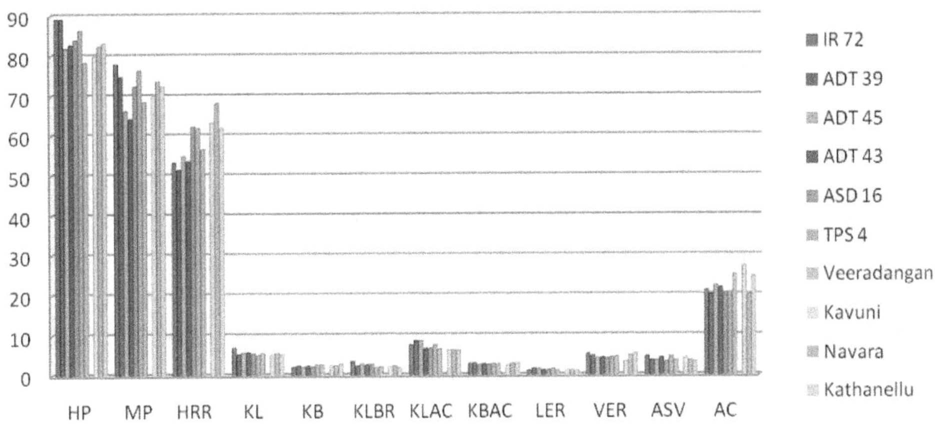

Figure 2. Mean performance of parents for nutritional traits

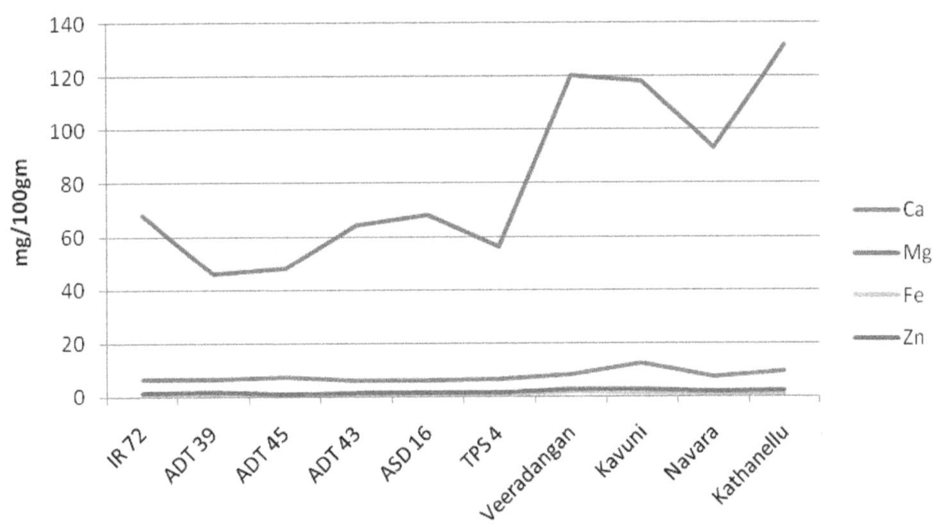

Volume expansion ratio was highest in Kathanellu (5.39) and lowest in Kavuni (3.40). Significant values were recorded in IR 72 (5.29), Navara (4.90) and ADT 39 (4.79). High alkali spreading value was observed in TPS 4 (4.66) and low in ASD 16 and Kathanellu (3.33). Amylose content was high in Kavuni (27.19) and low in ADT 39 and ASD 16 (20.11). Significant amylose content were recorded in Kavuni (27.19), Veeradangan (25.09) and Kathanellu (24.59). With regard to nutritional traits, calcium content was high in Kavuni (12.30 mg/100 g) and low in ADT 43 (6.03 mg/100 g). Veeradangan (8.26 mg/100 g) and Kathanellu (9.20

mg/100 g) recorded significantly higher value for calcium content. Among the ten parents, the highest magnesium content was observed in Kathanellu (131.59 mg/100 g) and ADT 39 (46.14 mg/100 g) recorded the minimum magnesium content. All the male parents *viz.*, Kathanellu (131.59 mg/100 g), Veeradangan (120.27 mg/100 g), Kavuni (118.04 mg/100 g) and Navara (92.93 mg/ 100 g) recorded significantly higher value for magnesium content. Iron content was highest (1.61 mg/100 g) in Veeradangan and lowest in ADT 45 (0.51 mg/100 g). Three male parents *viz.*, Veeradangan (1.61 mg/100 g), Kavuni (1.32 mg/100 g) and Navara (0.96 mg/100 g) recorded significant iron content except Kathanellu (0.77 mg/100 g). With regard to zinc content highest was recorded in Kavuni (2.79 mg/100 g) and lowest in ADT 45 (0.91 mg/100 g). Significant zinc content were recorded in Kavuni (2.79 mg/100 g) Veeradangan (2.73 mg/100 g) and Kathanellu (2.14 mg/100 g).

MEAN PERFORMANCE OF F_3 POPULATION AND PARENTS

Mean performance of selected F_3 plants (20 plants) of two cross combination *viz.*, IR 72 x Veeradangan and ADT 39 x Kavuni along with their parents for grain quality and nutritional traits are presented in Tables 3 and 4.

The parent 1, IR 72 (6.63 mm) recorded significantly higher mean values than the grand mean. Among the twenty selected F_3 plants kernel length ranged from 5.39 mm to 6.54 mm and maximum was recorded by plant 16 while minimum was recorded by plant 7. Nine plants in IR 72 x Veeradangan had significantly positive values for kernel length. For kernel breadth, the parent 2, Veeradangan (2.61 mm) recorded significantly higher mean values than the grand mean (2.30 mm). The plant 13 had the lowest kernel breadth 2.21 mm and plant 7 (2.41 mm) had the highest kernel breadth. Eleven out of 20 selected F_3 plants were found to have significantly higher mean values than the grand mean value (2.30 mm). The parent 1, IR 72 (3.20) recorded significantly higher mean value for kernel L/B ratio. The highest kernel L/B ratio was recorded by plant 18 (2.92), plant 13 (2.74), plant 15 (2.73), plant 10 (2.72), plant 16 (2.71), plant 11 (2.67), plant 6 (2.66) and plant 12 (2.66). The plant 7 showed the lowest kernel L/B ratio of 2.23. Out of 20 selected F_3 plants, eight plants were recorded significantly higher mean values than the grand mean (2.60).

For kernel length after cooking the parent 1, IR 72 (8.90 mm) recorded significantly higher mean value. Among the twenty selected F_3 plants kernel length after cooking ranged from 6.64 to 8.40 mm. The maximum was recorded by plant 15 and minimum by plant 7. Plant 15, plant 18, plant 6, plant 16, plant 5, plant 9, plant 19, plant 17, plant 11 and plant 10 had significantly higher kernel length after cooking than the grand mean (7.51 mm). The parent 2 Veeradangan (2.94 mm)

Table 3. Mean performance of selected F_3 plants of the cross (IR 72 x Veeradangan) for grain quality and nutritional traits

Genotypes	KL (mm)	KB (mm)	KLBR	KLAC (mm)	KBAC (mm)	LER (mm)	BWER (mm)	ASV	AC (%)	Ca (mg/100g)	Mg (mg/100g)	Fe (mg/100g)	Zn (mg/100g)	SPY (g)
Parent 1	6.63*	2.07	3.20*	8.90*	2.53	1.35*	1.22*	3.66	20.44	6.46	68.30	0.67	1.33	35.30
Parent 2	5.53	2.61*	2.11	6.73	2.94*	1.21	1.12	2.00*	25.15*	8.29*	120.63*	1.61	2.92*	39.62
Selected F_3 Plants														
Plant 1	5.69	2.23	2.55	6.74	2.63	1.18	1.18*	4.00	19.26	7.03*	92.73*	0.78	1.93*	37.60
Plant 2	5.64	2.25	2.50	6.86	2.64	1.21	1.17*	2.00*	23.39*	6.37	97.63*	0.73	1.53	38.76
Plant 3	6.14*	2.35*	2.61	7.14	2.77*	1.16	1.18*	3.00	24.39*	5.39	84.58*	1.03*	1.53	42.48
Plant 4	6.16*	2.38*	2.59	7.41	2.75*	1.20	1.15	3.00	23.46*	6.61	94.80*	0.72	1.98*	41.37
Plant 5	5.75	2.27	2.53	7.83*	2.60	1.30*	1.14	3.00	23.04*	6.75	86.42*	0.84*	1.63	41.18
Plant 6	6.24*	2.34*	2.66*	8.24*	2.72*	1.32*	1.16	3.00	19.25	6.05	74.63	0.85*	1.96*	36.29
Plant 7	5.39	2.41*	2.23	6.64	2.82*	1.23	1.17*	3.00	22.21	6.14	83.49*	0.83*	1.77	38.00
Plant 8	5.71	2.31*	2.47	6.78	2.73*	1.19	1.18*	4.00	20.87	7.39*	64.33	0.94*	1.95*	32.30
Plant 9	5.96	2.31*	2.58	7.83*	2.60	1.31*	1.12	2.00*	21.85	6.79*	71.40	0.86*	1.86*	31.94
Plant 10	6.34*	2.33*	2.72*	7.59*	2.64	1.20	1.13	4.00	23.01*	7.65*	93.59*	0.56	1.96*	42.64
Plant 11	6.35*	2.38*	2.67*	7.69*	2.67	1.21	1.12	3.00	23.41*	6.80*	62.88	0.65	1.88*	41.60
Plant 12	5.93	2.23	2.66*	7.28	2.64	1.23	1.18*	4.00	23.24*	6.40	71.85	0.53	1.56	28.67
Plant 13	6.06*	2.21	2.74*	7.34	2.62	1.21	1.18*	4.00	22.16	7.18*	73.18	0.84*	1.72	29.02
Plant 14	5.69	2.23	2.55	6.68	2.64	1.17	1.18*	2.00*	22.71	6.23	81.89*	0.70	1.82	39.09
Plant 15	6.40*	2.34*	2.73*	8.40*	2.67	1.31*	1.14	3.66	22.79	6.18	81.68*	0.62	1.51	32.40
Plant 16	6.54*	2.41*	2.71*	8.20*	2.86*	1.25*	1.19*	3.00	23.09*	6.12	61.43	0.73	1.74	36.09
Plant 17	5.84	2.38*	2.45	7.76*	2.63	1.32*	1.10	3.00	22.33	6.43	82.66*	0.85*	1.96*	41.80
Plant 18	6.53*	2.23	2.92*	8.38*	2.60	1.28*	1.16	2.00*	18.47	6.13	91.69*	0.91*	1.62	39.56
Plant 19	5.62	2.22	2.52	7.78*	2.70	1.38*	1.21*	4.00	18.45	7.39*	73.29	0.74	1.83	34.26
Plant 20	5.73	2.26	2.52	6.93	2.67	1.21	1.17*	2.33*	23.00*	6.38	61.58	0.63	1.93*	39.22
Grand mean	5.99	2.30	2.60	7.51	2.68	1.25	1.16	3.07	22.09	6.64	80.67	0.80	1.82	37.23
SE	0.021	0.007	0.02	0.014	0.021	0.007	0.007	0.113	0.219	0.077	0.169	0.014	0.014	-
CD (5%)	0.07	0.02	0.04	0.16	0.06	0.03	0.02	0.34	0.63	0.22	0.49	0.03	0.05	-

Table 4. Mean performance of selected F_3 plants of the cross (ADT 39 x Kavuni) for quality and nutritional traits in rice

Genotypes	KL (mm)	KB (mm)	KLBR	KLAC (mm)	KBAC (mm)	LER (mm)	BWER (mm)	ASV	AC (%)	Ca (mg/100g)	Mg (mg/100g)	Fe (mg/100g)	Zn (mg/100g)	SPY (g)
Parent 1	6.23*	2.28	2.73*	8.60*	2.85*	1.38*	1.25*	3.00	20.13	6.29	61.54	0.54	1.62	32.05
Parent 2	5.14	2.35	2.18	6.34	2.67	1.23	1.13	2.00*	26.53*	12.29*	118.52*	1.35*	3.01*	32.86
Selected F_3 Plants														
Plant 1	5.13	2.36	2.17	7.44*	2.70	1.45*	1.14	3.00	20.12	9.82*	78.22	0.75	1.86	34.51
Plant 2	5.23	2.26	2.31*	6.93	2.65	1.32	1.17*	3.00	21.13	7.87	67.76	0.93	1.73	32.14
Plant 3	5.16	2.24	2.30*	6.46	2.55	1.25	1.13	2.00*	20.30	9.45*	66.47	0.61	1.80	33.82
Plant 4	5.37*	2.23	2.40*	7.35*	2.73	1.37*	1.22*	2.66	22.61	8.37	76.71	0.85	2.16*	31.16
Plant 5	5.15	2.26	2.27	6.83	2.74	1.32	1.21*	2.33*	21.73	6.89	84.49*	1.25*	1.83	38.75
Plant 6	5.24	2.31	2.26	6.90	2.78*	1.31	1.19*	3.00	21.62	10.36*	74.47	1.05*	2.05*	32.27
Plant 7	5.21	2.33	2.23	7.81*	2.72	1.49*	1.16	3.00	20.92	8.76	87.70*	1.31*	1.76	21.34
Plant 8	5.20	2.20	2.36*	6.76	2.55	1.30	1.16	3.00	23.34*	8.21	88.70*	1.04*	1.83	28.74
Plant 9	5.17	2.45*	2.11	7.02	2.76*	1.35	1.12	3.00	23.98*	9.15*	53.38	0.64	1.84	21.44
Plant 10	5.15	2.44*	2.11	6.90	2.73	1.34	1.11	2.66	24.95*	10.39*	69.51	1.03*	1.76	31.61
Plant 11	5.17	2.29	2.25	7.12	2.59	1.37*	1.13	3.00	23.79*	9.16*	94.25*	0.93	1.74	28.56
Plant 12	5.25	2.33	2.25	7.36*	2.76*	1.40*	1.18*	3.00	20.79	7.62	87.58*	0.84	2.14*	31.85
Plant 13	5.13	2.34	2.18	6.36	2.74	1.24	1.17*	3.00	21.64	8.86*	85.87*	0.94	1.43	33.38
Plant 14	5.25	2.36	2.22	7.03	2.82*	1.34	1.19*	2.66	20.80	8.70	71.84	1.16*	1.93*	32.36
Plant 15	5.13	2.40*	2.14	7.12	2.76*	1.39*	1.15	2.33*	24.65*	8.47	66.26	0.96	1.73	37.82
Plant 16	5.12	2.42*	2.12	7.22*	2.79*	1.40*	1.15	3.00	20.93	10.34*	70.33	1.22*	1.82	33.56
Plant 17	5.22	2.40*	2.17	7.02	2.70	1.34	1.12	3.00	21.18	8.87*	92.78*	0.81	2.15*	29.55
Plant 18	5.21	2.39*	2.18	7.10	2.69	1.36*	1.12	3.00	23.52*	8.39	84.63*	1.33*	1.66	35.52
Plant 19	5.20	2.30	2.25	7.26*	2.66	1.39*	1.15	2.33*	21.64	6.46	76.84	0.84	1.75	33.47
Plant 20	5.18	2.39*	2.16	7.02	2.74	1.35	1.14	2.33*	22.14	8.43	92.88*	0.94	1.83	36.79
Grand mean	5.24	2.33	2.24	7.09	2.71	1.35	1.16	2.74	22.20	8.76	79.58	0.97	1.88	31.98
SE	0.014	0.021	0.021	0.028	0.021	0.007	0.007	0.183	0.233	0.035	1.732	0.014	0.028	-
CD (5%)	0.05	0.06	0.06	0.08	0.07	0.02	0.03	0.54	0.68	0.10	4.94	0.04	0.08	-

recorded significantly higher mean value for kernel breadth after cooking. A total of six selected F_3 plants were significant when compared to the grand mean (2.68 mm). The highest mean value was shown by plant 16 (2.86 mm) and the lowest was exhibited by plant 5 (2.60 mm). For linear elongation ratio the parent 1, IR 72 (1.35) recorded significantly higher mean values than the grand mean (1.25). Mean value for twenty selected F_3 plants ranged from 1.16 (plant 3) to 1.38 (plant 19).

The parent 1, IR 72 (1.22) recorded significant breadth wise expansion ratio. Among the twenty selected F_3 plants breadth wise expansion ratio ranged from 1.10 to 1.21 and the maximum was recorded by plant 19 and minimum was recorded by plant 17. Eleven F_3 plants were found to be significant for breadth wise expansion ratio. For alkali spreading value the parent 2, Veeradangan (2.00) recorded significantly lesser mean values than the grand mean value. The mean value of selected F_3 plants ranged from 2.00 to 4.00. Out of twenty selected F_3 plants, five had significantly lesser mean values than the grand mean (3.07). The significantly lesser alkali spreading value was recorded by five selected F_3 plants *viz.*, plant 2, plant 9, plant 14, plant 18 and plant 20.

For amylose content the parent 2, Veeradangan (25.15) recorded significant amylose content. The mean value of selected F_3 plants ranged from 18.45 to 24.39 and maximum was recorded by plant 3 and minimum was recorded by plant 19. Plant 3, plant 4, plant 11, plant 2, plant 12, plant 16, plant 5, plant 10 and plant 20 showed significantly higher mean values than the grand mean (22.09). The parent 2, Veeradangan (8.29 mg/100 g) recorded significant calcium content. The selected F_3 plants, plant 3 had the lowest calcium content of 5.39 mg/ 100 g while plant 10 recorded the highest value of 7.65 mg/100 g. Seven out of twenty plants *viz.*, plant 10, plant 8, plant 19, plant 13, plant 1, plant 11 and plant 9 had significantly higher calcium content than the grand mean value. For magnesium content parent 2, Veeradangan (120.63 mg/100 g) recorded significantly higher mean values. Among the selected F_3 plants magnesium content ranged from 61.43 to 97.63 mg/100 g and maximum was recorded by plant 2 and minimum was recorded by plant 16. Out of twenty selected F_3 plants eleven were found to have significant mean values.

For iron content none of the parents showed significant value. The mean values of selected F_3 plants ranged from 0.53 to 1.03 mg/100 g and maximum was recorded by plant 3 and minimum was recorded plant 12. The highest value of 1.03 mg/100 g was expressed by plant 3 followed by plant 8, plant 18, plant 9, plant 17, plant 6, plant 5, plant 13 and plant 7. The parent 2, Veeradangan (2.92 mg/100 g) recorded significantly higher mean value for zinc content. Nine selected F_3 plants were significant when compared to the grand mean value. The highest mean value was shown by plant 4 (1.98 mg/100 g) and the lowest was exhibited by plant 15 (1.51 mg/100 g). The range for single plant yield was from 28.67 to 42.64 g. The highest mean value shown by plant 10 and the lowest was exhibited by plant 12.

The parent 1, ADT 39 (6.23 mm) recorded significantly higher mean values than the grand mean for kernel length. Among the twenty selected F_3 plants kernel length ranged from 5.12 mm to 5.37 mm and maximum was recorded by plant 4 and minimum was recorded by plant 16. For kernel breadth, none of the parents showed significant value. The plant 8 had the lowest kernel breadth 2.20 mm and plant 9 (2.45 mm) had the highest kernel breadth. Seven out of twenty selected F_3 plants were found to have significantly lesser mean values than the grand mean value (2.33 mm). The parent 1, ADT 39 (2.73) recorded significantly higher mean values for kernel L/B ratio. The highest kernel L/B ratio was recorded by plant 4 (2.40), plant 8 (2.36), plant 2 (2.31) and plant 3 (2.30). The plant 9 and 10 showed the lowest kernel L/B ratio of 2.11. Out of twenty selected F_3 plants, four plants were recorded significantly higher mean values than the grand mean (2.24).

For kernel length after cooking the parent 1, IR 72 (8.60 mm) recorded significantly higher mean values than the grand mean (7.09 mm). Among the twenty selected F_3 plants kernel length ranged from 6.36 to 7.81 mm. The maximum was recorded by plant 7 and minimum by plant 13. Plant 7, plant 1, plant 12, plant 4, plant 12, plant 16 and plant 19 had significantly higher kernel length after cooking than the grand mean (7.09 mm). The parent 1, ADT 39 (2.85 mm) recorded significantly higher mean value. A total of five selected F_3 plants were significant when compared to the grand mean (2.71 mm). The highest mean value was shown by plant 14 (2.82 mm) and the lowest was exhibited by plant 3 (2.55 mm). For linear elongation ratio the parent 1, ADT 39 (1.38) recorded significantly higher mean values than the grand mean (1.35). Mean value for twenty selected F_3 plants ranged from 1.24 (plant 13) to 1.49 (plant 7). Nine selected F_3 plants showed significantly higher values than the grand mean (1.35). The parent 1, ADT 39 (1.25) recorded significant breadth wise expansion ratio. Among the twenty selected F_3 plants breadth wise expansion ratio ranged from 1.11 to 1.22 and the maximum was recorded by plant 4 and minimum was recorded by plant 10. Seven F_3 plants were found to be significant for breadth wise expansion ratio. For alkali spreading value the parent 2, Kavuni (2.00) recorded significantly lesser mean values than the grand mean value. The mean value of selected F_3 plants ranged from 2.00 to 3.00. Out of twenty selected F_3 plants, five plants *viz.*, plant 3, plant 5, plant 15, plant 19 and plant 20 had significantly lesser mean values than the grand mean (2.74).

For amylose content parent 2, Kavuni (26.53) recorded significant amylose content. The mean value of selected F_3 plants amylose content ranged from 20.12 to 24.95 and maximum was recorded by plant 10 and minimum was recorded by plant 1. Plant 15, plant 9, plant 11, plant 18 and plant 8 showed significantly higher mean values than the grand mean (22.20). The parent 2, Kavuni (12.29 mg/100 g) recorded significant calcium content. The selected F_3 plants, plant 19 had the lowest calcium content of 6.46 mg/100 g while plant 10 recorded the highest value of 10.39

mg/100 g. Nine out of twenty plants *viz.*, plant 10, plant 6, plant 16, plant 4, plant 3, plant 11, plant 9, plant 17 and plant 13 had significantly higher calcium content than the grand mean value. For magnesium content parent 2, Kavuni (118.52 mg/100 g) recorded significantly higher mean values than the grand mean value. Among the selected F_3 plants Magnesium content ranged from 53.38 to 94.25 mg/100 g and maximum was recorded by plant 11 and minimum was recorded by plant 9. Out of twenty selected F_3 plants nine, were found to have significant mean values.

With regard to iron content the parent 2, Kavuni (1.35 mg/100 g) showed significant value for iron content. The mean values of selected F_3 plants had a range from 0.61 to 1.33 mg/100 g and maximum was recorded by plant 18 and minimum was recorded plant 3. The highest value of 1.33 mg/100 g was expressed by plant 18 followed by plant 7, plant 5, plant 16, plant 14, plant 6, plant 8 and plant 10. For zinc content the parent 2, Kavuni (3.01 mg/100 g) recorded significantly higher mean values than the grand mean value. A total of four F_3 plants were significant when compared to the grand mean value. The highest mean value was shown by plant 4 (2.16 mg/100 g) and the lowest was exhibited by plant 13 (1.43 mg/100 gm). The F_3 plant *viz.*, plant 4 (2.16 mg/100 g), plant 17 (2.15 mg/100 g), plant 12 (2.14 mg/100 g) and plant 6 (2.05 mg/100 g). The range for single plant yield was from 21.34 to 38.75 g. The highest single plant yield was recorded mean value shown by plant 5 and the lowest was exhibited by plant 7.

GENETIC VARIABILITY PARAMETERS FOR GRAIN QUALITY AND NUTRITIONAL TRAITS IN PARENTS

Calcium content ranged from 6.03 (ADT 43) to 12.30 mg/100 g (Kavuni) with a grand mean of 7.54 mg/100 g. Magnesium content showed the range from 46.14 (ADT 39) to 131.59 mg/100 g (Kathanellu) with a grand mean of 81.36 mg/100 g. Iron content varied from 0.51(ADT 45) to 1.61 mg/100 g (Veeradangan) with a grand mean of 0.80 mg/100 g. Zinc content varied from 0.91 (ADT 45) to 2.79 mg/100 g (Kavuni) with a grand mean of 1.71 mg/100 g.

Genetic variability parameters on F_3 population (20 selected F_3 plants) of two cross combination *viz.*, IR 72 x Veeradangan and ADT 39 x Kavuni along with their parents for grain quality and nutritional traits are presented in Tables 5, 6, and 7 and Figures 3, 4, and 5.

Kernel Length

For kernel length, IR 72 x Veeradangan in F_3 population showed wide range of variability and ranged from 5.39 to 6.54 mm whereas, ADT 39 x Kavuni in F_3

Table 5. Genetic variability parameters for grain quality and nutritional traits in parents

Characters	Range		Grand Mean	Coefficient of Variation (%)		Heritability (%)	Genetic Advance as Percent of Mean
	Minimum	Maximum		Phenotypic (PCV)	Genotypic (GCV)		
Hulling percentage (H %)	78.30	89.11	83.59	4.57	4.31	89.03	8.38
Milling percentage (M %)	64.09	77.83	71.56	6.24	6.04	93.78	12.06
Head rice recovery (HRR %)	51.38	68.13	58.63	9.51	9.30	95.55	18.73
Kernel length (KL-mm)	4.96	6.82	5.50	9.84	9.40	91.29	18.51
Kernel breadth (KB- mm)	2.01	2.81	2.34	11.94	11.61	94.61	23.27
Kernel L/B ratio (KLBR)	1.83	3.39	2.38	19.73	19.61	98.80	40.16
Kernel length after cooking (KLAC-mm)	6.20	8.53	7.05	13.26	12.88	94.35	25.77
Kernel breadth after cooking (KBAC-mm)	2.49	3.00	2.75	6.70	6.16	84.69	11.69
Linear elongation ratio	1.10	1.64	1.29	14.88	14.66	94.06	29.76
Volume expansion ratio (VER)	3.40	5.39	4.54	13.23	12.98	96.30	26.25
Alkali spreading value	3.33	4.66	3.93	17.64	10.14	33.08	12.02
Amylose content (AC %)	20.11	27.19	22.29	11.48	11.06	92.77	21.95
Calcium content (mg/100g)	6.03	12.30	7.54	25.98	25.86	97.12	53.04
Magnesium content (mg/100g)	46.14	131.59	81.36	39.24	39.14	99.50	80.43
Iron content (mg/100g)	0.51	1.61	0.80	49.25	48.26	96.02	92.43
Zinc content (mg/100g)	0.91	2.79	1.71	39.57	36.57	83.00	67.67

population exhibited range from 5.12 to 5.37 mm with a grand mean of 5.99 and 5.24 mm respectively. The phenotypic and genotypic coefficient of variation for this trait in IR 72 x Veeradangan was 6.10 and 6.05 respectively. In the cross ADT 39 x Kavuni, the phenotypic and genotypic coefficients of variation was 4.38 and 4.34 respectively. High heritability (88.44 per cent) and moderate genetic advance (12.37) as per of mean was noticed in IR 72 x Veeradangan whereas, in ADT 39 x Kavuni registered high heritability (91.17) with low genetic advance (8.86) as per cent of mean.

Table 6. Genetic variability parameters of F_3 population of the cross (IR 72 x Veeradangan) for grain quality and nutritional traits in rice

Traits	Range		Grand Mean	Coefficient of Variation (%)		Heritability (%)	Genetic Advance as Percent of Mean
	Minimum	Maximum		Phenotypic (PCV)	Genotypic (GCV)		
KL (mm)	5.39	6.54	5.99	6.10	6.05	88.44	12.37
KB (mm)	2.21	2.41	2.30	4.65	4.60	77.57	9.36
Kernel L/B ratio	2.23	2.92	2.60	8.36	8.30	91.65	16.99
KLAC (mm)	6.64	8.40	7.51	8.87	8.77	83.80	17.87
KBAC (mm)	2.60	2.86	2.68	3.74	3.49	86.97	6.70
LER (mm)	1.16	1.38	1.25	5.48	5.28	92.91	10.49
BER (mm)	1.10	1.21	1.16	2.89	2.50	72.21	4.48
ASV	2.00	4.00	3.07	25.38	24.48	93.02	48.64
AC (%)	18.45	24.39	22.09	8.52	8.34	95.83	16.83
Ca (mg/100g)	5.39	7.65	6.64	10.86	10.64	95.58	20.41
Mg (mg/100g)	61.43	97.63	80.67	17.91	17.86	93.96	36.79
Fe (mg/100g)	0.53	1.03	0.80	27.56	27.42	95.03	56.22
Zn (mg/100g)	1.51	1.98	1.82	16.67	16.59	98.99	34.00

Kernel Breadth

With regard to kernel breadth, the range of variability was from 2.21 to 2.41 mm for IR 72 x Veeradangan in F_3 population whereas it ranged from 2.20 to 2.45 mm for ADT 39 x Kavuni in F_3 population. IR 72 x Veeradangan (2.30 mm) and ADT 39 x Kavuni (2.33 mm) registered high and low grand mean values respectively for this trait. The phenotypic and genotypic coefficients of variation for kernel breadth in IR 72 x Veeradangan was 4.65 and 4.60 respectively. In the cross ADT 39 x Kavuni, the phenotypic and genotypic coefficient of variation was 3.20 and 2.79 respectively. In the cross IR 72 x Veeradangan, high heritability of 77.57 per cent and low genetic advance 9.36 as per cent of mean was noticed.

Kernel L/B Ratio

For kernel L/B ratio, IR 72 x Veeradangan (2.23 to 2.92) exhibited wide range of variability followed by ADT 39 x Kavuni (2.11 to 2.40) in F_3 population with a

Table 7. Genetic variability parameters of F_3 population of the cross (ADT 39 X Kavuni) for grain quality and nutritional traits in rice

Traits	Range		Grand Mean	Coefficient of Variation (%)		Heritability (%)	Genetic Advance as Percent of Mean
	Minimum	Maximum		Phenotypic (PCV)	Genotypic (GCV)		
KL (mm)	5.12	5.37	5.24	4.38	4.34	91.17	8.86
KB (mm)	2.20	2.45	2.33	3.20	2.79	75.88	5.01
Kernel L/B ratio	2.11	2.40	2.24	6.11	5.87	92.38	11.63
KLAC (mm)	6.36	7.81	7.09	6.80	6.77	83.97	13.88
KBAC (mm)	2.55	2.82	2.71	3.22	2.73	71.81	4.77
LER (mm)	1.24	1.49	1.35	4.71	4.63	84.50	9.37
BER (mm)	1.11	1.22	1.16	3.40	2.88	72.22	5.05
ASV	2.00	3.00	2.74	16.24	10.95	45.45	15.20
AC (%)	20.12	24.95	22.20	8.00	7.78	91.60	15.60
Ca (mg/100g)	6.46	10.39	8.76	15.69	15.67	95.80	32.25
Mg (mg/100g)	53.38	94.25	79.58	17.98	17.58	95.60	35.42
Fe (mg/100g)	0.61	1.33	0.97	23.94	23.77	96.55	48.61
Zn (mg/100g)	1.43	2.16	1.88	16.40	16.19	97.47	32.93

grand mean of 2.60 and 2.24 respectively. With regard to kernel L/B ratio, IR 72 x Veeradangan showed low phenotypic and genotypic coefficients of variation of 8.36 and 8.30 respectively. Low phenotypic coefficient of variation (6.11) and genotypic coefficient of variation (5.87) was recorded in ADT 39 x Kavuni. In the cross IR 72 x Veeradangan, high heritability of 91.65 per cent with moderate genetic advance 16.99 as per cent of mean was noticed. ADT 39 x Kavuni recorded high heritability of 92.38 per cent with moderate genetic advance 11.63 as per cent of mean.

Kernel Length after Cooking

Wide range of variability was found in IR 72 x Veeradangan (6.64 to 8.40 mm) whereas, ADT 39 x Kavuni (6.36 to 7.81mm) was noticed in F_3 population with a grand mean of 7.51 mm and 7.09 mm respectively. The phenotypic and genotypic coefficients of variation for this trait in IR 72 x Veeradangan was 8.87 and 8.77 respectively. In the cross ADT 39 x Kavuni, the phenotypic and genotypic coefficient of variation were 6.80 and 6.77 respectively. High heritability (83.80 per

Figure 3. Genetic variability parameters for grain quality and nutritional traits for parents

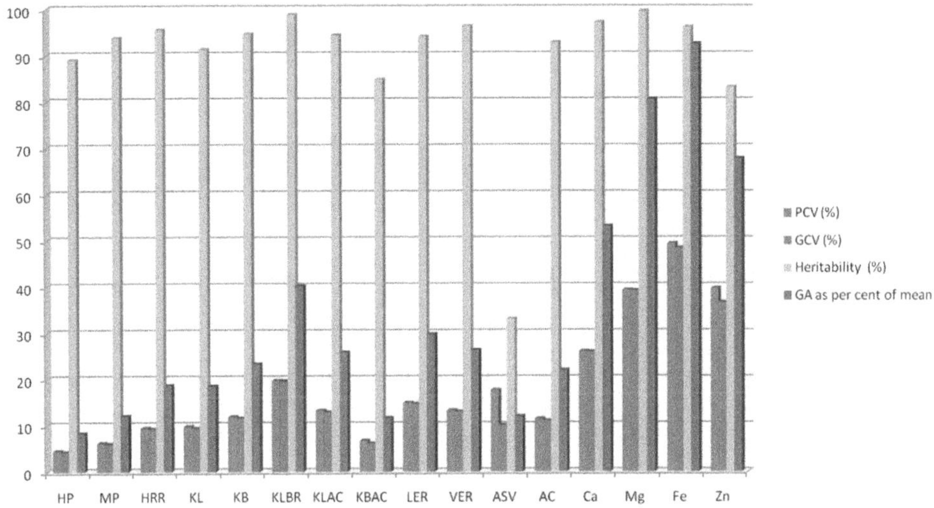

Figure 4. Genetic variability parameters of F3 generation of the cross (IR 72 x Veeradangan) for grain quality and nutritional traits

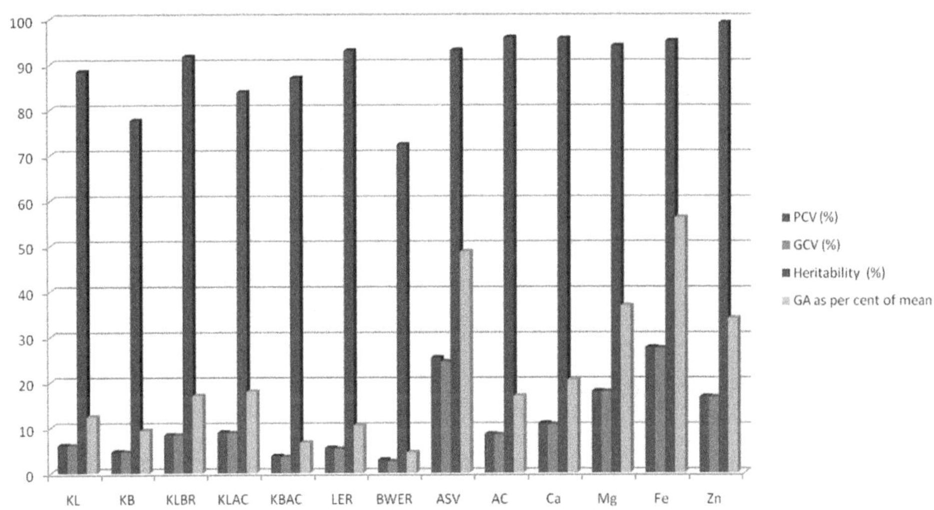

cent) and moderate genetic advance (17.87) as per cent of mean was noticed in IR 72 x Veeradangan whereas, the cross ADT 39 x Kavuni registered high heritability (83.97 per cent) with moderate genetic advance (13.88) as per cent of mean.

Figure 5. Genetic variability parameters of F3 generation of the cross (ADT 39 x Kavuni) for grain quality and nutritional traits

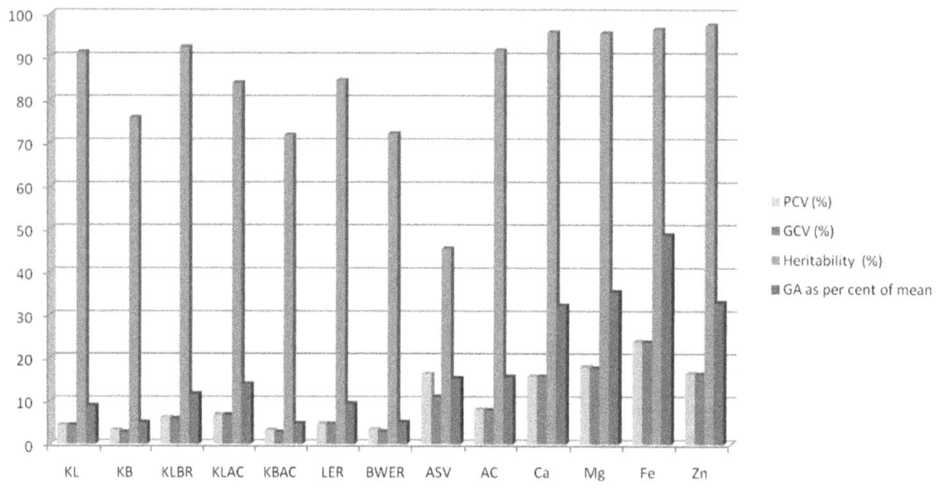

Kernel Breadth after Cooking

For kernel breadth, ADT 39 x Kavuni in F_3 population recorded wide range of variability (2.55 to 2.82 mm) where as low range of variability was observed in IR 72 x Veeradangan in selected F_3 population (2.60 mm to 2.86 mm) with a grand mean of 2.71 and 2.68 mm respectively. With regard to kernel breadth after cooking, IR 72 x Veeradangan showed low phenotypic and genotypic coefficients of variation of 3.74 and 3.49 respectively. The coefficients of phenotypic and genotypic variation were 3.22 and 2.73 respectively in ADT 39 x Kavuni. In the cross IR 72 x Veeradangan, high heritability of 86.97 per cent with low genetic advance 6.70 as per cent of mean was noticed. ADT 39 x Kavuni recorded high heritability of 71.81 per cent with low genetic advance 4.77 as per cent of mean.

Linear Elongation Ratio

For Linear elongation ratio the crosses IR 72 x Veeradangan (1.16 to 1.38) and ADT 39 x Kavuni in F_3 population (1.24 to 1.49) exhibited low range of variability. Linear elongation ratio registered low variability in two crosses with a grand mean of 1.25 and 1.35 mm respectively. The coefficient of variation due to phenotype and genotype were 5.48 and 5.28 respectively in IR 72 x Veeradangan. In the cross ADT 39 x Kavuni, the phenotypic and genotypic coefficient of variation was 4.71 and 4.63 respectively. High heritability (92.91 per cent) and moderate genetic advance (10.49) as per cent of mean was noticed in the cross IR 72 x Veeradangan whereas, the cross ADT 39 x Kavuni registered high heritability (84.50) with low genetic advance (9.37) as per cent of mean.

Breadth Wise Expansion Ratio

Low range of variability was observed in both the F_3 population of the two crosses. The grand mean 1.16 was found to be same in both the crosses. The two crosses recorded low phenotypic and genotypic coefficients of variation along with high heritability and low genetic advance as per cent of mean. The phenotypic and genotypic coefficients of variation for breadth wise expansion ratio in IR 72 x Veeradangan was 2.89 and 2.50 respectively. In the cross ADT 39 x Kavuni the phenotypic and genotypic coefficients of variation was 3.40 and 2.88 respectively. High heritability (72.21 per cent) and low genetic advance (4.48) as per cent of mean noticed in IR 72 x Veeradangan whereas, in ADT 39 x Kavuni registered high heritability (72.22) with low genetic advance (5.05) as per cent of mean.

Alkali Spreading Value

Generally low range of variability was observed for this trait. High grand mean value was observed for IR 72 x Veeradangan in F_3 population (3.07) while low grand mean value was observed for ADT 39 x Kavuni in F_3 population (2.74). With regard to alkali spreading value, IR 72 x Veeradangan showed high phenotypic and genotypic coefficients of variation of 25.38 and 24.48 respectively. Moderate phenotypic and genotypic coefficient of variation of 16.24 and 10.95 respectively was registered in cross ADT 39 x Kavuni. In the cross IR 72 x Veeradangan, high heritability of 93.02 per cent with high genetic advance 48.64 as per cent of mean was noticed. ADT 39 x Kavuni recorded moderate heritability (45.45 per cent) and genetic advance (15.20) as per cent of mean for this trait.

Amylose Content

Wide range of variability was found in ADT 39 x Kavuni (20.12 to 24.95) and IR 72 x Veeradangan (18.45 to 24.39) in F_3 population. ADT 39 x Kavuni exhibited grand mean value (22.20%) and mean value was observed in IR 72 x Veeradangan (22.09%). The phenotypic and genotypic coefficient of variations for amylose content in IR 72 x Veeradangan was 8.52 and 8.34 respectively. In the cross ADT 39 x Kavuni, the phenotypic and genotypic coefficients of variation were 8.00 and 7.78 respectively. High heritability (95.83 per cent) and moderate genetic advance (16.83) as per of mean noticed in IR 72 x Veeradangan whereas, in ADT 39 x

Kavuni registered high heritability (91.60 per cent) with moderate genetic advance (15.60) as per cent of mean.

Calcium Content

ADT 39 x Kavuni in F_3 population depicted wide range of variability and its ranged from 6.46 to 10.39 mg/100 g while it was from 5.39 to 7.65 mg/100 g in IR 72 x Veeradangan F_3 population. High mean value was observed in ADT 39 x Kavuni (8.76 mg/100 g) while low mean value was noticed in IR 72 x Veeradangan (6.64 mg/100 g). The estimates of phenotypic and genotypic coefficient of variations were 10.86 and 10.64 respectively in IR 72 x Veeradangan. Moderate phenotypic coefficient of variation (15.69) and genotypic coefficient of variation (15.67) were recorded in ADT 39 x Kavuni. In the cross IR 72 x Veeradangan, high heritability of 95.58 per cent with high genetic advance 20.41 as per cent of mean was noticed. ADT 39 x Kavuni recorded high heritability and genetic advance as per cent of mean 95.80 and 32.25 respectively.

Magnesium Content

Among the two crosses, IR 72 x Veeradangan in selected F_3 population recorded wide range of variability and its ranged from 61.43 to 97.63 mg/100 g with a mean value of 80.67 mg/100 g whereas, ADT 39 x Kavuni in F_3 population revealed the low range of variability and its ranged from 53.38 to 94.25 mg/100 g with a mean value of 79.58 mg/100 g. The phenotypic and genotypic coefficients of variation for magnesium content in IR 72 x Veeradangan were 17.91 and 17.86 respectively. In the cross ADT 39 x Kavuni the phenotypic and genotypic coefficient of variations were 17.98 and 17.58 respectively. High heritability (93.96 per cent) and moderate genetic advance (36.79) as per cent of mean noticed in cross IR 72 x Veeradangan whereas, cross ADT 39 x Kavuni registered high heritability (95.60 per cent) with low genetic advance (35.42) as per cent of mean.

Iron Content

For iron content, IR 72 x Veeradangan in F_3 population showed wide range of variability and its ranged from 0.53 to 1.03 mg/100 g with a grand mean of 0.80 mg/100 g whereas, ADT 39 x Kavuni in F_3 population exhibited low range of variability and its ranged from 0.61 to 1.33 mg/100 g and from with a grand mean value of 0.97 mg/100 g. With regard to iron content, IR 72 x Veeradangan showed high phenotypic and genotypic coefficients of variation of 27.56 and 27.42 respectively. High phenotypic coefficient of variation of 23.94 and genotypic coefficient of variation of 23.77 was recorded in ADT 39 x Kavuni. In the cross IR 72 x Veeradangan, high heritability of 95.03 per cent with high genetic advance 56.22 as per cent of mean was noticed. ADT 39 x Kavuni recorded high heritability and genetic advance as per cent of mean 96.55 and 48.61 respectively.

Zinc Content

Wide range of variability was found in ADT 39 x Kavuni (1.43 to 2.16 mg/100 g) and in IR 72 x Veeradangan (1.51 to 1.98 mg/100 g) in F_3 population. ADT 39 x Kavuni recorded high grand mean value (1.88 mg/100 g) while low grand mean value was observed in IR 72 x Veeradangan (1.82 mg/100 g). This trait recorded the phenotypic and genotypic coefficient of variation of 16.67 and 16.59 respectively for the cross IR 72 x Veeradangan. In the cross ADT 39 x Kavuni, the phenotypic and genotypic coefficient of variations were 16.40 and 16.19 respectively. High heritability (98.99 per cent) and genetic advance (34.00) as per cent of mean were noticed in IR 72 x Veeradangan whereas; in ADT 39 x Kavuni registered high heritability (97.47 per cent) with high genetic advance (32.93) as per cent of mean was observed.

FUTURE BREEDING PROGRAMME OF THE PRESENT MATERIAL

Selection of parents based on a combination of parameters would increase the probability of success in any breeding programme. It would be highly appropriate that, the parameter such as *per se* performance is taken into account at the time of selection of parents. Further, the nature of gene action governing the inheritance of characters has also to be given due weightage as it is going to decide the future course of breeding procedures.

Minerals are essential for normal metabolic functions and are required components in balanced diet. Brown rice is an excellent source of minerals. Since, all the four medicinal landraces studied were of brown and black rices, they could be the best source for minerals especially calcium and magnesium. Calcium is the essential element required for the formation and maintenance of skeleton and teeth. It is required for normal contraction of muscle to make limbs move, contraction of heart for its normal function, nervous activity and blood clotting. Based on the available information on retention of calcium by the human body in long term balance studies, the suggested level of intake for the adult male and growing children is between 0.4 and 0.6 g/day. Magnesium plays an important in cardiovascular disease. Magnesium and calcium shares many of the properties of absorption and tissue distribution. When comparing the high yielding varieties and landraces for calcium content, the landrace Kavuni had high calcium content followed by Veeradangan, while Kathanellu had high magnesium content. High calcium and magnesium contents could be helpful in improving muscle activity in patients suffering from muscle disorders (Deepa et al, 2008). For iron content maximum was registered by the landrace Kavuni, Veeradangan and Navara and for zinc content Kavuni ranks first followed by Veeradangan, Kathanellu and Navara. Zinc is an important element performing a range of functions in the body as it is a co-factor for a number of enzymes. Iron and zinc are very important limiting trace elements in rice grains. Finding out the rice genotypes having higher contents of these micronutrients is the need of the hour (Zhang et al, 2005 & Zhang et al, 2012). Comparing the released varieties the land races had double the amount of magnesium, iron and zinc contents. According among hybrids, IR 72 x Veeradangan, ADT 39 x Kavuni and ADT 45 x Kavuni can be recommended for recombination breeding in order to select a better genotype in later generations or in segregating population for yield coupled with high macro and micronutrient contents.

CONCLUSION

From this study, it was clear that among six hybrids, IR 72 x Veeradangan, ADT 39 x Kavuni and ADT 45 x Kavuni exhibited high heterosis for single plant yield over the standard check ADT 43 with relatively high nutritive contents. Hence these three hybrids were adjusted as best hybrids for heterosis breeding programme. Among the F_3 progenies of the cross IR 72 x Veeradangan, based on mean performance and significant registered eight plants *viz.,* plant 3, 4, 6, 8, 9, 10, 11 and plant 18 were having high grain quality with desirable nutrient content besides high single plant yield. In ADT 39 x Kavuni nine plants *viz.,* plant 4, 5, 6, 7, 8, 10, 11, 12 and plant 14 were having good grain quality characters with desirable nutrient contents. These selected plants in the above two crosses may be further advanced to later generations so as to select the best segregants for high single plant yield coupled with more nutritive content and grain quality.

REFERENCES

Das, T., & Das, A. K. (2014). Inventory of the traditional rice varieties in farming system of southern Assam: A case study. *Indian Journal of Traditional Knowledge.*, *13*(1), 157–163.

Deepa, G., Singh, V., & Naidu, K. A. (2008). Nutrient composition and physico-chemical properties of Indian medicinal rice – Njavara. *Food Chemistry*, *106*(1), 165–171. doi:10.1016/j.foodchem.2007.05.062

Latha, M., Abdul Nizar, M., Abraham, Z., Joseph John, K., Asokan Nair, R., Mani, S., & Dutta, M. (2013). Rice landraces of Kerala State of India: A documentation. *International Journal of Biodiversity and Conservation.*, *5*(4), 250–263.

Lockie & Carpenter. (2011). *Agriculture, Biodiversity and Markets. Livelihoods and agroecology in comparative perspective.* London: Earthscan publishers.

Nadesapanicker, A. K., Gopi, G., & Prajeesh, P. (2010). Genetic Erosion and Degradation of Ecosystem Services of Wetland Rice Fields: A Case Study From Western Ghats, India.

Rajukkannu, K., Sathya, A., & Quintal, O. (2009). The diversity of traditional rice varieties in India-A focus on Tamil Nadu. PANAP. Rice sheets, Penang, Malaysia. 1-11.

Season & crop report. (2012). Chennai: Department of Economics and Statistics, Government of India.

Walker, C. L. F., & Black, R. F. (2007). Functional Indicators for Assessing Zinc Deficiency. *Food and Nutrition Bulletin*, *23*(3), 454–479. doi:10.1177/15648265070283S305

Welch, R. M., & Graham, R. D. (2004). Breeding for micronutrients in staple food crops from a human nutrition perspective. *Journal of Experimental Botany*, *55*(396), 353–364. doi:10.1093/jxb/erh064 PMID:14739261

Zhang, J., Cao, Y. L. K. B., Wu, L., & Xu, S. (2012). Iron and Zinc accumulation trend in a Japonica rice grains after anthesis. *Afr. J. Agric. Res.*, *7*(8), 1312–1316.

Zhang, M. W., Guo, B. J., & Peng, Z. M. (2005). Genetic effects of grain characteristics of *indica* black rice and their uses on indirect selections for some mineral element content in grains. *Genetic Resources and Crop Evolution*, *52*(8), 1121–1128. doi:10.1007/s10722-004-6114-0

ADDITIONAL READING

Chimmili, S. R. (2012). Genetic analysis for nutritive traits using medicinal land races of rice (*Oryza sativa* L.). *M.Sc. (Ag.) Thesis* (Unpubl.), TNAU, Coimbatore.

Nayak, A. R., Chaudhary, R., & Reddy, J. N. (2003). Genetic variability and correlation study among quality characters in scented rice. *Agric. Sci. Digest*, *23*(3), 175–178.

Rajeswari, S., Robin, S., Chandirakala, R., Premalatha, N., & Muthuramu, S. (2010). Genetic analysis and character association of quality in rice. *Oryza*, *47*(2), 86–90.

Subbulakshmi, K. (2013). Genetic analysis for yield and quality traits in rice (*Oryza sativa* L). *M.Sc. (Ag.) Thesis* (Unpubl.) TNAU, Coimbatore.

Chapter 7
Antioxidants as Functional Foods in Metabolic Syndrome

Abishek B. Santhakumar
Charles Sturt University, Australia

Indu Singh
Griffith University, Australia

ABSTRACT

In the recent years, there has been a great deal of attention in investigating the disease preventive properties of functional foods. Particularly, impact of the antioxidant property of functional foods in reducing the risk or progression of chronic diseases has gained considerable interest amongst researchers and practitioners. Free radicals such as reactive oxygen species are generated in the body by exposure to a number of physiochemical or pathological mechanisms. It is imperative to preserve a balance between the levels of free radicals and antioxidants for routine physiological function, a disparity of which would accelerate oxidative stress. Increased oxidative stress and associated consequences in metabolic disorders such as obesity, cardiovascular diseases and diabetes has warranted the need for exogenous antioxidant concentrates derived from natural foods to alleviate the adverse effects. This chapter provides an overview on the efficacy of functional foods in reducing free radical-mediated damage in metabolic syndrome.

DOI: 10.4018/978-1-5225-0607-2.ch007

INTRODUCTION

Food not only provides the essential nutrients needed for life but also other bioactive components necessary for disease prevention and maintenance of good health. Elaborate research on the role of physiologically active food components derived from plants (phytochemicals) and animal (zoochemicals) have led to the development of a new class of foods known as functional foods. The term functional foods was first introduced in Japan during the mid-1980s and were known as Foods for Specified Health Use (FOSHU), which comprised foods that would enhance human health, in addition to being nutritious. For this reason, functional foods are defined as a group of foods or food ingredients that have a beneficial effect on human health and/or help in reducing the risk of chronic disorders beyond the widely accepted nutritional functions.

Metabolic syndrome is a collection of at least three of five precursors such as high fasting glucose, elevated triacylglycerol, high blood pressure, low high density lipoprotein (HDL) or abdominal obesity (Ford, Giles, & Dietz, 2002). Metabolic syndrome is associated with the risk of developing chronic conditions such as diabetes, cardiovascular diseases and obesity which are major health concerns in developed as well as developing nations (Alberti, Zimmet, Shaw, & Group, 2005). Oxidative stress plays one of the central roles in the pathogenesis of such conditions. Extensive research during the past decade has demonstrated that free radicals, particularly, reactive oxygen species (ROS) and reactive nitrogen species (RNS) are an important contributor to the damage caused by oxidative stress (Apel & Hirt, 2004). There is increased oxidative stress due to conditions such as diabetes, which impairs muscle glucose uptake, by damaging the blood vessel walls by oxidising lipids and in turn activating platelets resulting in thrombosis and other cardiac complications (Maritim, Sanders & Watkins, 2003). We will discuss this mechanism in detail later in the chapter. The results of many epidemiological studies have demonstrated a protective role of antioxidants through a diet rich in fruits and vegetables against the development and progression of metabolic syndromes. We will now deliberate the role of antioxidants as functional foods in reducing oxidative stress thereby reducing the risk or progression of metabolic dysfunction.

FREE RADICALS AND OXIDATIVE STRESS

A chemical reaction in which the electrons get transferred from a substance to an oxidizing agent is known as oxidation, which in turn produces free radicals (any independently existing chemical species having one or more unpaired electrons), which produced in excess, ultimately results in oxidative stress. Oxidation reactions are an essential part of normal metabolism as oxygen is the ultimate electron acceptor in the electron flow system that produces adenosine triphosphate – ATP, source of energy in body. Problems may arise when electron flow and energy production become uncoupled followed by the increased production of oxygen free radicals like ROS. It is a known fact that molecular oxygen can be reduced to water. The intermediate steps involved in this reduction of molecular oxygen are the formation of free radicals such as superoxide anions, hydrogen peroxide and hydroxyl radicals. Once these radicals are formed, they can react with each other or with another molecule depending on its concentration. The increase in such pro-oxidants is directly involved in pathogenesis or as a result of an aerobic metabolic process. The body continually battles to maintain levels of pro-oxidants and antioxidants to reduce the occurrence of chronic diseases. Nevertheless, reduced concentration of endogenous antioxidants to neutralise the released free radicals results in severe oxidative stress consequently leading to cell damage and death.

All forms of life maintain a reducing environment within their cells. Enzymes that maintain the reduced state through a constant input of metabolic energy preserve the cellular redox environment. Disturbances in this normal redox state can cause toxic effects through the production of peroxidase and free radicals that damage components of the cell such as lipids and DNA. ROS are continuously produced within the cell as a result of mitochondrial electron transfer processes or as byproducts of the activity of enzymes including xanthine oxidase (catalyze the oxidation of xanthine to uric acid), lipoxygenases (catalyze polyunsaturated fatty acids to lipoxidase) and cyclooxygenases (involved in platelet activation and inflammation) (Szocs, 2004). They can also be generated as a consequence of the intracellular metabolism of foreign compounds, toxins, drugs or because of exposure to environmental factors such as excessive iron salts or ultraviolet radiation (Ichihashi et al., 2003). External sources of oxidative stress include ageing, smoking, alcohol consumption, and environmental pollution, all of which increase production of free radicals more than required for normal body metabolism. Endogenous antioxidants are hence not sufficient to neutralize them. Other sources of ROS are activated white blood cells such as macrophages and neutrophils that contain membrane bound enzymes, like nicotinamide adenine dinucleotide phosphate-oxidase (NADPH) oxidase complex, which are able to generate superoxide radicals and hydrogen peroxide (Rosen, Pou, Ramos, Cohen, & Britigan, 1995). ROS play various constructive roles *in vivo*, being involved in energy production, phagocytosis, cell growth and intercellular signaling regulation. However, they may also be highly damaging, as they can attack biological macromolecules, namely, lipids, proteins and DNA; induce oxidation and cause membrane damage, enzyme inactivation; and DNA damage (Halliwell & Gutteridge, 1999; Valko, Izakovic, Mazur, Rhodes, & Telser, 2004). ROS include free radicals such as superoxide ($^{\bullet}O_2^-$), hydroxyl ($^{\bullet}OH$), peroxyl ($^{\bullet}RO_2$), hydroperoxyl ($^{\bullet}HRO_2^-$)

as well as nonradical species such as hydrogen peroxide (H_2O_2) and hydrochlorous acid (HOCl). RNS include free radicals like nitric oxide (•NO) and nitrogen dioxide ($•NO_2^-$), as well as nonradicals such as peroxynitrite ($ONOO^-$), nitrous oxide (HNO_2) and alkyl peroxynitrates (RONOO). Of these reactive molecules, $•O_2^-$, •NO and $ONOO^-$ are the most widely studied species and play important roles in the obesity, diabetes related cardiovascular complications. Possible exogenous routes of alleviation of such damage caused due to free radicals will now be discussed.

ANTIOXIDANTS AS FUNCTIONAL FOODS

The term "antioxidant" refers to any molecule capable of stabilizing or deactivating free radicals before they attack cells. These are the primary antioxidants. There are also molecules deserving the "antioxidant" term, because they act as chelating agents binding metal ions – redox activity (Percival, 1998). This chapter will focus on specific natural dietary antioxidant functional foods e.g. polyphenols, which may be instrumental in the reduction of metabolic disorders.

Polyphenols are a class of phytochemical functional components present in abundance in a variety of both plant and animal diets. The foods rich in polyphenols include berries, apples, grapes, plums, pears, and vegetables such as celery, parsley, cabbage and more. They are also present in high concentrations in tea and wine. Significant research interest has developed over the years to evaluate the potential of polyphenol compounds as antioxidant functional foods in reducing the risk or side effects of metabolic disorders. This information is also backed up by strong evidence in literature emphasizing on the protective effects of phenolic compounds (Gammon et al., 2013; Giampieri et al., 2015; Norberto et al., 2013; Abishek Bommannan Santhakumar et al., 2015; Singh, Turner, Sinclair, Li, & Hawley, 2007; Yao, Xu, Zhang, & Lu, 2013). Table 1 outlines the common fruits and vegetables known to contain large quantities of phenolic or bioactive compounds and encompasses disease preventative properties.

STRUCTURE OF PHENOLIC FUNCTIONAL FOODS

It has been established that there are more than 8000 phenolic structures out of which 4000 have been identified as flavonoids. Though polyphenols are chemically characterised as plant phenolics based on the phenolic structure these compounds possess, there are many subdivisions or subgroups of phenolic compounds. In addition, polyphenols have also been classified subject to its biological function and source of origin. On the basis of structure alone, they are broadly classified as

Table 1. Common functional foods and their bioactive ingredients

Functional Food	Functional Component	Physiologic Effect
Broccoli	Sulforaphen, diindolylmethane, flavonols	Anti-carcinogenic, DNA repair
Olive leaf	Oleuropein, hydroxytyrosol, other polyphenols	Anti-thrombotic, anti-ageing, anti-inflammatory
Kiwifruit seed oil	Omega-3 fatty acid	Anti-thrombotic, anti-inflammatory, anti-proliferative
Berries	Flavonoids (anthocyanin), other polyphenols, phenolic acids	Anti-thrombotic, anti-inflammatory, anti-ageing
Turmeric	Curcumin	Anti-microbial, anti-inflammatory, anti-fungal
Plums & prunes	Flavonoids (anthocyanin), other polyphenols	Anti-thrombotic, anti-inflammatory
Grapes, wine	Flavonoids, resveratrol	Anti-thrombotic, lipid lowering, neuro-protective
Purple carrot	Anthocyanins, other polyphenols	Anti-inflammatory, lipid lowering
Garlic, onion,	Allyl sulphur, quercetin	Anti-diabetic
Green tea, black tea	Catechins, polyphenols, quercetin	Anti-atheromatous, anti-thrombotic, improves endothelial function, anti-proliferative
Parsley, Celery	Flavones	Anti-inflammatory, lipid lowering
Ginseng	Eleutherosides	Anti-diabetic
Grapefruit	Flavanones	Lipid lowering, anti-microbial
Chia seeds	Flavonol aglycones/kaempferol	Reduction in lipid peroxidation

phenolic acids, flavonoids, polyphenolic amides and other polyphenols. Phenolic acids are further classified as cinnamic acid or benzoic acid derivatives. Flavonoids possess a C6-C3-C6 structural backbone (Figure 1) with the two C6 units (Ring A and Ring B) having a phenolic nature while polyphenolic amides have an N-containing functional substituent attached. Variations in the chromane ring (Ring C) are responsible for further subdivisions as anthocyanins, flavonols, flavanones or flavones (Tsao, 2010). The above mentioned structural properties are strongly linked to their *in vivo* functional capabilities such as antioxidant activities. Polyphenol by virtue of its structural and functional moieties suppress the generation of free radicals by blunting the active species and precursors of free radicals. More frequently they act as chain breakers i.e. by acting as direct scavengers in lipid peroxidation reactions by donating an electron to the free radical and becoming stable. In addition to its role in free radical scavenging, they also play an important role in the chelation of metal ions. For example, chelation of metal ions such as Fe^{2+} by polyphenols re-

Figure 1. Backbone structure of phenolic functional foods

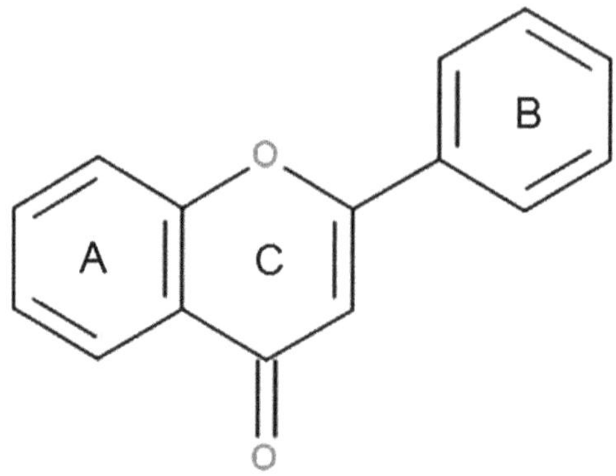

duces oxidation caused by hydroxyl radicals (Kim, Ham, Shigenaga, & Han, 2008). It is therefore important to understand the mechanism/s underlying oxidative-stress induced metabolic dysfunction to investigate the structure-activity relationship.

OXIDATIVE STRESS IN METABOLIC DISORDERS

Increasing evidence suggests the involvement of oxidative stress in the pathogenesis of metabolic conditions such as diabetes (type 1 and 2) and obesity. Oxidation of glucose, glycation of proteins and the oxidative degradation of the glycated proteins are responsible for the disproportionate formation of free radicals in diabetes (Maritim, Sanders, & Watkins, 2003). Imbalance in antioxidant defence and free radical production leads to cellular and enzymatic damage, increased lipid peroxidation and progression of insulin resistance. The oxidative stress related changes *in vivo* in diabetes can be effectively measured by evaluating biomarkers of oxidative stress such as lipid peroxidation, glutathione levels, superoxide dismutase, non-enzymatic glycosylated proteins etc. (Maritim et al., 2003).

Although the outstanding pathological feature in cardiovascular disease is the deposition of cholesterol esters from lipoproteins in arteries, the circulating concentrations of these lipoproteins remain a poor predictor of the disease. This has encouraged research into finding the pathological mechanisms or stimulant in facilitating the deposition of these lipoproteins in the vascular intima. Most of the cholesterol in atherosclerotic lesions is made up of low density lipoproteins (LDL). Oxidatively modified form of LDL (ox-LDL) is susceptible to macrophage attack and conversion to cholesterol-laden foam cells, a characteristic early histological evidence of atherosclerosis. Especially in obesity, circulating ox-LDL is considerably increased accelerating this process (Van Guilder, Hoetzer, Greiner, Stauffer,

& Desouza, 2006). The bioactive inner layer of vasculature, endothelium, is important in maintaining hemostasis or regulating vascular tone permeability. ROS have been implicated in several mechanisms in contributing to endothelial dysfunction, for example, in reduction of nitric oxide, a potent vasodilator (Wink et al., 1993). Figure 2 shows the mechanism of involvement of free radicals in the pathogenesis of metabolic disorders such as obesity, diabetes and cardiovascular diseases.

Functional Foods in Obesity-Related Vascular Dysfunction

The alarming increase in the number of overweight and obese individuals is recognised as one of the serious growing public health concerns. Overweight and obese individuals are associated with significantly increased mortality rate from cardiovascular disorders, strokes. In addition to hyperlipidaemia, the additional risk factors in such individuals include smoking, diabetes, hypertension and other metabolic conditions (A. B. Santhakumar, Bulmer, & Singh, 2014). Besides obesity's association with cardiovascular diseases, evidence from clinical and epidemiological studies has established its link with insulin resistance and diabetes. The mechanistic understanding of the relationship between obesity and metabolic disorders has been a widely debated topic. Oxidative stress either systemically or within vasculature is one of the hypotheses to explain the progression of vascular dysfunction (arterial and venous) in humans. Lipid peroxidation is considered as a major contributor to the development of atherosclerotic plaque inside arteries (Lakshmi, Padmaja, Kup-

Figure 2. Underlying mechanism in oxidative stress induced metabolic dysfunction

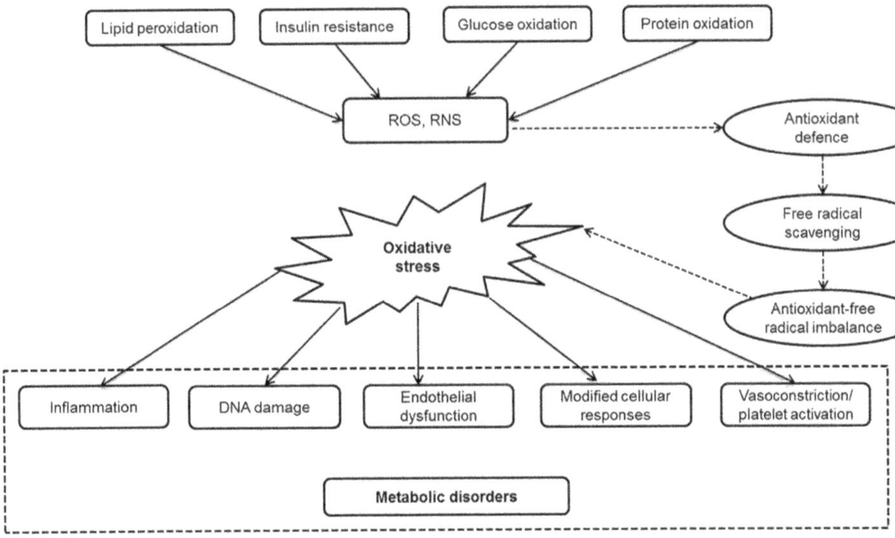

pusamy, & Kutala, 2009). The oxidised lipids derived from increased plasma LDL deposits on atherosclerotic lesions consequently lead to vessel occlusion. Other contributing factors to the build-up of the plaque in addition to oxidation of LDL are platelet hyper-activation/aggregation, tissue factor expression, impaired fibrinolysis, increased cytokine production including tumour necrosis factor, and other oxidative enzymes inside the vasculature. Figure 3 elucidates the mechanisms involved in the progression of atherosclerotic plaques and thrombosis in general during increased oxidative stress states such as in obesity or dyslipidaemia.

Some of the common functional foods or ingredients associated with improvement of body weight regulation include: fibre-rich food, low glycaemic index starchy food, caffeine, capsaicin, green tea, nuts, non-caloric sweeteners, and nuts. Some of the target functions of such foods are satiety, energy intake, body fat, and energy expenditure (Myrie, Jones, & Saarela, 2011). Functional foods rich in polyphenols have been demonstrated to reduce the progression of atherosclerosis or thrombus formation by virtue of its antioxidant property. The different target pathways utilised by polyphenols include:

Figure 3. Atherosclerotic progression in metabolic disorders. The major instigators of atherosclerotic plaque development are a) increased lipid peroxidation due to increased circulatory free fatty acids, b) cholesterol-laden foam cells, c) platelet activation and aggregation, and d) release of inflammatory cytokines. ox-LDL, oxidative-low density lipoprotein; IL-6, interleukin-6; TNF-α, tumour necrosis factor-α; EC, endothelial cells; RBC, red blood cells

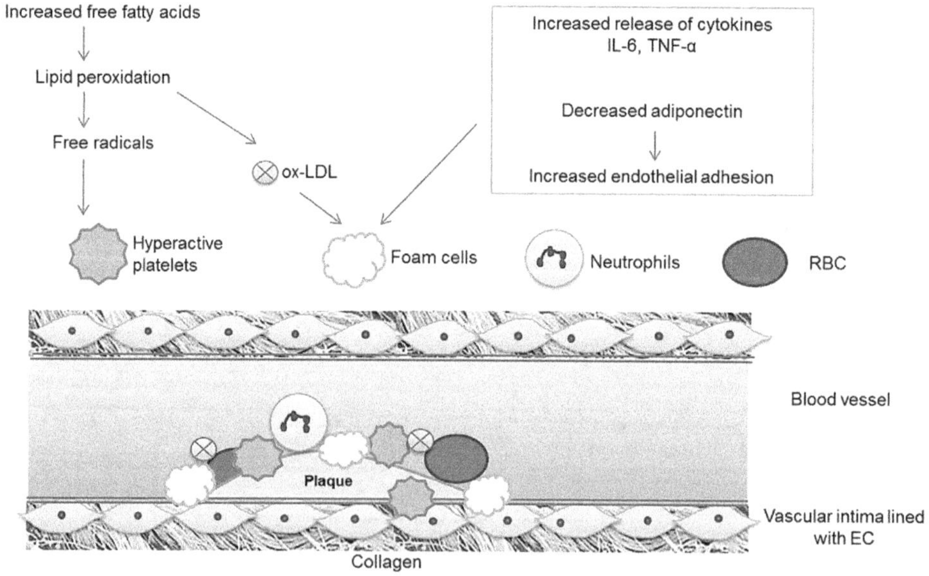

1. **Reduction of Foam Cell Formation:** By alleviating free radical mediated increase in ox-LDL and by down-regulation of CD36, the macrophage scavenger receptor (Lakshmi et al., 2009)
2. **Reduction of Platelet Hyperactivity:** By blunting platelet activation receptors on platelet surface, inhibition of platelet aggregation (Alvarez-Suarez et al., 2014; Duttaroy & Jorgensen, 2004; Erlund et al., 2008; Abishek Bommannan Santhakumar et al., 2015)
3. **Reduction of Inflammation:** By lowering inflammatory cytokines, increasing adiponectin, and endothelial nitric oxide synthase (Biesalski, 2007)
4. **Reduction of Fibrinogen Levels:** By potentially blunting tissue factor activation (Di Santo et al., 2003)

Functional Foods in Diabetes

Diabetes especially type 2 diabetes mellitus (T2DM) is one of the fastest growing endocrine disorders causing public health concern worldwide. Genetic background and environmental influences such as sedentary life style and diet, promotes insulin resistance and is considered as an early manifestation to diabetes. Diabetes-induced metabolic dysfunction induces platelet hyper-activation, release of pro-inflammatory cytokines, activation of endothelial cells through increased oxidative stress and non-enzymatic oxidation of fatty acids and glycation compounds (Maritim et al., 2003; A. B. Santhakumar et al., 2014). Increased free radical production also results in protein kinase C (PKC – an enzyme involved in several signal transduction cascades) isoform activation, thereby reducing the production of potent vasodilators such as nitric oxide and endothelial nitric oxide synthase (eNOS) (Ganz & Seftel, 2000).

It has been suggested by a number of dietary intervention trials that 90% of T2DM cases can be prevented by increasing physical activity, consumption of a diet rich in antioxidants and moderate weight loss. However, mechanistic and physiological involvement of functional foods in reducing incidence of diabetes or its complications is still a widely debated topic. Some of the examples of functional foods or ingredients that can potentially be considered for improving insulin sensitivity and glucose metabolism include: low glycaemic index starchy foods, wholegrain, low-saturated fat foods, fruits and vegetables rich in antioxidants and polyphenols (Myrie et al., 2011). Benefits of polyphenols in T2DM have generally been attributed to its broad antioxidant activity and its ability to blunt signalling proteins (Manach, Scalbert, Morand, Remesy, & Jimenez, 2004; Pandey & Rizvi, 2009). In addition to this, several *in vitro* trials have identified its potential in modulating metabolic enzymes, gene expression, simultaneous signalling pathways and nuclear receptors (Maritim et al., 2003). Phenolic functional foods have been associated with alleviating fasting and postprandial hyperglycaemia by moderating disaccharides such as α-amylase and α-glucosidase hence limiting polysaccharide digestion consequently reducing the absorption of simple sugars (Matsui et al., 2002). In addition, phenolic foods have been instrumental in:

1. Improving glucose uptake by intestinal epithelial cells (Johnston, Sharp, Clifford, & Morgan, 2005).
2. Promoting hepatic glucokinase activity which promotes glucose utilisation (Hanhineva et al., 2010).
3. Protecting pancreatic β-cells from gluco-toxicity (Lapidot, Walker, & Kanner, 2002) .
4. Improving insulin secretion (Jayaprakasam, Vareed, Olson, & Nair, 2005).

Phenolic compounds such as catechins, epi-catechins, isoflavones, tannic acid and chlorogenic acid have been associated with reducing S-Glut-1 mediated intestinal transport of glucose (Dembinska-Kiec, Mykkanen, Kiec-Wilk, & Mykkanen, 2008). Resveratrol, a phenolic compound has been shown to significantly reduce diabetic associated changes in the kidney and improve renal function in diabetic rats (Chen, Chi, Chuang, & Su, 2007). Quercetin in a recent study also exhibited protective effects on lipid peroxidation and inhibition of antioxidant system in diabetics (Mishra & Rizvi, 2012). Ferulic acid abundant in fruits and vegetables has been associated with anti-diabetic activity by lowering blood glucose and significantly increasing plasma insulin levels (Jung, Kim, Hwang, & Ha, 2007).

BIOAVAILABILITY

Bioavailability is the amount or proportion of a nutrient that is digested, absorbed and metabolised through regular biochemical pathways. The bioavailability of functional foods greatly varies and is independent of the amount ingested. The most abundant functional food in our day to day diet does not necessarily have the best biochemical profile. There are a number of factors which are responsible for affecting the bioavailability of these foods.

1. The native form of the nutrient is an important consideration. For e.g. majority of the polyphenols are present in the form of glycosides or esters and cannot be readily absorbed. They will have to be broken down by intestinal microflora or gastric secretions before being absorbed by the gastric epithelium. Furthermore, during the process of absorption, the phenolic functional foods undergo extensive modifications (glucuronidation, sulfation, and methylation) making it challenging to identify all the active metabolites to accurately measure

its biological activity. Hence, it is the chemical structure and composition that decides on the bioavailability, extent of absorption and not its concentration.

2. Site of absorption is another important factor to consider when evaluating the bioavailability of phenolic functional foods *in vivo*. Some compounds are well absorbed in the gastric epithelium while others in different sites of the digestive tract (D'Archivio, Filesi, Vari, Scazzocchio, & Masella, 2010).
3. Interaction with other compounds in the diet such as fats, alcohol, proteins, and carbohydrates can affect their absorption potential. Metabolites of phenolic foods circulate in the blood bound to proteins, particularly albumin. This binding is strongly dependant on the chemical structure of the functional phenolic. Therefore, this binding could possibly have consequences on the rate of clearance and regulation to tissues and cells (Manach et al., 2004). Interaction with certain therapeutics, particularly cholesterol lowering or hypertension drugs has negative consequences by generation of harmful intermediates and modifying bioavailability (Galli, 2007).
4. Host-related factors such as intestinal dysfunction or systemic conditions.
5. Other external factors such as environment, rainfall, yield, type of culture, and processing can affect the overall content of functional components.

The accumulation and concentration of phenolic functional foods into tissues and cells is vital to confer their disease preventative properties. Polyphenols are known to penetrate cells and tissues of the liver and intestine. The excretion of phenolic foods has been observed to be through both bile, in the case of large conjugated metabolites, and urine for smaller conjugates. Both, amount of ingestion and bioavailability is essential for functional foods to exert its health beneficial properties.

BIOMARKERS

Implementation of multiple long term dietary intervention trials to establish the health promoting properties of a particular functional food is neither cost effective nor feasible. Hence, standardised methods to evaluate its merits need to be established. Identification of reliable and sensitive biomarkers will be valuable in adequately evaluating the true effect of foods or its components/metabolites and for identifying diseases where oxidative stress in involved. A biomarker should be able to a) identify biological changes in response to intake or changes to physiology or exposure b) calculate the modification of a particular analyte or tissue within the physiology hence leading to change in health or disease risk. This is easier said than done due to a number of impeding factors such as retention time, maximum bioavailable concentration, and other factors discussed in the previous bioavailability section.

In general, the most effective biomarkers demonstrated are the ones with a long-term consequence such as reduction in disease risk or improvement in health status. However a few markers may be immediate such as those associated with mental or physical performance. Several invasive and semi-invasive means of evaluating oxidative stress are available such as tissue biopsies, plasma, urine, cerebrospinal fluid and synovial fluid (Dalle-Donne, Rossi, Colombo, Giustarini, & Milzani, 2006). Due to the difficulty in obtaining invasive samples such as cerebrospinal or synovial fluid, recent studies have focussed on non-invasive procedures to assess oxidative stress biomarkers. Plasma or urine biomarkers of oxidative stress such as malondialdehyde, glutathione, iso-prostanes and acrolein have been instrumental in the diagnosis of a number of oxidative stress related pathological conditions (Dalle-Donne et al., 2006). It has also been extensively used as a biomarker of oxidative stress post functional food consumption to evaluate its free radical scavenging properties and to assess its ability in reducing the risk factors leading to metabolic syndromes. Exhaled breath condensate has also been recently used to assess oxidative stress related inflammatory lung diseases (Carpagnano et al., 2003). The development of new, more accurate oxidative stress biomarkers is limited due to the easy access to tissues in patient cohorts hence restricting research to animal models.

Therefore successful development of antioxidant therapeutics to reduce the risk of oxidative stress mediated metabolic disorders remains a key objective.

FUTURE RESEARCH DIRECTIONS

Development of successful antioxidant therapies for metabolic disease prevention is crucial, the attainment of which is possible through large-scale, controlled, randomised dietary intervention and epidemiological trials. Some of the considerations include:

1. Understanding the pharmacokinetics and bioavailability of functional food intake in the population being studied to evaluate its protective effects.
2. Choice of accurate biomarkers to reflect, validate or disprove the scientific analysis.
3. In-depth understanding of the underlying mechanism of action of the functional food under study.
4. Potential interactions with other food components and metabolic enzymes or co-factors.
5. Designing *in vitro* or pilot trials to reflect physiologically attainable concentrations.
6. Consideration of genetic, environmental and technologic factors.
7. Processing of the dietary products to retain maximum effective concentration of active antioxidants.

CONCLUSION

Increasing evidence continues to emerge that the consumption of functional foods or its constituents have profound physiological and disease preventative effects. Nevertheless, it should be considered that these functional foods or its components need to be considered as a fraction of a nutritious diet and not in isolation. In spite of these foods exhibiting disease lowering effects, or health promoting benefits, they cannot be considered as the gold standard in associated treatment. Considerable interest needs to be instigated on the benefits of functional foods as complementary therapy thereby reducing side-effects or resistance to certain drugs. Strategies should be devised to enhance the understanding of consumers that there is no food as good or bad, but only good or bad diets. As new discoveries are made in this area, the updated information needs to appropriately reach consumers in order to make informed decisions.

REFERENCES

Alberti, K. G. M., Zimmet, P., Shaw, J., & Group, I. E. T. F. C. (2005). The metabolic syndrome—a new worldwide definition. *Lancet*, *366*(9491), 1059–1062. doi:10.1016/S0140-6736(05)67402-8 PMID:16182882

Alvarez-Suarez, J. M., Giampieri, F., Tulipani, S., Casoli, T., Di Stefano, G., Gonzalez-Paramas, A. M., & Battino, M. (2014). One-month strawberry-rich anthocyanin supplementation ameliorates cardiovascular risk, oxidative stress markers and platelet activation in humans. *The Journal of Nutritional Biochemistry*, *25*(3), 289–294. doi:10.1016/j.jnutbio.2013.11.002 PMID:24406274

Apel, K., & Hirt, H. (2004). Reactive oxygen species: Metabolism, oxidative stress, and signal transduction. *Annual Review of Plant Biology*, *55*(1), 373–399. doi:10.1146/annurev.arplant.55.031903.141701 PMID:15377225

Biesalski, H. K. (2007). Polyphenols and inflammation: Basic interactions. *Current Opinion in Clinical Nutrition and Metabolic Care*, *10*(6), 724–728. doi:10.1097/MCO.0b013e3282f0cef2 PMID:18089954

Carpagnano, G. E., Kharitonov, S. A., Resta, O., Foschino-Barbaro, M. P., Gramiccioni, E., & Barnes, P. J. (2003). 8-Isoprostane, a marker of oxidative stress, is increased in exhaled breath condensate of patients with obstructive sleep apnea after night and is reduced by continuous positive airway pressure therapy. *Chest*, *124*(4), 1386–1392. doi:10.1378/chest.124.4.1386 PMID:14555570

Chen, W. P., Chi, T. C., Chuang, L. M., & Su, M. J. (2007). Resveratrol enhances insulin secretion by blocking K(ATP) and K(V) channels of beta cells. *European Journal of Pharmacology*, *568*(1-3), 269–277. doi:10.1016/j.ejphar.2007.04.062 PMID:17573071

D'Archivio, M., Filesi, C., Vari, R., Scazzocchio, B., & Masella, R. (2010). Bioavailability of the polyphenols: Status and controversies. *International Journal of Molecular Sciences*, *11*(4), 1321–1342. doi:10.3390/ijms11041321 PMID:20480022

Dalle-Donne, I., Rossi, R., Colombo, R., Giustarini, D., & Milzani, A. (2006). Biomarkers of oxidative damage in human disease. *Clinical Chemistry*, *52*(4), 601–623. doi:10.1373/clinchem.2005.061408 PMID:16484333

Dembinska-Kiec, A., Mykkanen, O., Kiec-Wilk, B., & Mykkanen, H. (2008). Antioxidant phytochemicals against type 2 diabetes. *British Journal of Nutrition, 99*, ES109-117.

Di Santo, A., Mezzetti, A., Napoleone, E., Di Tommaso, R., Donati, M. B., De Gaetano, G., & Lorenzet, R. (2003). Resveratrol and quercetin down-regulate tissue factor expression by human stimulated vascular cells. *Journal of Thrombosis and Haemostasis*, *1*(5), 1089–1095. doi:10.1046/j.1538-7836.2003.00217.x PMID:12871381

Duttaroy, A. K., & Jorgensen, A. (2004). Effects of kiwi fruit consumption on platelet aggregation and plasma lipids in healthy human volunteers. *Platelets*, *15*(5), 287–292. doi:10.1080/09537100410001710290 PMID:15370099

Erlund, I., Koli, R., Alfthan, G., Marniemi, J., Puukka, P., Mustonen, P., & Jula, A. et al. (2008). Favorable effects of berry consumption on platelet function, blood pressure, and HDL cholesterol. *The American Journal of Clinical Nutrition*, *87*(2), 323–331. PMID:18258621

Ford, E. S., Giles, W. H., & Dietz, W. H. (2002). Prevalence of the metabolic syndrome among US adults: Findings from the third National Health and Nutrition Examination Survey. *Journal of the American Medical Association*, *287*(3), 356–359. doi:10.1001/jama.287.3.356 PMID:11790215

Galli, F. (2007). Interactions of polyphenolic compounds with drug disposition and metabolism. *Current Drug Metabolism*, *8*(8), 830–838. doi:10.2174/138920007782798180 PMID:18220564

Gammon, C. S., Kruger, R., Minihane, A. M., Conlon, C. A., von Hurst, P. R., & Stonehouse, W. (2013). Kiwifruit consumption favourably affects plasma lipids in a randomised controlled trial in hypercholesterolaemic men. *The British Journal of Nutrition*, *109*(12), 2208–2218. doi:10.1017/S0007114512004400 PMID:23151354

Ganz, M. B., & Seftel, A. (2000). Glucose-induced changes in protein kinase C and nitric oxide are prevented by vitamin E. *American Journal of Physiology. Endocrinology and Metabolism*, *278*(1), E146–E152. PMID:10644549

Giampieri, F., Forbes-Hernandez, T. Y., Gasparrini, M., Alvarez-Suarez, J. M., Afrin, S., Bompadre, S., & Battino, M. et al. (2015). Strawberry as a health promoter: An evidence based review. *Food & Function*, *6*(5), 1386–1398. doi:10.1039/C5FO00147A PMID:25803191

Halliwell, B., & Gutteridge, J. M. C. (1999). Free radicals in biology and medicine. In Free radicals in biology and medicine (3rd ed.). Clarendon Press.

Hanhineva, K., Torronen, R., Bondia-Pons, I., Pekkinen, J., Kolehmainen, M., Mykkanen, H., & Poutanen, K. (2010). Impact of dietary polyphenols on carbohydrate metabolism. *International Journal of Molecular Sciences*, *11*(4), 1365–1402. doi:10.3390/ijms11041365 PMID:20480025

Ichihashi, M., Ueda, M., Budiyanto, A., Bito, T., Oka, M., Fukunaga, M., & Horikawa, T. et al. (2003). UV-induced skin damage. *Toxicology*, *189*(1-2), 21–39. doi:10.1016/S0300-483X(03)00150-1 PMID:12821280

Jayaprakasam, B., Vareed, S. K., Olson, L. K., & Nair, M. G. (2005). Insulin secretion by bioactive anthocyanins and anthocyanidins present in fruits. *Journal of Agricultural and Food Chemistry*, *53*(1), 28–31. doi:10.1021/jf049018+ PMID:15631504

Johnston, K., Sharp, P., Clifford, M., & Morgan, L. (2005). Dietary polyphenols decrease glucose uptake by human intestinal Caco-2 cells. *FEBS Letters*, *579*(7), 1653–1657. doi:10.1016/j.febslet.2004.12.099 PMID:15757656

Jung, E. H., Kim, S. R., Hwang, I. K., & Ha, T. Y. (2007). Hypoglycemic effects of a phenolic acid fraction of rice bran and ferulic acid in C57BL/KsJ-db/db mice. *Journal of Agricultural and Food Chemistry*, *55*(24), 9800–9804. doi:10.1021/jf0714463 PMID:17973443

Kim, E. Y., Ham, S. K., Shigenaga, M. K., & Han, O. (2008). Bioactive dietary polyphenolic compounds reduce nonheme iron transport across human intestinal cell monolayers. *The Journal of Nutrition*, *138*(9), 1647–1651. PMID:18716164

Lakshmi, S. V., Padmaja, G., Kuppusamy, P., & Kutala, V. K. (2009). Oxidative stress in cardiovascular disease. *Indian Journal of Biochemistry & Biophysics*, *46*(6), 421–440. PMID:20361706

Lapidot, T., Walker, M. D., & Kanner, J. (2002). Antioxidant and prooxidant effects of phenolics on pancreatic β-cells in vitro. *Journal of Agricultural and Food Chemistry*, *50*(25), 7220–7225. doi:10.1021/jf020615a PMID:12452635

Manach, C., Scalbert, A., Morand, C., Remesy, C., & Jimenez, L. (2004). Polyphenols: Food sources and bioavailability. *The American Journal of Clinical Nutrition*, *79*(5), 727–747. PMID:15113710

Maritim, A. C., Sanders, R. A., & Watkins, J. B. III. (2003). Diabetes, oxidative stress, and antioxidants: A review. *Journal of Biochemical and Molecular Toxicology*, *17*(1), 24–38. doi:10.1002/jbt.10058 PMID:12616644

Matsui, T., Ebuchi, S., Kobayashi, M., Fukui, K., Sugita, K., Terahara, N., & Matsumoto, K. (2002). Anti-hyperglycemic effect of diacylated anthocyanin derived from Ipomoea batatas cultivar Ayamurasaki can be achieved through the alpha-glucosidase inhibitory action. *Journal of Agricultural and Food Chemistry*, *50*(25), 7244–7248. doi:10.1021/jf025913m PMID:12452639

Mishra, N., & Rizvi, S. I. (2012). Quercetin modulates Na(+)/K(+) ATPase and sodium hydrogen exchanger in type 2 diabetic erythrocytes. *Cellular and Molecular Biology (Noisy-Le-Grand)*, *58*(1), 148–152. PMID:23273205

Myrie, S., Jones, P., & Saarela, M. (2011). Functional foods and obesity. In *Functional foods: concept to product*, (pp. 234-260).

Norberto, S., Silva, S., Meireles, M., Faria, A., Pintado, M., & Calhau, C. (2013). Blueberry anthocyanins in health promotion: A metabolic overview. *Journal of Functional Foods*, *5*(4), 1518–1528. doi:10.1016/j.jff.2013.08.015

Pandey, K. B., & Rizvi, S. I. (2009). Plant polyphenols as dietary antioxidants in human health and disease. *Oxidative Medicine and Cellular Longevity*, *2*(5), 270–278. doi:10.4161/oxim.2.5.9498 PMID:20716914

Percival, M. (1998). Antioxidants. *Clinical Nutrition Insight*, *31*, 1–4.

Rosen, G. M., Pou, S., Ramos, C. L., Cohen, M. S., & Britigan, B. E. (1995). Free radicals and phagocytic cells. *The FASEB Journal*, *9*, 200–209. PMID:7540156

Santhakumar, A. B., Bulmer, A. C., & Singh, I. (2014). A review of the mechanisms and effectiveness of dietary polyphenols in reducing oxidative stress and thrombotic risk. *Journal of Human Nutrition and Dietetics*, *27*(1), 1–21. doi:10.1111/jhn.12177 PMID:24205990

Santhakumar, A. B., Kundur, A. R., Fanning, K., Netzel, M., Stanley, R., & Singh, I. (2015). Consumption of anthocyanin-rich Queen Garnet plum juice reduces platelet activation related thrombogenesis in healthy volunteers. *Journal of Functional Foods*, *12*(0), 11–22. doi:10.1016/j.jff.2014.10.026

Singh, I., Turner, A. H., Sinclair, A. J., Li, D., & Hawley, J. A. (2007). Effects of gamma-tocopherol supplementation on thrombotic risk factors. *Asia Pacific Journal of Clinical Nutrition*, *16*(3), 422–428. PMID:17704022

Szocs, K. (2004). Endothelial dysfunction and reactive oxygen species production on ischemia/reperfusion and nitrate tolerance. *General Physiology and Biophysics*, *23*, 265–295. PMID:15638116

Tsao, R. (2010). Chemistry and biochemistry of dietary polyphenols. *Nutrients*, *2*(12), 1231–1246. doi:10.3390/nu2121231 PMID:22254006

Valko, M., Izakovic, M., Mazur, M., Rhodes, C. J., & Telser, J. (2004). Role of oxygen radicals in DNA damage and cancer incidence. *Molecular and Cellular Biochemistry*, *266*(1/2), 37–56. doi:10.1023/B:MCBI.0000049134.69131.89 PMID:15646026

Van Guilder, G. P., Hoetzer, G. L., Greiner, J. J., Stauffer, B. L., & Desouza, C. A. (2006). Influence of metabolic syndrome on biomarkers of oxidative stress and inflammation in obese adults. *Obesity (Silver Spring, Md.)*, *14*(12), 2127–2131. doi:10.1038/oby.2006.248 PMID:17189537

Wink, D. A., Hanbauer, I., Krishna, M. C., DeGraff, W., Gamson, J., & Mitchell, J. B. (1993). Nitric oxide protects against cellular damage and cytotoxicity from reactive oxygen species. *Proceedings of the National Academy of Sciences of the United States of America*, *90*(21), 9813–9817. doi:10.1073/pnas.90.21.9813 PMID:8234317

Yao, S.-L., Xu, Y., Zhang, Y.-Y., & Lu, Y.-H. (2013). Black rice and anthocyanins induce inhibition of cholesterol absorption in vitro. *Food & Function*, *4*(11), 1602–1608. doi:10.1039/c3fo60196j PMID:24056583

Chapter 8
Exploring the Potentials of Antioxidants in Retarding Ageing

Minu Kesheri
Shridhar University, India

Swarna Kanchan
Shridhar University – Pilani, India

Rajeshwar P. Sinha
Banaras Hindu University, India

ABSTRACT

In retrospect to the rise in the occurrence of ageing related disorders and the ever-lasting desire to overcome ageing, exploring the causes, mechanisms and therapies to curb ageing becomes relevant. Reactive Oxygen Species (ROS) are commonly generated during normal growth and development. However abiotic and biotic stresses enhance the level of ROS which in turn pose the threat of oxidative stress. Ability to perceive ROS and to speedily commence antioxidant defenses is crucial for the survival as well as longevity of living cells. Therefore living organisms are bestowed with antioxidants to combat the damages caused by oxidative stress. This chapter aims to elucidate an overview of the process of ageing, generation and enhancement of reactive oxygen species, damages incurred by oxidative stress, its amelioration strategies, therapeutic and biotechnological potentials of antioxidants and various sources of bioactive compounds significant in retardation of aging process.

DOI: 10.4018/978-1-5225-0607-2.ch008

INTRODUCTION

As postulated by the free radical theory of aging, exogenous administration of antioxidants may extend the lifespan of organisms provided that the main culprit behind the unavoidable aging is oxidative stress caused by imbalanced free radical reactions. Oxidative stress refers to the imbalance between oxidants and antioxidants in favor of oxidants. The term 'oxidative stress' may be visualized under four categories:

1. Enhanced ROS production leading to increased oxidative load;
2. The potential for uncontrolled oxidation due to rates of production exceeding rates of metabolism;
3. Oxidative damage to cellular components; causing
4. The buildup of injured cellular components that somehow lead to loss of function and eventual death (Foyer & Noctor, 2003).

Emergence of 'nutrigerontology', a new scientific discipline that encompasses biogerontology, medicine, and dietetics emphasizes the severity of the need to curb the increasing rise in prevalence of aging-related diseases in recent decades (Verburgh, 2015). Even if antioxidant supplementation is receiving growing attention and is increasingly adopted in western countries, supporting evidence is still scarce. Extensive exploration of literature is still needed for better evaluation of the potential benefits from antioxidant supplementation. Organisms with high adaptability and ubiquitous presence such as cyanobacteria are bestowed with arsenals against reactive oxygen species in order to cope with various endogenous as well as exogenous stresses comprising of four lines of defense mechanisms. First line of defense is avoidance strategy which includes mat formation, migration, alterations in morphology, enclosure of filaments in amorphous silica matrices and synthesis of extracellular polysaccharides. Second line of defense encompasses scavengers which includes enzymatic and non enzymatic antioxidants. The presence of enzymatic and non-enzymatic antioxidants as natural arsenal against multiple stresses has been reported in various cyanobacterial species at their natural habitat (Kesheri, Richa & Sinha, 2011; Kesheri, Kanchan, Richa & Sinha, 2014). Third line of defense includes screening by compounds such as biopterin glucoside and photoprotective compounds. Fourth line of defense comprises of repair and resynthesis mechanisms. An enhanced understanding of oxidation mechanisms pertaining to aging process would facilitate understanding the physiological and biochemical processes involved in ageing phenomenon. The determination of reliable markers of oxidative damage and antioxidant status is a burgeoning area of research demanding extensive exploration. Moreover literature regarding the identification of a therapeutic porthole in which an eventual antioxidant supplementation may be beneficial is also scarce and requires a deeper knowledge of the antioxidant molecules which in several conditions act as pro-oxidants. In the present chapter, after a preliminary introduction to the free radical theory of aging and the underlying principle of antioxidant supplementation as an anti-aging intervention, an outline of evidence relating antioxidant supplementations with clinical conditions characteristic of older age (cardiovascular disease, Alzheimer's disease, cancer, hyperlipidemia) will be discussed. Studies evaluating whether antioxidant supplementation might improve major outcomes of interest will also be explored. This chapter in a nutshell presents an overview of advanced as well as basic concepts regarding causes of ageing, generation of reactive oxygen species, causes of enhancement of free radicals, damages caused by increased oxidants and free radicals; amelioration strategies for oxidative stress; therapeutic and biotechnological potentials of antioxidants and various sources of bioactive compounds significant in retardation of aging process. Thus this chapter would surely enhance and help readers to understand the basics as well as advanced development in exploring the potentials of antioxidants in retarding ageing.

BACKGROUND

Biogerontological insights may be explored for dietary recommendations in order to retard the risk of various aging-related diseases that are on the rise in both developed and developing countries. There are numerous medical fields where aging-related diseases are common. Some of them are cardiology (atherosclerosis, diastolic dysfunction, ventricular hypertrophy, and high blood pressure), endocrinology (related with type 2 diabetes), neurology (dealing with Alzheimer's disease, stroke, and Parkinson's disease), ophthalmology (comprising of cataract, aging-related macular degeneration), oncology (mainly cancer), and rheumatology (dealing with osteoporosis, sarcopenia, frailty). It would be paramount to discuss about aging itself, and not only discussing aging-related diseases without emphasis on aging (biogerontology) and nutrigerontology (Verburgh, 2015).

Reactive oxygen species are commonly generated during normal growth and development. However abiotic and biotic stresses are known to increase the amount of ROS which consequently pose the threat to oxidative stress. Although aging is a multifactorial process, yet it has been observed that oxidative stress is one of the main factors influencing cellular longevity. Moreover, oxidative damage significantly contributes to factors which aid in the onset of age related degenerative diseases. The "Free Radical Theory of Aging" (Harman, 1956), commonly termed recently as the oxidative damage theory of ageing, seems to provide a crucial facet of inherent biological unsteadiness observed in living organisms (Kirkwood & Kowald 2012; Gladyshev, 2014). Factors influencing longevity has grown recently, thereby being the major reason of death associated with comorbidities connected to age and oxidative stress. Superoxide dismutase 2 (Mn-SOD or SOD2) has been shown to protect against oxidative stress, a main factor influencing cellular longevity (De Carvalho & De Mesquita, 2013). Therefore in retrospect to the benefits of mankind in the present scenario, it seems pertinent to explore the sources for mass production of antioxidants and other functional foods that serve for retarding the process of ageing. A better understanding of the aging process and subsequent practical, clinical, and nutritional arenas shall minimize healthcare expenses related with aging. It also increases working potential and amplifies economical competiveness.

AN OVERVIEW OF AGEING PROCESS

Aging, a sophisticated process of biology, can be described as the accumulation of various deleterious alterations occurring at cellular level with growing age that are responsible for the increased risk of disease and death. Aging is an inescapable natural process by which almost all (with few exceptions) multicellular organisms and unicellular organisms, including protozoa, yeast, and bacteria are known to be affected (Książek, 2010; Lin & Austriaco, 2014). In light of the aging population and the parallel rise in aging-related diseases, it becomes pertinent to explore the intriguing mechanisms, causes, consequences and their sources of mitigation.

Various existing theories pertaining to aging such as immune theory, nerve-endocrine theory and heredity theory are prevelant. However the most acknowledged theory among them is the free radical theory which states that free radicals, especially oxygen-derived free radicals such as $\bullet O_2^-$, $\bullet OH$ and H_2O_2, are the main culprit behind the damage of biomolecules resulting in alterations to the biology of the cell and thereby causing organismal aging. Two major pathways associated with aging process are the insulin/insulin-like growth factor signaling (IIS) pathway (Bartke, Sun & Longo, 2013) and mammalian or mechanistic target of rapamycin (mTOR) pathway (Johnson, Rabinovitch & Kaeberlein, 2013). These pathways are basically nutrient-sensing pathways that are activated by nutrients such as carbohydrates (Bartke et al., 2013) and amino acids (Wullschleger, Loewith, & Hall, 2006). Rapamycine, a pharmacological mTOR inhibitor is known to extend the lifespan by 9% and 14% in male and female mice respectively (Harrison et al., 2009). Occurrence of 20% increase in the median lifespan has been illustrated in mice expressing mTOR at 25% of wild-type mice (Wu et al., 2013). Restricting superfluity of amino acids in diet is advantageous since aging-related pathways like mTOR are activated by amino acids (Efeyan, Zoncu & Sabatini, 2012). An increase in lifespan as a result of reduced mTOR activation was reported in mice fed on low-protein diets (5% to 15% protein) that live up to 150 weeks as compared to mice fed on a high-protein diet (50% protein) that lived up to 100 weeks (Solon-Biet et al., 2014). Amino acids threonine and valine in case of yeast cells were reported to activate Tor1 (the yeast orthologue of mTOR) that was considered as the culprit behind promoting aging (Mirisola et al., 2014).

Synchronization of knowledge from the biogerontological field with nutritional science and medicine would aid in curbing the rapidly increasing epidemic of aging-related and metabolic diseases, accelerated by unhealthy lifestyle of normal as well as aging population. It has been observed that senescent-like preadipocytes and insulin resistant adipocytes are less efficient in handling and processing fatty acids, causing ectopic fatty acid deposition and thus contributing to heart disease, fatty liver disease, and stroke (Tchkonia et al., 2010; Stout et al., 2014). The role of specific proteins targeted by fatty acids and their potential role in aging remains a matter of delima (Hou & Taubert, 2012; Hansen, Flatt & Aguilaniu, 2013), however when the mTOR and IIS pathway in preadipocytes get overstimulated owing to the nutrients like carbohydrates and amino acids then it leads to their alteration into senescent-like preadipocytes. These preadipocytes secrete proinflammatory compounds stimulating insulin resistance in surrounding adipose cells.

Caloric restriction has been reported to enhance cardiometabolic parameters. This causes a decrease in both atherosclerosis and diastolic dysfunction (Fontanaet al., 2004; Meyer et al., 2006; Heilbronn et al., 2006) thus retarding aging-related diseases. Fasting renders tumor cells more vulnerable to chemotherapy thereby improving regeneration of the immune system following chemotherapy (Lee et al., 2012; Cheng et al., 2014).

Little amounts of toxic or hormetic substances may be crucial in inducing cellular stress resistance mechanisms, such as upregulation of heat shock proteins (hsps), enzymatic antioxidants, or detoxification enzymes of phase II. The reason why high doses of extracorporeal antioxidants exemplified by vitamin A, vitamin E along with beta-carotene are not beneficial in retarding the aging process or increasing lifespan (Bjelakovic, Nikolova, Gluud, Simonetti & Gluud, 2007) lies in the fact that high doses of antioxidants downregulate cellular stress resistance proteins since high levels of antioxidants signal minimal need for the production of antioxidants. Significantly reduced lifespan in voles administered with antioxidant supplementation under controlled conditions may be due to feedback mechanism of antioxidants signaling minimal need for their own production (Selman, McLaren, Collins, Duthie & Speakman, 2013). Thus various parameters regarding aging would be discussed in detail in the subsequent sections.

REACTIVE OXYGEN SPECIES: PARADOX AS WELL AS CHALLENGE

From time immemorial, the everlasting desire to overcome aging has been observed in human beings. Although oxygen is vital to life, yet this essential element may contribute to human aging and illness in the form of reactive oxygen species. This presents both a paradox and a challenge since we are obliged to live with its presence despite the fact that it poses a major threat to our lives. Despite their destructive activity, ROS are also referred to as second messengers in a variety of cellular processes including tolerance to environmental stresses (Yan, Tsuichihara, Etoh & Iwai, 2007). A fragile equilibrium between ROS production and scavenging decides whether ROS will act as damaging or signaling molecule. Due to the multifunctional roles of ROS, it is necessary that there is a tight control on level of ROS. It was demonstrated that ROS have a role in cell signaling, including; apoptosis; gene expression; and the activation of cell signaling cascades (Hancock, Desikan & Neill, 2001). ROS can serve as both intra- and inter-cellular messengers. Cyanobacteria are believed to be the first one to introduce oxygen into the initially reducing atmosphere by oxygenic photosynthesis and thereby being the main primary producers of organic matter at that time. Oxygen accumulation permitted the development of aerobic organisms that used oxygen as a powerful electron acceptor. However it posed a challenge to survive the detrimental effects of oxygen on the systems that had originally evolved in an anoxic environment. ROS attack molecules by capturing electrons, thereby modifying their chemical structures and altering their functions. Thus ROS damage cell structures such as carbohydrates, nucleic acids, lipids, and proteins. ROS damage cells leading to pathological changes associated with aging (Kadwe, Bhamre, Naukudkar & Barhate, 2015).

Atomic oxygen with two unpaired electrons in separate orbits in its outer electron shell makes oxygen susceptible to development of radical. The sequential addition of electrons leads to the formation of a number of reactive oxygen species (ROS). On the basis of presence and absence of unpaired electrons, ROS are classified into two groups. First group comprises of free radicals which contain one or more unpaired electrons. Nonradical forms created when two free radicals share their unpaired electrons comprise the second group. Thus, reactive oxygen species include hydrogen peroxide, hydroxyl radical and the superoxide anion which is both ion and radical.

ROS are commonly generated during growth and development as well as during normal cell metabolism related with processes involving redox reactions. For example, in chloroplasts and mitochondria during during photosynthesis and respiration respectively. When oxygen comes in contact with metabolic systems it can be transformed into more reactive and toxic forms. Formation of singlet oxygen ($^1O_2$)

subsequently kindles the subsequent production of ROS which may comprise of (H_2O_2), superoxide anion (O_2), hydroxyl (OH^-), and perhydroxyl radicals (O_2H).

OXIDATIVE STRESS

Besides spontaneous errors in biochemical processes, reactions of metabolites such as sugars and reactive aldehydes, the reactions of free radicals and other reactive oxygen species form the major source of damages incurred by oxidative stress (Rattan, Kryzch, Schnebert, Perrier & Nizard, 2013). Abiotic and biotic stresses are known to augment the level of ROS subsequently leading to oxidative stress.

Site-specific amino acid modifications, fragmentation, aggregation, altered electrical charge and amplified inclination towards proteolysis are some of the consequences of oxidative damages caused in proteins. Amino acids containing sulfur and thiol groups are considered as susceptible sites for oxidative attack. Reactive oxygen may lead to the formation of disulphide bridges. Reduction of both disulphide bridges and methionine sulphoxide derivatives formed as a result of oxidative damage may be accomplished in microbial systems by thioredoxin and thioredoxin reductase (Farr & Kogoma, 1991). Some of the free radical attack on proteins is irreversible in nature. For example, destruction of enzymatic functions as a result of oxidation of iron-sulphur centres by superoxides (Gardner & Fridovich, 1991) and formation of bityrosine products as a result of cross-linking of tryptophan (Davies, 1987).

The reactions of oxygen free radicals with polyunsaturated lipids are the most frequent consequence of oxygen radical production in plant cells. The peroxidation reactions differ among the fatty acids on the basis of number and position of the double bonds on the acyl chain present in the lipid bilayer membrane (Frankel, 1985). Unsaturated fatty acids produce distinctly different products than the hydroxyl radical upon oxidative attack (Bradley & Min, 1992). Differences in composition pose hindrances in understanding the effect of free radical reactions on the presence of specific lipid-soluble, membrane antioxidants such as phenols, flavonoids and quinines. UV irradiation supposed to be the culprit behind multilevel oxidative stress, may lead to morphological changes, variation in pigment composition, influence adaptive mechanisms, impair photosynthesis and decrease bioproductivity (Vass et al., 1996). Imbalance in the production and reduction monodehydroascorbate radical (MDA) may be due to UV-B irradiation. This further causes an enhanced light-induced MDA signal. UV-B radiation is visualized as a threat leading to the production of ROS that subsequently plays significant role in demolishing the native structure of proteins, DNA and other biological molecules (Sinha, Klisch, Gröniger & Häder, 1998).

DNA seems to be a weak link in a cell's ability to tolerate oxygen free radical attack. DNA is effective in binding metals that are involved in Fenton reactions. DNA is less tolerant to damages; therefore the cell has a number of DNA repair enzymes (Beyer, Imlay & Fridovich, 1991). Compartmentalization of DNA in the nucleus in the eukaryotes may probably be a reason to avoid oxidative damage from sites of redox reactions occurring in the cell. It is observed that ionizing radiations play significant role in generation of ROS. These ROS further generate numerous lesions in DNA resulting in deletions, mutations and lethal genetic discripencies. This has been illustrated that both the sugar and the base moieties are susceptible to oxidation thereby causing base degradation, single strand breakage, and cross-linking to protein (Imlay & Linn, 1986). Degradation of the base produces numerous products, comprising of adenine ring-opened and -saturated products; 8-hydroxy-guanine, hydroxymethyl urea, urea, thymine glycol and thymine. The oxidation of the sugar moiety by the hydroxyl radical leads to single strand breaks. One of the consequences of hydroxyl radical attack on either DNA or its associated proteins seems to be the cross-linking of DNA to protein (Oleinick, Chiu, Ramakrishnan, & Xue, 1986). The peroxidation reactions in membrane lipids are terminated when the carbon or peroxy radicals cross-link to form conjugated products that are not radicals, such as those shown in the following reactions:

$$R^{\cdot} + R^{\cdot} \rightarrow R\,R$$

$$R^{\cdot} + ROO^{\cdot} \rightarrow ROOR$$

$$ROO^{\cdot} + ROO^{\cdot} \rightarrow ROOR + O_2$$

Typically high molecular weight, cross-linked fatty acids and phospholipids accumulate in peroxidised membrane lipid samples. Singlet oxygen can react readily with unsaturated fatty acids producing a complex mixture of hydroperoxides. The lipid hydroperoxide (ROOH) is unstable in the presence of Fe or other metal catalysts because ROOH participates in a Fenton reaction leading to the formation of reactive alkoxy radicals:

$$ROOH + Fe^{2+} \rightarrow OH^{-} + RO\bullet + Fe^{3+}$$

Therefore, in the presence of Fe, the chain reactions not only propagate but get amplified too.

Figure 1. Role of antioxidants in scavenging free radicals and curbing oxidative damage

Superoxide Dismutase (SOD); Catalase (CAT); Ascorbate peroxidase (APX); Glutathione Reductase (GR); Dehydroascorbate reductase (DHAR); Monodehydroascorbate reductase (MDHAR).

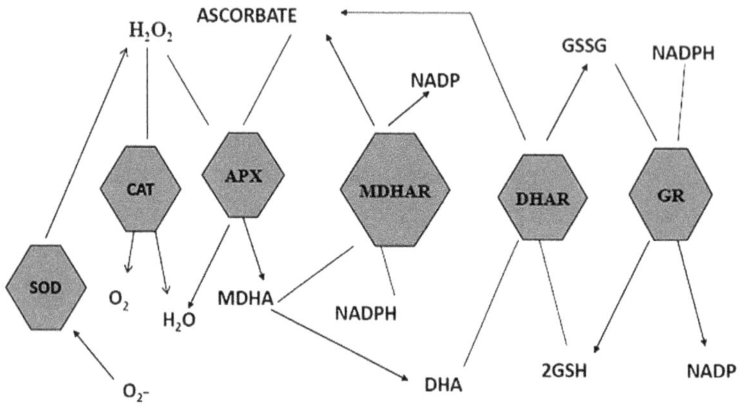

ANTIOXIDANTS AS SCAVENGERS OF ROS

Antioxidants prevent or retard the oxidation of easily oxidisable biomolecules. These biomolecules which are prone to oxidative damage are lipids, proteins or DNA. Antioxidants counteract free radicals and thereby check oxidative damage (Becker, Nissen & Skibsted, 2004; Ratnam, Ankola, Bhardwaj, Sahana & Kumar, 2006). Antioxidants are involved in the prevention of cellular damage that serves as common pathway for cancer, aging and a variety of diseases (Kadwe et al., 2015). Scavenging of ROS has been reported to follow Halliwell-Asada cycle (Halliwell & Gutteridge, 1989). Antioxidants are found to be natural arsenal against multiple stresses scavenging free radicals (Figure 1) and thereby preventing oxidative stress, which can otherwise damage DNA, RNA, proteins and lipids resulting in an increased risk for cardiovascular disease, cancer, autism and other diseases. Antioxidants can be broadly categorized as enzymatic and non enzymatic antioxidants.

ENZYMATIC ANTIOXIDANTS

Among all the antioxidative enzymes, superoxide dismutase serves to be the first line of defense against nascent oxygen species which mitigates the toxic effect of superoxide ion. On the basis of metal cofactor there are three distinct types of SOD. These are the copper/zinc (Cu/Zn-SOD), the manganese (Mn-SOD) and the iron (Fe-SOD) isozymes (Figure 2). Prokaryotic cells and many eukaryotic algae contain

Figure 2. 3D structure of Fe-superoxide dismutase from the thermophilic cyanobacterium Thermosynechococcus elongatus (Pdb id: 1MY6)

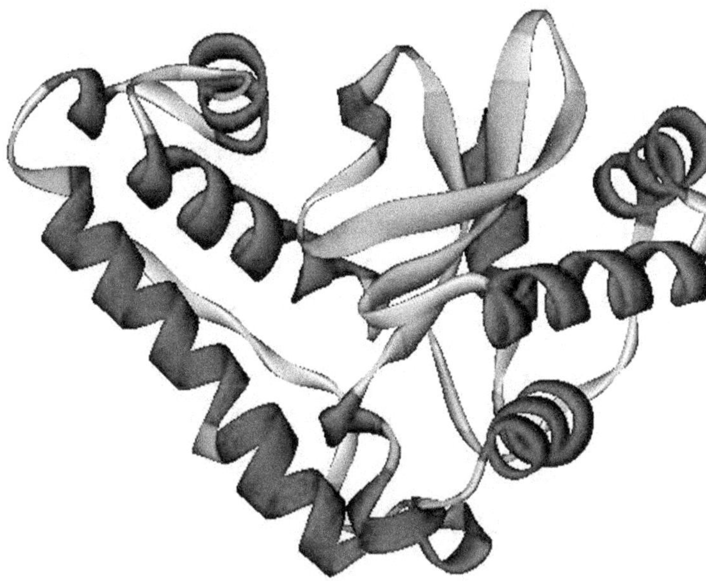

only Mn-SOD and Fe-SOD isozymes and are believed to be the ancient forms. SOD is considered as a major biomarker of defense against oxidative stress (Priya et al., 2010). It is seen that the activity of SOD increases with increasing stress. On the basis of presence and absence of ascorbate peroxidase, the cyanobacteria may be classified into two groups. First group include those cyanobacteria that scavenge hydrogen peroxide with the peroxidase utilizing a photoreductant as the electron donor. The second group comprise of those which scavenge hydrogen peroxide by the action of catalase enzyme. Ascorbate is regenerated either via monodehydroascorbate reductase, or glutathione and dehydroascorbate reductase.

Glutathione reductase (GR) enzyme catalyzes the reduction of GSSG to GSH using NADPH as the reducing cofactor. GR is essential for maintaining high GSH/GSSG ratios in cells (Williams, 1976). In particular, it is a key enzyme in the glutathione-ascorbate cycle, which functions in peroxide scavenging and protection against other oxidative processes (Foyer & Halliwell, 1976).

A protective function, analogous to that that of the chloroplast enzyme was assigned to NADPH-glutathione reductase (EC 1.6.4.2) that was purified from the filamentous cyanobacterium *Anabaena* sp. strain 7119 (Serrano, Rivas & Losada, 1984). Glutathione reductase (GR) has been shown to play a role in the protection mechanism which removes oxygen radical in N_2-fixing cyanobacterium *Nostoc muscorum* (Karni, Moss & Tel-Or, 1984). *Solanum lycopersicum* has been reported to be a good source of GR (Figure 3). Recent trends emphasize that tertiary structure prediction is emerging arena of bioinformatics which may be significant in filling up large vacuum between the available number of protein sequences of antioxidants and the known experimentally solved structures (Kesheri, Kanchan, Chowdhury & Sinha, 2015; Priya, Kesheri, Sinha & Kanchan, 2016). Cyanobacterial GR has been found to show remarkable thermostability. They do so by retaining secondary structure upon reaching higher temperatures as high as 80° C in *Spirulina maxima* (Domínguez, Hernández-Arana, Mendoza- Hernández, & Rendón, 1997). GR has already been purified from the cyanobacterium *Anabaena* PCC 7120 and a 3Kb genomic DNA fragment containing the coding sequence for the GR gene (*gor*) was identified and cloned by polymerase chain reaction. Sequences of selected peptides isolated from proteolyzed GR served as the basis for this identification (Jiang, Hellman, Sroga, Bergman & Mannervik, 1995). *Glycine max* is considered as source of another prominent enzymatic antioxidant ascorbate peroxidase (Figure 4).

NON-ENZYMATIC ANTIOXIDANTS

Non-enzymatic antioxidants can be divided into two general classes:

1. Non polar solvent soluble carotenoids and membrane associated tocopherols;
2. Polar solvent soluble reductants such as ascorbic acid, glutathione, and phycobiliproteins.

Phycobiliproteins are reported to be used in the measurement of peroxy radical damage (DeLange & Glazer, 1989). Phycobiliproteins have antimicrobial, antioxidant, anti-inflammatory, neuroprotective and hepatoprotective properties (Richa et al., 2011). In addition, they are being extensively used as natural colorants in food and cosmetics. Phycobiliproteins have been reported to be used as fluorescent neoglycoproteins. Nowadays probes for single particle fluorescence used for imaging fluorescent applications in clinical and immunological analyses significantly use phycobiliproteins. There are four ways in which carotenoids can protect the photosystems. The first method being reacting with lipid peroxidation products terminating chain reactions. Scavenging singlet oxygen and dissipating the energy as heat forms the second significant way of protection by carotenoids. Thirdly the protection by carotenoids is offered by reacting with triplet or excited chlorophyll molecules to prevent formation of singlet oxygen. Dissipating excess excitation energy through the xanthophyll cycle forms the fourth way of protection by the carotenoids. The tripeptide glutathione is a major antioxidant and a low-molecular-weight non-proteinous thiol compound which mainly in its reduced form acts as an intracellular reductant (Galhano, Peixoto & Gomes-Laranjo, 2011).

Figure 3. Crystal structure of S-nitrosoglutathione reductase from tomato (Solanum lycopersicum) (Pdb Id: 4DL9)

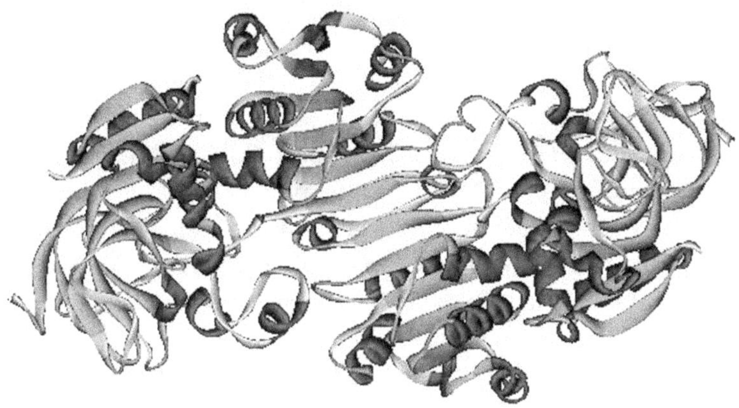

Figure 4. 3D structure of ascorbate peroxidase from soybean (Glycine max) cytosol (Pdb id: 1oag)

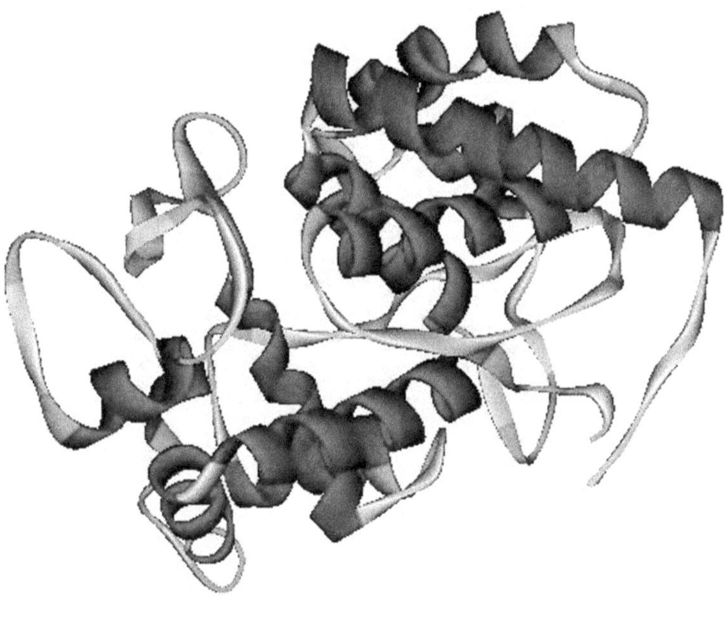

PHYCOBILIPROTEINS

Cyanobacteria are photosynthetic prokaryotic producers of pigments such as chlorophyll, carotenoids and phycobiliproteins (Prasanna et al., 2010). In algae and cyanobacteria, the phycobiliproteins are constituents of supramolecular complexes named phycobilisomes, whose physiological function is to capture light for photosynthesis.

Phycobilins have a linear tetrapyrrole structure. This characteristic structure of phycobilins resembles that of biliverdin and bilirubin. Phycobilins are also expected to have antioxidant activity similar to that of biliverdin and bilirubin. *Spirulina platensis*, is known to prevent peroxidation of linoleic acid by involving phycobilin pigments (Hirata, Tanaka, Ooike, Tsunomura & Sakaguchi, 2000). Similarly *Leptolyngbya* sp. possess antioxidant property owing to the presence of c-phycocyanin (Figure 5). I*n vitro* experiments regarding lipid peroxidation using phosphatidylcholine liposomes depicted that scavenging of ROS by phycocyanobilin which are scattered extracellularly, subdued the radical initiation for peroxidation of unsaturated lipid molecules. Phycobiliprotein also serve as potential pro-oxidant. Phycocyanin possesses radical scavenging activity in dark environments. However it leads to the production of hydroxylradicals in light environments. Surfactants, urea, and alkaline completely diminish hydroxyl radical production as a result of denaturation of phycocyanin proteins although radical scavenging activity still remains (Zhou et al., 2005). Therefore, it is possible that phycobilin, itself, functions as an antioxidant while protein-bound phycobilin functions as a pro-oxidant.

Figure 5. Crystal structure of c-phycocyanin from Leptolyngbya sp. n62dm (pdb id:4lle)

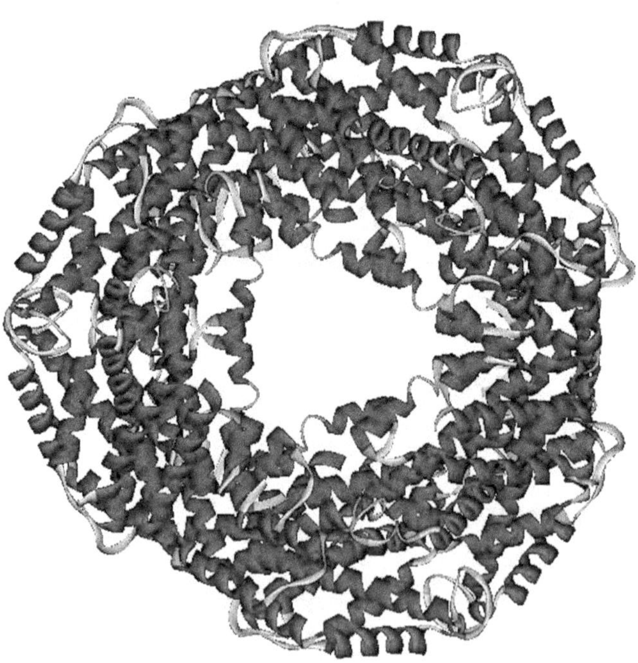

Phycobiliproteins are reported to be used in the measurement of peroxy radical damage (DeLange & Glazer, 1989). *Spirulina* may serve as an effective antioxidant for humans owing to the antioxidative characteristics of phycobilins reported in it (Hirata et al., 2000). Based on their response to light quantity, cyanobacteria can alter their phycobilisomes size and number; it can also change the phycoerythrin and/or phycocyanin levels (Tandeu de Marsac et al., 1988) by a process called as chromatic adaptation. Low light intensities are known to stimulate phycobilisomes production consequently leading to increase in the size of rod structure (Lonneborg, Lind, Kalla, Gustafsson & Öquist, 1985; Melis et al., 1985). Phycoerythrins are highly sensitive to alterations in factors like pH, salt, temperature, water stress and light (Sarada, Pillai & Ravishankar, 1999; Sun, Wang, Chen & Gong, 2003; Martinez-Oyanedel, Contreras-Martel, Bruna & Bunster, 2004).

TOCOPHEROL

Tocopherol is a non-polar solvent soluble organic molecule. It is only synthesized by oxygen-evolving phototrophs including some cyanobacteria and all green algae and plants (Threlfall & Whistance, 1971, Collins & Jones, 1981). Alpha (α), beta (β), gamma (γ) and delta (δ) tocopherols comprise a group of lipophilic molecules that are collectively termed as vitamin E. They differ in the number and position of methyl groups on the chromanol ring. Tocopherols serve as scavengers of various ROS and lipid oxidation byproducts, thus preventing the lipid peroxidation chain reactions in membranes (Kamal-Eldin & Appelqvist, 1996). D-alpha-tocopherol a naturally-occurring form of vitamin E plays crucial role in stabilization of biological membranes particularly those with elevated amounts of polyunsaturated fatty acids. Being a potent peroxyl radical scavenger, d-alpha-Tocopherol inhibits noncompetitively cyclooxygenase activity in many tissues, resulting in a decrease in prostaglandin production (Figure 6). A shielding role of tocopherol against photooxidative damage in photosystem II has been reported in *Chlamydomonas reinhardtii* (Trebst, Depka, Jager & Oettmeier, 2004). The major functions of tocopherols comprise of antioxidation, membrane stabilization, intracellular signaling and cyclic electron transport around photosystem II (Fryer, 1992; Hess, 1993; Munné-Bosch & Alegre 2002). Inhibiting angiogenesis and tumor dormancy by suppressing vascular endothelial growth factor (VEGF) gene transcription (NCI04) is also one of the known functions of Vitamin E. The antioxidant property of tocopherol is the result of its ability to quench both singlet oxygen and peroxides.

Figure 6. Structure of d-alpha-Tocopherol (Pubchem id: 14985)

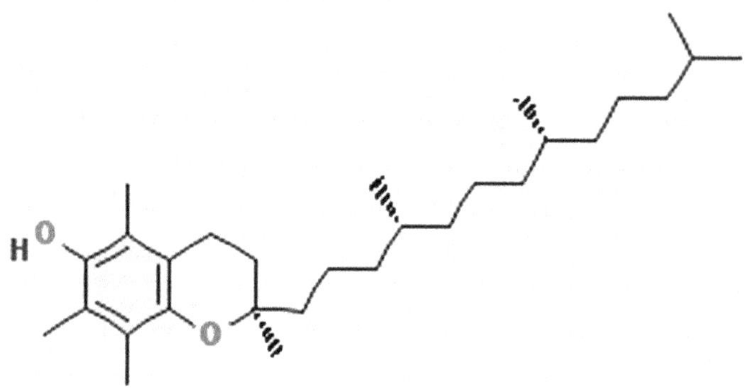

CAROTENOIDS

Carotenoids are lipophilic tetraterpenoids that occur in many microorganisms (Britton, Liaaen-Jensen & Pfander, 2004). Carotenoids act as a competitive inhibitor for the formation of singlet oxygen. This is aided considerably due to their proximity to chlorophyll in the light harvesting complex. This method of protection is especially critical as light intensity increases above saturation levels (Demmig-Adams & Adams, 1992).

Carotenoids commonly have three absorption bands covering the region between 400 and 500 nm. Their strongly hydrophobic nature is due to the presence of long unsaturated alkene chain. This enables them to localize and function in biomembranes. Common structural character of carotenoids is characterized by long π-conjugated polyene structure with numerous methyl substituents. This forms the unique chromophore of carotenoids. Many kinds of carotenoids have cyclohexene end groups at one side or both sides.

In terms of its antioxidant properties carotenoids possess the potential to shield the photosystems. Reacting with lipid peroxidation products and terminating chain reactions serve as the first way of protection offered by carotenoids. Scavenging singlet oxygen and dissipating the energy as heat is also a means of protection by carotenoids. Protection by carotenoids is also offered by reacting with triplet or excited chlorophyll molecules to prevent formation of singlet oxygen. Dissipating excess excitation energy through the xanthophyll cycle is also one of the criteria adopted by carotenoids to curb the ill effects of oxidative stress. Carotenoids may augment α-tocopherol in scavenging peroxy radicals (Burton & Ingold, 1984).

Both carotenoids and their glycosides function as photo-protectants. Lutein and zeaxanthin possess extremely low IC50values (50% inhibitory concentration) against

$O^{2-\bullet}$, $OH^{\bullet}$, and lipid peroxide as compared to typical antioxidants, such as ascorbic acid and Trolox (Sindhu, Preethi & Kuttan, 2010). Hydrophobicity of carotenoids isextremely high. Therefore their IC50values for scavenging against hydrophobic ROS such as DPPH radical are generally lower than those against hydrophilic ROS, such as ABTS radicals. On the contrary, hydrophilic antioxidants, such as ascorbic acid and Trolox, show the opposite tendency.

About 600 different carotenoids have been identified from cyanobacteria, bacteria, fungi, phytoplankton, macroalgae, plants and animals (Polivka & Sundström 2004; Grynbaum et al., 2005). Animals are devoid of the ability to synthesize carotenoids endogenously and thus have to take up these compounds through their diets (Moeller, Gilroy, Williamson & Grad, 2005). A considerable augmentation in the outer-membrane carotenoids echinenone and myxoxanthophyll was illustrated in the cyanobacterium *Nostoc commune* upon exposure to UV-B irradiation (Ehling-Schulz, Bilger & Scherer, 1997). The photosynthetic activity revealed by cyanobacterium *Synechococcus* sp. was found to be more tolerant against UV-B radiation when having increased amounts of endogenous carotenoids caused by genetic manipulation (Götz, T., Windhovel, U., Böger, P. & Sandmann, 1999). A small increase in carotenoid content was found in a *Oscillatoria* sp. strain BG 091600, following exposure to UV-A irradiance of 10 W/m^2 (Wachi et al., 1995). Diadinoxanthin, diatoxanthin and β-carotene were found to be induced in phytoplankton under high PAR and UVR (Smith et al., 1992) and they may play a role in reducing photoinhibition of photosynthesis (Brown et al., 1999). It seems that the beneficial aspects of carotenoids in UV light protection lies in their capacity to act as quenchers of photosensitization products and also as inhibitors of free radical reactions (Demmig-Adams & Adams, 1992), rather than with their ability to screen out UV radiation (Gao & Gracia-Pichel, 2011).

ß-carotene is formed by the cyclization of lycopene. Xanthophylls are formed as a result of mixed function oxidases introducing hydroxyl groups to the carotene molecule (Pallett & Young, 1993). Another carotenoid, zeaxanthin, has been implicated in the dissipation of thermal energy. Zeaxanthin facilitates the conversion of triplet to singlet chlorophyll more proficiently than ß-carotene. The xanthophyll cycle there occurs reversible conversion of the xanthophylls between two forms, violaxanthin and zeaxanthin.

GLUTATHIONE

The tripeptide glutathione is a major antioxidant and a low-molecular-weight non-proteinous thiol compound which is widely distributed in most living cells. In cyanobacterial cells, glutathione mainly in its reduced form acts as an intracellular reductant (Galhano et al., 2011). Reduced glutathione (GSH) together with its disulfide oxidized form (GSSG) acts as a free radical scavenger, an arsenal against oxidizing molecules and harmful xenobiotics, maintains the cellular redox balance, and provides the basis for GSH stress signaling (Meister 1989; Peña-Llopis, Peña, Sancho, Fernández-Vega & Ferrando, 2001; Blokhina & Fagerstedt, 2010). GSH is synthesized in the cell cytosol *via* two ATP-requiring enzymatic steps. The first step is the formation of γ-glutamylcysteine from L-glutamate and L-cysteine. The formation of GSH from γ-glutamylcysteine and glycine forms the second step. The first step is catalyzed by γ-glutamylcysteine synthetase (EC 6.3.2.2, GCS), whereas the second step is catalyzed by glutathione synthetase (EC 6.3.2.3, GS). The initial step of GSH biosynthesis usually forms the rate-limiting step. GSH biosynthesis is regulated by feed-back competitive inhibition by GSH and the availability of L-cysteine (DeLeve & Kaplowitz, 1991). Glutathione (GSH), a nonribosomal thiol tripeptide, is found in virtually all eukaryotic cells. However, its production in prokaryotes is confined to cyanobacteria and proteobacteria and a few strains of Gram-positive bacteria. GSH plays an essential role in numerous cellular functions, protection against oxidative stress being one of them. GSH has been reported to be a part of shielding process against (ROS), osmotic shock, acidic conditions, toxic chemicals, and heavy metals. The investigations on *Synechocystis* sp. indicate a strong similarity of the sub-cellular distribution of glutathione and cysteine in cyanobacteria and plastids of plants providing a deeper insight into glutathione metabolism in bacteria (Bernd, Ana, Lucija & Hrvoje, 2010). Although little is known about the roles of glutathione in cyanobacteria, it was elucidated that conditions promoting growth stimulate glutathione biosynthesis in *Synechocystis* sp. PCC 6803 (Cameron & Pakrasi, 2010). It has been reported that the structural gene for glutathione synthetase (*gshB*) is involved in the biosynthesis of glutathione in *Synechococcus* sp. PCC 7942 (Okumura, Masamoto & Wada, 1997).

SOURCES OF ANTI-AGING SUBSTANCES

Apart from macronutrient content (carbohydrates, proteins, or fats) of a diet, micronutrient content can also influence metabolism and aging related disorders. Blueberries containing anthocyanidins are elucidated to have improved insulin sensitivity and a lower risk of type 2 diabetes (Muraki et al., 2013). Research on total phenolic contents of red wine displayed a good correlation ($p < 0.01$) with antioxidant properties emphasizing on predominant role of phenols in antioxidant activity (Büyüktuncel, Porgal & Çolak, 2014). Accoring to the French paradox, although high amount of consumption of saturated fat diet is reported in South-Western France yet there are relatively few incidences of coronary heart diseases and cardiovascular diseases.

This was correlated to some extent with the regular consumption of red wine, which contains high levels of resveratrol (Marchal, Pifferi & Aujard, 2013). First isolated from the roots of white hellebore (*Veratrum grandiflorum, O. Loes*) and later on from the roots of *Polygonum cuspidatum* (or *Fallopia japonica*), a plant used in traditional Chinese and Japanese medicine (Timmers, Auwerx & Schrauwen, 2012), resveratrol belongs to polyphenolic compounds that are distinguished as phytoalexin which stimulates cell defenses in plants.

Mass production of intracellular polysaccharides extracted from *Lepista sordida* mycelium by submerged fermentation emphasized its potent antioxidant activity. It is known for being potential dietary supplement retarding aging and attenuate age-related diseases in humans (Zhong et al., 2013). The anti-aging effect of polysaccharides extracted from *Athyrium multidentatum* extraordinarily improved the activities of antioxidative enzymes and lessened the product of lipid peroxide (Liu, Sheng, Qi & Zhang, 2015).

Fasting blood glucose levels and lower glycated HbA1c concentrations were reported to be improved by extracts from cinnamon in patients suffering from type-2 diabetes (Lu et al., 2012). Intake of high amounts of natural antioxidants in the form of natural products rich in vitamins, carotenoids, phenolics in everyday diet of human beings can serve to protect against cardiovascular diseases, cataract, cancer and aging-related disorders (Steffen et al., 2003). Cacao which forms the main ingredient of dark chocolate is reported to be associated with increased insulin sensitivity and a reduced risk of cardiovascular disease (Buitrago-Lopez et al., 2011). It has been observed in people of higher age group that cacao can slow down the progress of mild cognitive impairment (Desideri et al., 2012). Phenolic compounds impart nutraceutical effects on human health apart from possessing antimicrobial, anticarcinogenic, and antioxidant properties (Seruga, Novak & Jakobek, 2011).

Hormesis elucidates that high doses of antioxidants do not retard ageing owing to the feedback mechanism signaling downregulation of antioxidant production. When compared to non-vegetarian diets, a vegetarian diet provides more plant-based proteins and lower methionine content, aiding in lifespan and health enhacement (McCarty, Barroso-Aranda & Contreras, 2009; Cavuoto & Fenech, 2012). Thus vegetarian diets are associated with reduced all-cause mortality.

FUTURE RESEARCH DIRECTIONS

Modulation of IIS and mTOR pathways genetically or nutritionally poses an innovative field of research in future since it can impact the rate of aging and postpone the advent of aging-related diseases. Thus the outcomes of future research may hopefully formulate a diet sourcing carbohydrates, amino acids, and fats in a such a way that cause pro-aging nutrient-sensing pathways such as the IIS and mTOR pathway to remain less activated. This may aid in extenuating the risk of aging-related diseases. Although the advantageous effects of antioxidant supplements seem undoubtful in cases of antioxidant deficiencies, yet gap in research regarding benefits of exogeneous administration of antioxidants in healthy persons needs to be bridged by future research in this field. Hormesis describing how small amounts of toxic substances can be beneficial by acting as inducers of cellular stress resistance mechanisms would widen a burgeoning field of research in the area of pharmacy. Future research would certainly focus on caloric restriction, balanced dose of antioxidants, carbohydrates, proteins and fats while devising healthier diets that lead to disease-free longer life span.

CONCLUSION

A comprehensive understanding of the aging process can help to better envisage the efficacy of diets and specific nutritional interventions. Imbalance of generation of reactive oxygen species leads to oxidative stress. According to free radical theory of ageing, if ROS are the main culprits behind ageing then administration of antioxidants may retard the process of ageing and ageing related diseases. However it has also been observed that hormetic substances in small quantities may induce the production of stress borne antioxidants. Antioxidants in general belong to either enzymatic or non enzymatic group. Thus judicial and balanced use of antioxidants along with required calories of food intake may extend the life span of living organisms.

ACKNOWLEDGMENT

Dr. Minu Kesheri and Swarna Kanchan are thankful to Shridhar University, Pilani, India for granting project (SU/RNC/BS/2015/001) and supporting the research work.

REFERENCES

Bartke, A., Sun, L. Y., & Longo, V. (2013). Somatotropic signaling: Trade-offs between growth, reproductive development, and longevity. *Physiological Reviews*, *93*(2), 571–598. doi:10.1152/physrev.00006.2012 PMID:23589828

Becker, E. M., Nissen, L. R., & Skibsted, L. H. (2004). Antioxidant Evaluation Protocols: Food Quality or Health Effects. *European Food Research and Technology*, *219*(6), 561–571. doi:10.1007/s00217-004-1012-4

Bernd, Z., Ana, T., Lucija, H., & Hrvoje, F. (2010). Subcellular distribution of glutathione and cysteine in cyanobacteria. *Protoplasma*, *246*(1-4), 65–72. doi:10.1007/s00709-010-0126-8 PMID:20349253

Beyer, W., Imlay, J., & Fridovich, I. (1991). Superoxide dismutases. *Progress in Nucleic Acid Research*, *40*, 221–253. doi:10.1016/S0079-6603(08)60843-0 PMID:1851570

Bjelakovic, G., Nikolova, D., Gluud, L. L., Simonetti, R. G., & Gluud, C. (2007). Mortality in randomized trials of antioxidant supplements for primary and secondary revention: Systematic review and meta-analysis. *Journal of the American Medical Association*, *297*, 842–857. doi:10.1001/jama.297.8.842 PMID:17327526

Blokhina, O., & Fagerstedt, K. V. (2010). Oxygen deprivation, metabolic adaptations and oxidative stress. In S. Mancuso & S. Shabala (Eds.), *Waterlogging Signaling and Tolerance in Plants* (pp. 119–147). Berlin: Springer-Verlag. doi:10.1007/978-3-642-10305-6_7

Bradley, D. E., & Min, D. B. (1992). Singlet oxygen oxidation of foods. *Critical Reviews in Food Science and Nutrition*, *31*(3), 211–236. doi:10.1080/10408399209527570 PMID:1571085

Britton, G., Liaaen-Jensen, S., & Pfander, H. (2004). *Carotenoids Handbook*. Birkhäuser Basel. doi:10.1007/978-3-0348-7836-4

Brown, B. E., Ambarsari, I., Warner, M. E., Fitt, W. K., Dunne, R. P., Gibb, S. W., & Cummings, D. G. (1999). Diurnal changes in photochemical efficiency and xanthophyll concentrations in shallow water reef corals: Evidence for photoinhibition and photoprotection. *Coral Reefs*, *18*(2), 99–105. doi:10.1007/s003380050163

Buitrago-Lopez, A., Sanderson, J., Johnson, L., Warnakula, S., Wood, A., Di-Angelantonio, E., & Franco, O. H. (2011). Chocolate consumption and cardiometabolic disorders: Systematic review and meta-analysis. *British Medical Journal*, *343*(1), d4488. doi:10.1136/bmj.d4488 PMID:21875885

Burton, G. W., & Ingold, K. U. (1984). ß-carotene: An unusual type of lipid antioxidant. *Science*, *224*(4649), 569–573. doi:10.1126/science.6710156 PMID:6710156

Büyüktuncel, E., Porgal, E., & Çolak, C. (2014). Comparison of Total Phenolic Content and Total Antioxidant Activity in Local Red Wines Determined by Spectrophotometric Methods. *Food and Nutrition Sciences*, *5*(17), 1660–1667. doi:10.4236/fns.2014.517179

Cameron, J. C., & Pakrasi, H. B. (2010). Essential Role of glutathione in acclimation to environmental and redox perturbations in the cyanobacterium *Synechocystis* sp. PCC 6803. *Plant Physiology*, *154*(4), 1672–1685. doi:10.1104/pp.110.162990 PMID:20935175

Cavuoto, P., & Fenech, M. F. (2012). A review of methionine dependency and the role of methionine restriction in cancer growth control and life-span extension. *Cancer Treatment Reviews*, *38*(6), 726–736. doi:10.1016/j.ctrv.2012.01.004 PMID:22342103

Cheng, C.-W., Adams, G. B., Perin, L., Wei, M., Zhou, X., Lam, B. S., & Longo, V. D. et al. (2014). Prolonged fasting reduces IGF-1/PKA to promote hematopoietic-stem-cell-based regeneration and reverse immunosuppression. *Cell Stem Cell*, *14*(6), 810–823. doi:10.1016/j.stem.2014.04.014 PMID:24905167

Collins, M. D., & Jones, D. (1981). Distribution of isoprenoid quinone structural types in bacteria and their taxonomic implications. *Microbiological Reviews*, *45*, 316–354. PMID:7022156

Davies, K. J. A. (1987). Protein damage and degradation by oxygen radicals. I. General aspects. *The Journal of Biological Chemistry*, *162*, 9895–9901. PMID:3036875

De Carvalho, M. D. C., & De Mesquita, J. F. (2013). Structural Modeling and In Silico Analysis of Human Superoxide Dismutase 2. *PLoS ONE*, *8*(6), e65558. doi:10.1371/journal.pone.0065558 PMID:23785434

DeLange, R. L., & Glazer, A. N. (1989). Phycoerythrin fluorescence based assay for peroxy radicals: A screen for biologically relevant protective agents. *Analytical Biochemistry*, *177*(2), 300–306. doi:10.1016/0003-2697(89)90056-0 PMID:2567129

DeLeve, L., & Kaplowitz, N. (1991). Glutathione metabolism and its role in hepatotoxicity. *Pharmacology & Therapeutics*, *52*(3), 287–305. doi:10.1016/0163-7258(91)90029-L PMID:1820580

Demmig-Adams, B., & Adams, W. W. (1992). Photoprotection and other responses of plants to high light stress. Ann. Rev. *Plant Physiology*, *43*, 599–626.

Desideri, G., Kwik-Uribe, C., Grassi, D., Necozione, S., Ghiadoni, L., Mastroiacovo, D., & Ferri, C. et al. (2012). Benefits in cognitive function, blood pressure, and insulin resistance through cocoa flavanol consumption in elderly subjects with mild cognitive impairment: The Cocoa, Cognition, and Aging (CoCoA) study. *Hypertension*, *60*(3), 794–801. doi:10.1161/HYPERTENSIONAHA.112.193060 PMID:22892813

Domínguez, A.R., & Hernández-Arana, A., Mendoza- Hernández, G. & Rendón, J.L. (1997). Thermal denaturation of glutathione reductase from cyanobacterium *Spirulina maxima*. *Biochemistry and Molecular Biology International*, *42*, 631–639. PMID:9247721

Efeyan, A., Zoncu, R., & Sabatini, D. M. (2012). Amino acids and mTORC1: From lysosomes to disease. *Trends in Molecular Medicine*, *18*(9), 524–533. doi:10.1016/j.molmed.2012.05.007 PMID:22749019

Ehling-Schulz, M., Bilger, W., & Scherer, S. (1997). UV-B induced synthesis of photoprotective pigments and extracellular polysaccharides in the terrestrial cyanobacterium *Nostoc commune*. *Journal of Bacteriology*, *179*, 1940–1945. PMID:9068639

Farr, S. B., & Kogoma, T. (1991). Oxidative stress responses in *Escherichia coli* and *Salmonella typhimurium*. *Microbiological Reviews*, *55*, 561–585. PMID:1779927

Foyer, C. H., & Halliwell, B. (1976). The presence of glutathione and glutathione reductase in chloroplasts: A proposed role in ascorbic acid metabolism. *Planta*, *133*(1), 21–25. doi:10.1007/BF00386001 PMID:24425174

Foyer, C. H., & Noctor, G. (2003). Redox sensing and signaling associated with reactive oxygen in chloroplasts, peroxisomes and mitochondria. *Physiologia Plantarum*, *119*(3), 355–364. doi:10.1034/j.1399-3054.2003.00223.x

Frankel, E. N. (1985). Chemistry of free radical and singlet oxidation of lipids. *Progress in Lipid Research*, *23*(4), 197–221. doi:10.1016/0163-7827(84)90011-0 PMID:6100997

Fryer, M. J. (1992). The antioxidant effects of thylakoid vitamin E (α-tocopherol). *Plant, Cell & Environment*, *15*(4), 381–392. doi:10.1111/j.1365-3040.1992.tb00988.x

Galhano, V., Peixoto, F., & Gomes-Laranjo, J. (2011). Exposure of the cyanobacterium *Nostoc muscorum* from Portuguese rice fields to Molinate: Effects on the antioxidant system and fatty acid profile. *Aquatic Toxicology (Amsterdam, Netherlands)*, *101*(2), 367–376. doi:10.1016/j.aquatox.2010.11.011 PMID:21216347

Gao, Q., & Garcia-Pichel, F. (2011). Microbial ultraviolet sunscreens. *Nature Reviews. Microbiology*, *9*(11), 791–802. doi:10.1038/nrmicro2649 PMID:21963801

Gardner, P. R., & Fridovich, I. (1991). Superoxide sensitivity of *Escherichia coli* 6-phosphogluconate dehydratose. *The Journal of Biological Chemistry*, *266*, 1478–1483. PMID:1846355

Gladyshev, V. N. (2014). The free radical theory of aging is dead. Long live the damage theory. *Antioxidants & Redox Signalling*, *20*(4), 727–731. doi:10.1089/ars.2013.5228 PMID:24159899

Götz, T., Windhovel, U., Böger, P., & Sandmann, G. (1999). Protection of photosynthesis against UV-B radiation by carotenoids in transformants of the cyanobacterium *Synechococcus* PCC 7942. *Plant Physiology*, *120*(2), 599–604. doi:10.1104/pp.120.2.599 PMID:10364412

Grynbaum, M. D., Hentschel, P., Putzbach, K., Rehbein, J., Krucker, M., Nicholson, G., & Albert, K. (2005). Unambiguous detection of astaxanthin and astaxanthin fatty acid esters in krill (*Euphausia superba* Dana). *Journal of Separation Science*, *28*(14), 1685–1693. doi:10.1002/jssc.200500152 PMID:16224962

Halliwell, B., & Gutteridge, J. M. C. (1989). *Free Radicals in Biology and Medicine*. Oxford, UK: Clarendon Press.

Hancock, J. T., Desikan, R., & Neill, S. J. (2001). Role of Reactive Oxygen Species in Cell Signaling Pathways. *Biochemical and Biomedical Aspects of Oxidative Modification*, *29*(2), 345–350. PMID:11356180

Hansen, M., Flatt, T., & Aguilaniu, H. (2013). Reproduction, fat metabolism, and life span: What is the connection? *Cell Metabolism*, *17*(1), 10–19. doi:10.1016/j.cmet.2012.12.003 PMID:23312280

Harman, D. (1956). Aging: A theory based on free radical and radiation chemistry. *Journal of Gerontology*, *11*(3), 298–300. doi:10.1093/geronj/11.3.298 PMID:13332224

Harrison, D. E., Strong, R., Sharp, Z. D., Nelson, J. F., Astle, C. M., Flurkey, K., & Miller, R. A. et al. (2009). Rapamycin fed late in life extends lifespan in genetically heterogeneous mice. *Nature*, *460*, 392–395. PMID:19587680

Hess, J. L. (1993). Vitamin E, α-tocopherol. In R. G. Alscher & J. L. Hess (Eds.), *Antioxidants in Higher Plants* (pp. 111–134). Boca Raton, FL: CRC Press.

Hirata, T., Tanaka, M., Ooike, M., Tsunomura, T., & Sakaguchi, M. (2000). Antioxidant activities of phycocyanobilin prepared from Spirulina platensis. *Journal of Applied Phycology*, *12*(3/5), 435–439. doi:10.1023/A:1008175217194

Hou, N. S., & Taubert, S. (2012). Function and regulation of lipid biology in caenorhabditis elegans aging. *Frontiers in Physics*, *3*, 143. PMID:22629250

Imlay, J. A., & Linn, S. (1986). DNA damage and oxygen radical toxicity. *Science*, *240*(4857), 1302–1309. doi:10.1126/science.3287616 PMID:3287616

Jiang, F., Hellman, U., Sroga, G. E., Bergman, B., & Mannervik, B. (1995). Cloning, sequencing, and regulation of the glutathione reductase gene from the cyanobacterium *Anabaena* PCC 7120. *The Journal of Biological Chemistry*, *270*(39), 22882–22889. doi:10.1074/jbc.270.39.22882 PMID:7559423

Johnson, S. C., Rabinovitch, P. S., & Kaeberlein, M. (2013). mTOR is a key modulator of ageing and age-related disease. *Nature*, *493*(7432), 338–345. doi:10.1038/nature11861 PMID:23325216

Kadwe, S. K., Bhamre, M. A., Naukudkar, V. J., & Barhate, M. D. (2015). Effect of antioxidants on free radicals. *International Journal of Pharmaceutical Research & Development*, *6*(12), 57–60.

Kamal-Eldin, A., & Appelqvist, L. (1996). The chemistry and antioxidant properties of tocopherols and tocotrienols. *Lipids*, *31*(7), 671–701. doi:10.1007/BF02522884 PMID:8827691

Karni, L., Moss, S. J., & Tel-Or, E. (1984). Glutathione reductase activity in heterocysts and vegetative cells of *Nostoc muscorum*. *Archives of Microbiology*, *140*(2-3), 215–217. doi:10.1007/BF00454930

Kesheri, M., Richa, & Sinha, R.P. (2011). Antioxidants as natural arsenal against multiple stresses in cyanobacteria. *International Journal Pharma and Bioscience*, *2*(2), B-168-B-187.

Kesheri, M., Kanchan, S., Chowdhury, S., & Sinha, R. P. (2015). Secondary and Tertiary Structure Prediction of Proteins: A Bioinformatic Approach. In Q. Zhu & A. T. Azar (Eds.), *Studies in Fuzziness and Soft Computing* (pp. 541–569). Springer Verlag. doi:10.1007/978-3-319-12883-2_19

Kesheri, M., Kanchan, S., Richa, , & Sinha, R. P. (2014). Isolation and in silico analysis of Fe-superoxide dismutase in the cyanobacterium Nostoc commune. *Gene*, *553*(2), 117–125. doi:10.1016/j.gene.2014.10.010 PMID:25303871

Kirkwood, T. B., & Kowald, A. (2012). The free-radical theory of ageing—older, wiser and still alive. *BioEssays*, *34*(8), 692–700. doi:10.1002/bies.201200014 PMID:22641614

Książek, K. (2010). Let's stop overlooking bacterial aging. *Biogerontology*, *11*(6), 717–723. doi:10.1007/s10522-010-9278-3 PMID:20440559

Lee, C., Raffaghello, L., Brandhorst, S., Safdie, F. M., Bianchi, G., Martin-Montalvo, A., & Longo, V. D. et al. (2012). Fasting cycles retard growth of tumors and sensitize a range of cancer cell types to chemotherapy. *Science Translational Medicine*, *4*(124), 124–127. doi:10.1126/scitranslmed.3003293 PMID:22323820

Lin, S. J., & Austriaco, N. (2014). Aging and cell death in the other yeasts, Schizosaccharomyces pombe and Candida albicans. *FEMS Yeast Research*, *14*(1), 119–135. doi:10.1111/1567-1364.12113 PMID:24205865

Liu, D., Sheng, J., Qi, H., & Zhang, W. (2015). Anti-aging activities of polysaccharides from *Athyrium multidentatum* (Doll.) Ching. *Journal of Chemical and Pharmaceutical Research*, *7*(1), 386–389.

Lonneborg, A., Lind, L. K., Kalla, S. R., Gustafsson, P., & Öquist, G. (1985). Acclimatation process in the light harvesting system of cyanobacterium *Anacystis nidulans* following a light shift from white light to red light. *Plant Physiology*, *78*(1), 110–114. doi:10.1104/pp.78.1.110 PMID:16664182

Lu, T., Sheng, H., Wu, J., Cheng, Y., Zhu, J., & Chen, Y. (2012). Cinnamon extract improves fasting blood glucose and glycosylated hemoglobin level in Chinese patients with type 2 diabetes. *Nutrition Research (New York, N.Y.)*, *32*(6), 408–412. doi:10.1016/j.nutres.2012.05.003 PMID:22749176

Marchal, J., Pifferi, F., & Aujard, F. (2013). Resveratrol in mammals: Effects on aging biomarkers, age-related diseases, and life span. *Annals of the New York Academy of Sciences*, *1290*(1), 67–73. doi:10.1111/nyas.12214 PMID:23855467

Martinez-Oyanedel, J., Contreras-Martel, C., Bruna, C., & Bunster, M. (2004). Stuctural-functional analysis of the oligomeric protein R-phycoerythrin. *Biological Research*, *37*(4), 733–745. doi:10.4067/S0716-97602004000500003 PMID:15586822

Mathis, P., & Kleo, J. (1973). The triplet state of ß-carotene and of analog polyenes of different length. *Photochemistry and Photobiology*, *18*(4), 343–346. doi:10.1111/j.1751-1097.1973.tb06431.x

McCarty, M. F., Barroso-Aranda, J., & Contreras, F. (2009). The low-methionine content of vegan diets may make methionine restriction feasible as a life extension strategy. *Medical Hypotheses*, *72*(2), 125–128. doi:10.1016/j.mehy.2008.07.044 PMID:18789600

Meister, A. (1989). Metabolism and function of glutathione. In D. Dolphin, R. Poulson, & R. Auramovic (Eds.), *Glutathione: chemical, biochemical, and medical aspects* (pp. 367–474). New York: John Wiley and Sons.

Melis, A., Mamdori, A., Glick, R. E., Ghirardi, M. L., McCauly, S. W., & Neal, P. J. (1985). The mechanism of photosynthetic membrane adaptation to environmental stress conditions; a hypothesis on the role of electron transport capacity and of ATP/NADPH pool in regulation of thylakoid membrane organization and function. *Physiologie Vegetale*, *23*, 757–765.

Mirisola, M. G., Taormina, G., Fabrizio, P., Wei, M., Hu, J., & Longo, V. D. (2014). Serine- and threonine/valine-dependent activation of PDK and Tor orthologs converge on Sch9 to promote aging. *PLOS Genetics*, *10*(2), e1004113. doi:10.1371/journal.pgen.1004113 PMID:24516402

Moeller, R. E., Gilroy, S., Williamson, C. E., Grad, G., & Sommaruga, R. (2005). Dietary acquisition of photoprotective compounds (mycosporine-like amino acids, carotenoids) and acclimation to ultraviolet radiation in a freshwater copepod. *Limnology and Oceanography*, *50*(2), 427–439. doi:10.4319/lo.2005.50.2.0427

Munné-Bosch, S., & Alegre, L. (2002). The function of tocopherols and tocotrienols in plants. *Critical Reviews in Plant Sciences*, *21*(1), 31–57. doi:10.1080/0735-260291044179

Muraki, I., Imamura, F., Manson, J. E., Hu, F. B., Willett, W. C., Van Dam, R. M., & Sun, Q. (2013). Fruit consumption and risk of type 2 diabetes: Results from three prospective longitudinal cohort studies. *British Medical Journal*, *347*(1), f5001. doi:10.1136/bmj.f5001 PMID:23990623

Okumura, N., Masamoto, N., & Wada, H. (1997). The *gshB* gene in the cyanobacterium *Synechococcus* sp. PCC 7942 encodes a functional glutathione synthetase. *Microbiology*, *143*(9), 2883–2890. doi:10.1099/00221287-143-9-2883 PMID:9308172

Oleinick, N. L., Chiu, S., Ramakrishnan, N., & Xue, L. (1986). The formation, identification, and significance of DNA-protein cross-links in mammalian cells. *British Journal of Cancer*, *55*, 135–140. PMID:3477283

Pallett, K. E., & Young, A. J. (1993). Caratenoids. In R. G. Alscher & J. L. Hess (Eds.), *Antioxidants in Higher Plants* (pp. 91–110). Boca Raton, FL: CRC Press.

Peña-Llopis, S., Peña, J. B., Sancho, E., Fernández-Vega, C., & Ferrando, M. D. (2001). Glutathione-dependent resistance of the European eel *Anguilla anguilla* to the herbicide molinate. *Chemosphere*, *45*(4-5), 671–681. doi:10.1016/S0045-6535(00)00500-2 PMID:11680763

Polivka, T., & Sundström, V. (2004). Ultrafast dynamics of carotenoid excited states- from solution to natural and artificial systems. *Chemical Reviews*, *104*(4), 2021–2071. doi:10.1021/cr020674n PMID:15080720

Prasanna, R., Sood, A., Jaiswal, P., Nayak, S., Gupta, V., Chaudhary, V., & Natarajan, C. et al. (2010). Rediscovering cyanobacteria as valuable sources of bioactive compounds. *Prikladnaia Biokhimiia i Mikrobiologiia*, *46*(2), 133–147. PMID:20391755

Priya, B., Sivaprasanth, R. K., Jensil, V. D., Uma, L., Subramanian, G., & Prabaharan, D. (2010). Characterization of manganese superoxide dismutase from a marine cyanobacterium *Leptolyngbya valderiana* BDU20041. *Saline Systems*, *6*(1), 1–10. doi:10.1186/1746-1448-6-6 PMID:20525290

Priya, P., Kesheri, M., Sinha, R. P., & Kanchan, S. (2016). Molecular dynamics simulations for Biological Systems. In W. B. A. Karâa & N. Dey (Eds.), *Biomedical Image Analysis and Mining Techniques for Improved Health Outcomes, Advances in Bioinformatics and Biomedical Engineering (ABBE) Series* (pp. 286–313). IGI Global. doi:10.4018/978-1-4666-8811-7.ch014

Ratnam, D. V., Ankola, D. D., Bhardwaj, V., Sahana, D. K., & Kumar, M. N. V. R. (2006). Role of Antioxidants in Prophylaxis and Therapy: A Pharmaceutical Perspective. *Journal of Controlled Release*, *113*(3), 189–207. doi:10.1016/j.jconrel.2006.04.015 PMID:16790290

Rattan, S. I., Kryzch, V., Schnebert, S., Perrier, E., & Nizard, C. (2013). Hormesis-based anti-aging products: A case study of a novel cosmetic. *Dose-Response*, *11*(1), 99–108. doi:10.2203/dose-response.11-054.Rattan PMID:23548988

Richa, Rastogi, R.P., Kumari, S., Singh, K.L., Kannaujiya, V.K., Singh, G., … Sinha, R.P. (2011). Biotechnological potential of mycosporine-like amino acids and phycobiliproteins of cyanobacterial origin. *Biotechnolgy Bioinformatics and Bioengineering*, *1*(2), 159–171.

Sarada, R., Pillai, M. G., & Ravishankar, G. A. (1999). Phycocyanin from *Spirullina* sp.: Influence of processing of biomass on phycocyanin yield, analysis of efficiency of extraction methods and stability studies on phycoyanin. *Process Biochemistry*, *34*(8), 795–801. doi:10.1016/S0032-9592(98)00153-8

Selman, C. J., McLaren, S., Collins, A. R., Duthie, G. G., & Speakman, J. R. (2013). Deleterious consequences of antioxidant supplementation on lifespan in a wild-derived mammal. *Biology Letters*, *9*(4), 20130432. doi:10.1098/rsbl.2013.0432 PMID:23825087

Serrano, A., Rivas, J., & Losada, M. (1984). Purification and properties of glutathione reductase from the cyanobacterium *Anabaena* sp. strain 7119. *Journal of Bacteriology*, *158*, 317–324. PMID:6425264

Seruga, M., Novak, I., & Jakobek, L. (2011). Determination of Polyphenols Content and Antioxidant Activity of Some Red Wines by Differential Pulse Voltammetry, HPLC and Spectrophotometric Methods. *Food Chemistry*, *124*(3), 1208–1216. doi:10.1016/j.foodchem.2010.07.047

Sindhu, E. R., Preethi, K. C., & Kuttan, R. (2010). Antioxidant activity ofcarotenoid luteinin vitroandin vivo. *Indian Journal of Experimental Biology*, *48*, 843–848. PMID:21341544

Sinha, R. P., Klisch, M., Gröniger, A., & Häder, D.-P. (1998). Ultraviolet absorbing/screening substances in cyanobacteria, phytoplankton and macroalgae. *Journal of Photochemistry and Photobiology. B, Biology*, *47*(2-3), 83–94. doi:10.1016/S1011-1344(98)00198-5

Smith, R. C., Prézelin, B. B., Baker, K. S., Bidigare, R. R., Boucher, N. P., Coley, T., & et, et al.. (1992). Ozone depletion: Ultraviolet radiation and phytoplankton biology in Antarctic waters. *Science*, *255*(5047), 952–959. doi:10.1126/science.1546292 PMID:1546292

Solon-Biet, S. M., McMahon, A. C., Ballard, J. W. O., Ruohonen, K., Wu, L. E., Cogger, V. C., & Simpson, S. J. et al. (2014). The ratio of macronutrients, not caloric intake, dictates cardiometabolic health, aging, and longevity inad libitum-fed mice. *Cell Metabolism*, *19*(3), 418–430. doi:10.1016/j.cmet.2014.02.009 PMID:24606899

Steffen, L. M., Jacobs, D. R., Stevens, J., Shahar, E., Carithers, T., & Folsom, A. R. (2003). Associations of WholeGrain, Refined-Grain, and Fruit and Vegetable Consumption with Risks of All-Cause Mortality and Incident Coronary Artery Disease and İschemic Stroke: The Atherosclerosis Risk in Communities (ARIC) Study. *The American Journal of Clinical Nutrition*, *78*, 383–390. PMID:12936919

Stout, M. B., Tchkonia, T., Pirtskhalava, T., Palmer, A. K., List, E. O., Berryman, D. E., & Kirkland, J. L. et al. (2014). Growth hormone action predicts ge-related white adipose tissue dysfunction and senescent cell burden in mice. *Aging*, *6*(7), 575–586. doi:10.18632/aging.100681 PMID:25063774

Sun, L., Wang, S., Chen, L., & Gong, X. (2003). Promising fluorescent probes from phycobiliproteins. *IEEE Journal of Select Topics in Quantam Electronics*, *9*(2), 177–188. doi:10.1109/JSTQE.2003.812499

Tandeau de Marsac, N., & Houmard, J. (1988). Complementary chromatic adaptation: Physiological conditions and action spectra. *Methods in Enzymology*, *167*, 318–328. doi:10.1016/0076-6879(88)67037-6

Tchkonia, T., Morbeck, D. E., Von Zglinicki, T., Van Deursen, J., Lustgarten, J., Scrable, H., & Kirkland, J. L. et al. (2010). Fat tissue, aging, and cellular senescence. *Aging Cell*, *9*(5), 667–684. doi:10.1111/j.1474-9726.2010.00608.x PMID:20701600

Threlfall, D. R., & Whistance, G. R. (1971). Biosynthesis of isoprenoid quinones and chromanols. In T. W. Goodwin (Ed.), *Aspects of Terpenoid Chemistry and Biochemistry* (pp. 357–404). London: Academic Press.

Timmers, S., Auwerx, J., & Schrauwen, P. (2012). The journey of resveratrol from yeast to human. *Aging*, *4*(3), 146–158. doi:10.18632/aging.100445 PMID:22436213

Trebst, A., Depka, B., Jager, J., & Oettmeier, W. (2004). Reversal of the inhibition of photosynthesis by herbicides affecting hydroxyphenylpyruvate dioxygenase by plastoquinone and tocopheryl derivatives in *Chlamydomonas reinhardtii*. *Pest Management Science*, *60*(7), 669–674. doi:10.1002/ps.847 PMID:15260297

Vass, I., Sass, L., Spetea, C., Bakou, A., Ghanatakis, D. F., & Petrouleas, V. (1996). UV-B inhibition of photosystem II electron transport system studied by EPR and chlorophyll florescence. Impairment of donor and acceptor side components. *Biochemistry*, *35*(27), 8964–8973. doi:10.1021/bi9530595 PMID:8688433

Verburgh, K. (2015). Nutrigerontology: Why we need a new scientific discipline to develop diets and guidelines to reduce the risk of aging-related diseases. *Aging Cell*, *14*(1), 17–24. doi:10.1111/acel.12284 PMID:25470422

Wachi, Y., Burgess, J. G., Iwamoto, K., Yamada, N., Nakamura, N., & Matsunaga, T. (1995). Effect of ultraviolet-A (UV-A) light on growth, photosynthetic activity and production of biopterin glucoside by the marine UV-A resistant cyanobacterium *Oscillatoria* sp. *Biochimica et Biophysica Acta*, *1244*(1), 165–168. doi:10.1016/0304-4165(94)00219-N PMID:7766653

Williams, C. H. Jr. (1976). Flavin containing dehydrogenases. In P. D. Boyer (Ed.), *The Enzymes* (pp. 89–173). New York: Academic Press.

Wu, J. J., Liu, J., Chen, E. B., Wang, J. J., Cao, L., Narayan, N., & Finkel, T. et al. (2013). Increased mammalian lifespan and a segmental and tissue-specific slowing of aging after genetic reduction of mTOR expression. *Cell Reports*, *4*(5), 913–920. doi:10.1016/j.celrep.2013.07.030 PMID:23994476

Wullschleger, S., Loewith, R., & Hall, M. N. (2006). TOR signaling in growth and metabolism. *Cell*, *124*(3), 471–484. doi:10.1016/j.cell.2006.01.016 PMID:16469695

Yan, J., Tsuichihara, N., Etoh, T., & Iwai, S. (2007). Reactive oxygen species and nitric oxide are involved in ABA inhibition of stomatal opening. *Plant, Cell & Environment*, *30*(10), 1320–1325. doi:10.1111/j.1365-3040.2007.01711.x PMID:17727421

Zhong, W., Liu, N., Xie, Y., Zhao, Y., Song, X., & Zhong, W. (2013). Antioxidant and anti-aging activities of mycelial polysaccharides from *Lepista sordida*. *International Journal of Biological Macromolecules*, *60*, 355–359. doi:10.1016/j.ijbiomac.2013.06.018 PMID:23811078

Zhou, Z. P., Liu, L. N., Chen, X. L., Wang, J. X., Chen, M., Zhang, Y. Z., & Zhou, B. C. (2005). Factors that affect antioxidant activity of C-phycocyanins from Spirulina platensis. *Journal of Food Biochemistry*, *29*(3), 313–322. doi:10.1111/j.1745-4514.2005.00035.x

KEY TERMS AND DEFINITIONS

Antioxidants: Substances which combat oxidative stress.

Carotenoids: Carotenoids act as a competitive inhibitor for the formation of singlet oxygen.

Glutathione: A tripeptide which is major antioxidant and a low-molecular-weight non-proteinous thiol.

Hormesis: How small amounts of toxic substances can be beneficial by acting as inducers of cellular stress resistance mechanisms.

Nutrigerontology: A new scientific discipline that encompasses biogerontology, medicine, and dietetics.

Oxidative Stress: The imbalance between oxidants and antioxidants in favor of oxidants.

Phycobiliproteins: The phycobiliproteins are constituents of supramolecular complexes known as phycobilisomes.

Superoxide Dismutase: Enzymatic antioxidant which is the first line of defense against nascent oxygen species which mitigates the toxic effect of superoxide ion.

Chapter 9
Food Allergy and Food Poisoning:
Toxicology on Culinary Sciences

Jose Iñaki Alava Marquinez
Basque Culinary Center, Mondragon University, Spain

Miguel Angel Lopez
Basque Culinary Center, Mondragon University, Spain

ABSTRACT

Taken into account data from which is considered a product not safe, estimate the safe level of a contaminant on food, for example, always have many unavoidable uncertainties. It cannot be overemphasized enough, that this also happens as in any other human activity. In most cases, we hope, to define as clearly as possible the eventual risk associated with particular conditions of exposure to a given substance in food. There are numerous toxic compounds that reside naturally in certain foods that unable these to be consumed above certain limits or even are fully prohibited in some other countries. Chapter starts with a clear explanation of differences and relationships between food allergy and food poisoning, continued with main allergens in food and main toxics. Finally, authors summarize different origins of toxins and allergens (natural from foods, from additives, pollutants and food processing).

DOI: 10.4018/978-1-5225-0607-2.ch009

INTRODUCTION

Nowadays food allergy is a public health problem and a matter of concern for consumers. This is firstly, due to the way that affects the quality of life of individuals who suffer them, because is often difficult to choose the right foods for diet. Keep in mind that sometimes symptoms can be serious, or even lead to death. Secondly, the importance of food allergies prevalence that has been observed in the recent years, despite the lack of concrete data to estimate the prevalence precisely is because, among other factors, the lack of uniformity of diagnostic methods and confusion regarding other adverse reactions to foods, it is estimated that between 1 and 3% of adults and between 4 and 6% of children have food allergies (CODEX, 2006).

This chapter reviews the general characteristics of food allergies and their current impact on society, based on a literature review of published literature.

It is known as food allergy a set of adverse reactions to food, due to their ingestion, or inhalation, proven immune pathogenesis. This only occurs in some individuals, maybe after taking small amounts of food not relating them with any physiological or pathophysiological effect. The term "food allergy" is being abused, improperly applied to any adverse reaction to a food or food additive, which is in fact a toxic effect.

Cooking related toxicology has achieved a leading state in recent years, as shown a considerable amount of information on social media (TV and news) and in different scientific journals and texts (Tareke et al, 2000; Berjia et al, 2014; Kima, 2015). Regarding the origin of toxins in the culinary, we can consider four main sources: natural, accidental / allergens, industrial and process generated. Although in some cases, toxins may belong to more than one of these categories simultaneously. Natural toxins can occasionally cause problems, because they can be found unexpectedly in foods with a higher concentration than usual, or toxic species can be confused with harmless ones as often happens with some herbs and plants. Accidental intoxication generally represents the greatest risk to health, unlike the previous ones, not the quantity, frequency, type of associated food is known, or how it came to food. Sometimes it is a little known toxic or popular use abroad as Tonka beans (Dolan et al, 2010) and difficulty to diagnose poisoning. Moreover, the presence of allergens in food is extremely difficult to control, despite the most advanced legislation (European) ((UE) Nº 1169/2011) is always possible the presence of uncontrolled allergens (Alcalá AESAN 2012). Industrial poisons are foreign substances to food, added in amounts known to achieve a particular purpose, such as additives or uncontrolled such as pollutants. These compounds are not safe, even some of them are potentially toxic to most consumers; who may have symptoms with varying intensity. However if additives were not used would be very difficult to have a wide variety and quantity of food in urban areas, which has concentrated the highest percentage of the population in recent years, demanding food for subsistence. Toxic generated by the process, are the result of the transformation of food through different stages of development; from cooking, stabilization, formulation, mixing, sterilization, transportation, etc. These toxins can result from such simple processes such as roast meats, doing different polycyclic aromatic hydrocarbons, many with mutagenic and carcinogenic molecules finally generated.

BACKGROUND

Some eats are inherently poisonous while others can lead to health conditions that sometimes prove fatal. From pre-hominids time to now every time that we eat something, we are suffering a (more or less) controlled risk to death. This risk will come, from the toxicity of the food eaten or from and adverse reaction of our organism to normal food composition. Obviously the age, sex, size and previous exposition, are factor that modulate the negative action of eaten food. Modern industrial processes, as well as culinary ones, introduce new molecules in our food-stock, creating new sceneries for food poisoning.

METABOLIC DIFFERENCES BETWEEN ALLERGY AND POISONING

In fact body reactions due to food intake may create a wide range of results. Adverse food reactions (food hypersensitivities,) include any abnormal reaction resulting from the ingestion of a food and might be the result of food intolerances (non-allergic food hypersensitivities) or food hypersensitivity/allergy (food allergy).

In many cases, differences between intolerance and a clear allergy are imperceptibles. Food intolerances (non-allergic food hypersensitivities) are adverse responses caused by some unique physiologic characteristic of the host, such as metabolic disorders. Food hypersensitivities/allergies are adverse immunologic. Toxic reactions might mimic food hypersensitivities and typically are due to factors inherent in a food, such as toxic contaminants (e.g., histamine in scombroid fish poisoning) or pharmacologic substances within the food, which can affect most healthy individuals when given in appropriate doses.

Food aversions also might mimic adverse food reactions but are not mounting a brisk protective response to dangerous pathogens (Sampson 2004).

The gastrointestinal immune response thus plays a pivotal role in maintaining protective immunity in health and a critical role in the pathogenesis of a wide variety of clinical disorders associated with food allergy (MacDonal & DiSabatino,

2009). Within both (food allergy and poisoning), food allergy reactions mediated by IgE immune pathogenesis (immediate hypersensitivity or allergic type) such as those produced by other immune mechanism known (non-IgE mediated reactions) are included. It is characteristic of the early presence of high titers of antibodies against IgE in food. (Bellanti et al, 2004) Also it can be found increased specific antibodies from other classes of immunoglobulins, immune complexes and most probably mediated immunity responses cells. The existence of a joint involvement, i.e. IgE mediated reactions partially and cells, in varying degrees are also possible. In any case, plus evidence of dependency between ingestion of a food and the appearance of symptoms, it is necessary that these altered immune parameters are directly involved in the pathophysiology responsible for the symptoms.

Some enteropathy such as celiac disease and enteropathy and other food protein enterocolitis (cow's milk, rice, chicken, soy, etc.) may be included within the concept of food allergy, because in them is proven or probably the existence of an underlying immune mechanism. Allergic reactions to foods must be distinguished from food intolerance reactions and toxic reactions to foods.

Food intolerance is a form of adverse reaction to a food or food additive in the pathogenesis does not exist or has not been demonstrated, unlike food allergy, immune-based mechanism. Senses, food intolerance and food allergy have been used and, sometimes, are still used indiscriminately and even with a similar meaning, which has favored the emergence of confusion when analyzing the pathogenic, clinical, diagnostic and therapeutic processes. Despite all, more than 20 years ago, for the first time was defined with a pathogenic base, the concepts used to describe adverse reactions to foods (Metcalfe, 1984), whose use, has allowed better communication in the scientific literature regarding the different reactions to food components.

Food intolerance reactions can occur by the following mechanisms:

- Enzymatic or metabolic, defects related to enzymes involved in the metabolism of food (Table 1).
- Pharmacological foods or intolerance due to the pharmacological action of chemical compounds naturally or added to food, such as caffeine, theobromine that may cause heart rhythm disturbances, tremor or migraine in certain individuals, even when ingested in moderate doses (Table 2).
- Finally, there is food intolerance called indeterminate, to denote any intolerance reaction whose mechanism is not clarified production. At last, most adverse reactions include food additives.

Toxic reactions caused by food (food poisoning), include those for foodborne diseases and produced by chemical or biological agents contained therein.

Table 1. Main food intolerances by enzymatic effect

Situation	Enzyme Deficiency
Disaccharidase deficiency	Lactose, sucrose
Galactosemia	Galactose-*1*-phosphate uridyl transferase
Hyperbilirubinemia	uridine diphosphate -epimerase
phenylketonuria	Fenilalanin-hidroxilasa
Alcohol intolerance	Aldehyde-dehydrogenase
Favism	*Glucose-6*-phosphate dehydrogenase

Table 2. Endogenous agents responsible for the pharmacological action of food

Vasoactive Amines	Diamines	Histamine
	Monoamines	Tyramine *Phenylalanine* Serotonin Dopamine
Methylxanthines		Caffeine Theobromine Theophylline
Others		Capsaicin Ethanol Myristin

Its main feature is that anyone can be susceptible to poisoning from these products, although the vast majority of them are not dangerous, because the amount that can be ingested in a normal diet is insufficient to cause any harm. Table 3 shows a classification of the agents capable of causing food poisoning. Some, such as additives or histamine may act by different mechanisms as poisoning agents.

Intolerance reactions and toxic reactions are characterized both by being dose-dependent. The clinical manifestations that occur are the more intense the higher amount of ingested food or food additive. This dose-response relationship cannot exist in allergic reactions, so that, in some of them, very small doses can lead to an exaggerated clinical response. Another peculiar feature is that toxic reactions can occur in any individual, whenever you eat food in sufficient quantity. Instead, both toxic and allergic reactions in intolerance, the onset of clinical manifestations before the ingestion of a particular product at a given dose is only in relation to individual characteristics, so that the same dose is perfectly tolerated by any other individual, otherwise healthy (Table 4). Probably small quantities of poisoning products (histamine-like), during the early development of immune system, are responsible of immunoglobulin's alterations in childhood and in correspondence early food allergy development (Taylor et al, 1984).

Issues, Controversies, Problems

Despite these differences, sometimes toxic reactions, intolerance or allergy can lead to very similar clinical pictures. This situation will occur when the agent responsible, in addition to a general pharmacological action, is acting on an individual who, for certain characteristics, has a response threshold decreased. It is also possible that

Table 3. Toxic food reactions

Due to Added Chemicals	
Agricultural chemicals Chemicals packaging Industrial chemicals	Insecticides, herbicides, fungicides, fertilizers Lead, tin, copper, cinc Polychlorides and biphenyl polibromuros, mercury
Due to Natural Contaminants	
Microorganisms Toxins	Campylobacter, Salmonella, Sighella Clostridium botulinum (botulism) Estaphylococcus aureus (staphylococcal intoxication) Neurotoxin dinoflagellate (ciguatera) Mycotoxins (ergotism, aflatoxins)
Due to Persistent Toxic Chemicals	
Dangerous at any dose	Poisonous animals Poisonous plants Poisonous mushrooms
Dangerous if ingested in Large Quantities	Cyanogenic Glycosides (plumlike) Latirógenos (almortas) Bociógenos (berros, nabos) Atropina (estramonio) Solanina (patata y tomate verdes)
By Generated Natural Toxicants	
	Histamine poisoning (scromboid)

Table 4. Differences and similarities between allergic reactions, intolerance reactions and toxic reactions to food

	Allergic Reaction	Intolerance Reaction	Toxic Reaction
Depending on the individual factors	(+)	(+)	
Depending on food factors	(-)	(-)	
Pathogeny	Inmunological	Diverse, non inmunological	Diverse, non inmunological
Examples	Urticaria	Lactose intolerance	Escombroid
	Anaphylaxis	Favism	Lathyrism
	Enteropathies	Galactosemia	Botulism
	Colitis	Phenylketonuria	Toxic Oil syndrome

the responsible agent, ex, histamine, also is a mediator of anaphylactic reactions, which may result in similar clinical pictures to them ("anaphylactoid reactions", "food pseudoallergy").

In contrast to the ingrained idea among laymen and even among some medical doctors, it is likely that food allergy constitutes only a quantitatively very small part of all the adverse reactions to foods. Data on prevalence of food allergy in the population are very limited in both children and adults, because the conceptual gap and the different diagnostic criteria used. If a method of controlled provocation is used to assess a possible adverse reaction to a food. No more than one third of the supposedly allergic children respond positively (Bock 1987) and less in the adult population (Jansen et al., 1994) (Young & Stoneham, 1994). Also, within the pediatric population, it appears that its incidence is higher in younger children.

Food Allergy

All foods can be potentially sensitizing. Its prevalence is related, among other factors, to feeding habits of the population studied. However, when excluding sensitizations with no clinical relevance, most patients respond only to few foods. Also, its prevalence may vary with age, associates regarding exposure to allergens and mainly to immunological and physiological processes of maturation factors. Approximately half of the cases of childhood food allergies are associated with animal allergens. In our environment, the child, the egg (protein clear) is the most common food allergen, followed by cow's milk and fish (Crespo et al., 1995). After that become dominated by sensitization to vegetables, such as nuts, fresh fruits, legumes and vegetables; frequently found in these patients, associated sensitization to pollens (Kany et al., 2001). Food allergens are water-soluble proteins or glycoproteins with a size between 10 and 70 kDal. and consequently more stable to heat, acid and proteases. In foods are often one or several main, major or larger and other secondary or minor allergens allergen and which are regarded as respectively allergens to which respond most immunologically sensitized patients or relevant food allergens to which respond only a few individuals. Some are characteristic of a particular food can be shared with other species of the same or close family (eg, fish, legumes) and others may be present even in phylogenetically distant families.

This usually correspond to proteins with similar function (profilin, Trophomyosins, serum albumins, etc.). Some are widespread, being known as "panallergens". These panallergens may be involved in the poly-sensibilities detected in many patients,

1. **Food Allergens of Animal Origin:**
   a. **Cow Milk:** Although, it has been demonstrated, various mammalian milks cause allergic reactions. Cow milk, is most common and best studied.

Milk human species, cow's milk, or a derivative formula are usually the first food that non-homologous individual receives in significant quantities. This means, that it is also the first food antigen which humans come into contact with in a usual way. Therefore, is not surprising that is, in the early childhood, the food that causes the greatest number of adverse reactions. In Spain, the incidence data of immediate allergy to cow's milk proteins (PLV) in infants varies between 0.4 and 1.9 per 100 (Sanz et al., 2001) (García et al., 2003).

Major allergen components include serum proteins in cow's milk (particularly, beta-lactoglobulin, alpha-lactalbumin and, to a less extent bovine serum albumin) and casein (alpha, beta and kappa). Comparing with purified proteins from cow's milk, it was observed that beta-lactoglobulin is the protein that more often induces clinical responses.

b. **Egg:** The egg is a widely consumed food worldwide and the leading cause of allergic reactions in children (Crespo et al.,1995). The light seems to be more allergenic than the yolk. Egg the major allergen present in the clear, is the ovomucoid (Gal d 1) (Bernhisel-Broadbent et al., 1994). Is a trypsin inhibitor and represents 10% of the protein content of the egg white. The main feature of ovomucoid is its extreme resistance to degradation by proteases and thermos-stability, so allergen resulting affected by cooking in minimal amounts. Another allergenic protein is egg white or ovotransferrin, conalbumin (Gal d 3) having homology with other iron binding proteins, such as serum transferrin and more labile than previously commented. Other allergen is white egg white lysozyme (Gal d 4), 14.3 kDa protein, composed of a single polypeptide chain linked by four disulfide bridges.

Also the yolk can have a major allergen paper, since the involvement of yolk livetins. In syndrome called "feather-egg" (Mandallaz et al., 1988), based on clinical observation of patients showed that starts with respiratory allergy awareness feathers and subsequently develops egg allergy (in adults), with some special features like its beginning at a later age, presence of asthma due to sensitization to feathers and a recognition profile egg allergens different. In children with this clinical framework, feathers sensitization, usually occur, previous to egg sensitization (Añibaro et al., 1997). These patients exhibit IgE antibodies to a protein of 65-70 kDa yolk, alpha-livetin, identified as chicken serum albumin and responsible for cross-reactivity.

c. **Fish:** Fish allergy is relatively common in countries where consumption is high, like Japan, Scandinavian countries and Spain. However, this distribution tends to change due to market entry of new food products derived from fish such as surimi, or by the use of fish oil rich in polyunsaturated fatty acids, given their beneficial effects on the cardiovascular system. The fish species most frequently involved in allergic reactions are gadiformes (cod, hake) and flatfish (flounder, rooster); less salmon, clupeiforms (sardine, anchovy) and tuna (Pascual et al., 1992).

The first purified and well-characterized allergen fish was Gad c 1 (previously designated as Allergen M), found in cod (*Gadus callarias*) (Aas 1966). This allergen belongs to a group of proteins known as parvalbumins muscle, which control the flow of calcium through the cell membrane and are only found in the muscle of fish and amphibians. Gad c 1 is very heat-stable and resistant to proteolysis. Allergenicity is considerably reduced in canned fish.

The structural similarity of different fish parvalbumins makes in sensitized patients very often to arise cross reactions (Pascual et al., 1992). However, the differences make its importance not alike in all species of fish. A third of those allergies to fish, tuna patients tolerate as albacore (*Thunnus alalunga*).

d. **Crustaceans and Mollusks:** Crustaceans have been recognized as a common cause of food hypersensitivity reactions. Their allergens are thermostable. In recent years described the existence of cross-reactivity between different species of crustaceans and less, but also relevant to other allergens present in insects and mites (Dermatophagoides spp.).

Shellfish can be gastropods such as snails, bivalves such as clams, mussels, oysters and cephalopods such as octopus and squid. The major allergen seems to be also tropomyosin and is often is associated with sensitization to shellfish (Leung et al., 1996).

2. **Food allergens of plant origin:**

a. **Vegetables:** Legumes are dicotyledonous plants botanical order of *Fabaces* comprising three families: *Mimosaceae, Papilionaceae* and *Cesalpiniaceae.* Major species responsible for allergic reactions (lentil, pea, pea, peanut, soybean, lupine) belonging to the *Papilionaceae* family, commonly known as legumes. The vegetables are among the food allergens that most often cause immediate allergy in children (Pereira et al., 2002). In Mediterranean countries the introduction of nuts, including peanuts, not done before 2 or 3 years, although in recent times the use of peanut, soybean and lupine as additives makes its consume earlier and also hidden-form, which could be contributing to the incidence of allergy to legumes.

Peanut (*Arachis hypogaea*) is responsible for many serious allergic reactions, whose frequency has not only increased in recent years, but also its appearance is earlier, partly due to increased consumption, possessing proteins Very versatile, easily digested and various presentations; aperitif, fresh, grilled, butter or an oil.

The peanut is the major food allergen in US and the leading cause of anaphylaxis. It is estimated that allergy in the general US population may be about 1%. According to some authors would be the major food allergen in children over three years (Bock and Atkins, 1989) but it is also rising at younger ages. In Europe, more specifically in Anglo-Saxon countries, their allergenic importance is increasing in recent years by the similarity of dietary patterns with the US, due to both changes in dietary habits (increased consumption of fast food, immigration and different dietary habits), and its role as hidden allergen. It has been found that roasting increases allergenicity, possibly due to changes in the molecular structure or enzyme function (Beyer et al., 2001).

In peanuts have been identified several major allergens in sensitized patients. The Ara h 1 allergen is a 63.5 kDa glycoprotein that has high homology with vicilins (storage proteins present in the seeds of many plants). The identification of this protein family may partly explain the wide immunological cross-reactivity between peanut and other legumes.

Soybean (*Glycine max*) is the basis of tofu, soybean paste and soy milk, also consumed fresh. It is common cause of adverse reactions, possibly helped by its wide use in the West as an additive and as a food supplement to enrich the protein content of other foods. Soy can be found in bread, cakes, ice cream, breakfast cereals, packet soups, canned tuna, hot dogs, sauces, Chinese food, etc. Also, their use in dietary formulas has been considered as a possible cause of sensitization in infants, sometimes with the presence of specific IgE to soy, but generally no demonstrable clinic for soybean (Cordle, 2004) (Martin, 2006).

Among the various allergens identified in soybeans, fractions with molecular weight 13-14 kDa and 25 kDa 22-, are the most powerful in three different groups except;whole soybean powder and shell, and have proven their allergenicity both inhalation and through the digestive tract (González et al., 1995).

The lentil (*Lens sculenta*) is the most consumed vegetable in Spain. In this country with a traditionally Mediterranean diet, lentils are legumes that most often cause IgE-mediated hypersensitivity, followed by chick-pea. They are the fourth or fifth leading cause of food allergy in the child population. In addition, half the cases begin between the first and third year of life, predominantly in the second year (Pereira et al., 2002).

In lentil described a protein band between 12 and 16 kDa, which would be called a gamma-Len c 1 vicilin subunit, and a weight of approximately 66 kDa, Len c 2, corresponding to a biotinylated seed protein.
Has been identified Len c 1 as a major allergen and Len c 2 as a minor allergen lentil (López-Torrejón et al., 2003). Len c 1 shows a 45% similarity with Ara h 1 Peanut allergen greater.

b. **Other Vegetables:** The chickpea (*Cicer arietinum*) is similarly important cause of allergic reactions in the East and in our environment, due to their high consumption. The bean (*Phaseolus vulgaris*) is native to Central and South America. There are many edible species and can be divided broadly into two types: those that are eaten with pods whose seeds are not developed (green beans) and those which only the seeds (beans, beans, pinto bean) are eaten. The lupine (*Lupinus sativus*) is used as a protein rich in pastries and other food for its high content of nitrogenous substances, fats and minerals. It has been identified as a hidden allergen responsible for anaphylactic reactions (Rojas-Hijazo et al., 2006). The pea (*Pisum sativum*) is an herbaceous legume from Asia. It is rich in proteins, lipids, lysine, vitamins A, B and E, phosphorus and calcium. In children ingestion is rare before 2 or 3 years. There have been rare allergic reactions to this legume.

c. **Cereals:** Described the major allergens in wheat flour, barley and rye are water soluble (albumins and globulins) and related symptoms are derived from no exposure inhalation and ingestion with (Houba et al., 1998).
The higher in baker's asthma allergen is a group of inhibitors of alpha-amylase. A 15-kDa allergen in wheat flour and other flour 14.5 kDa barley inhibitors trypsin / alpha-amylase have been identified. Also, homodimeric 25 kDa proteins of rye and barley have been isolated. Swallowed allergy to wheat and other cereals is rare in the West (Crespo et al., 1995a). Regarding intake, has been identified, frequently involved in sensitization to wheat flour in children with atopic dermatitis and more recently been shown that the alpha-amylase inhibitor is a wheat allergen relevant allergenic protein of 50 kDa Patients who experience hypersensitivity reactions with wheat protein intake (Palosou, 2003).
The major allergens of rice (Oryza sativa) have been identified as albumins 14 to 16 kDa molecular weight, belonging to the family of inhibitors of trypsin / alpha-amylase (Alvarez et al., 1995). They have also identified a lipid transfer protein as a major allergen in individuals with corn clinical signs after ingestion (Pastorello et al, 2000).

d. **Gluten:** The term "gluten"as a fraction of proteins from wheat, rye, barley, and oats, or crossed varieties and derivatives thereof and which is insoluble in water and in 0.5 M NaCl Prolamines form the gluten fraction which can be extracted with a 40-70 percent ethanol. The prolamin from wheat is gliadin, from rye is secalin, barley hordein and oats avenin. Oats currently appears separated from the three cereals referred to above and it may not be disease-inducing like other cereals (rice, corn), although this phenomenon is correlated with possibly fewer oats contains prolamine proportionally to the others mentioned cereals.

According to their amino acid sequences, the gliadins are subdivided into alpha, gamma and omega-gliadins and are rich in proline and glutamine. These prolamins are harmful to certain individuals and their intake triggers them celiac disease .It is often said that these patients have "gluten sensitivity". Prolamin content of gluten is generally reduced by 50 percent (Codex 2006).

e. **Fruits and Vegetables:** In the Mediterranean area fruits are a common cause of food allergy, particularly of oral allergy syndrome. They have been identified only in a few clinical studies species, causing IgE mediated allergy. The family *Rosaceae* (apple, pear, peach, albarcoque, plum, cherry) and *Cucurbitaceae* (melon, watermelon, cucumber, pumpkin, zucchini) have received special attention in clinical studies as well as bananas (family *Musaceae*) and kiwi (family *Actinidiaceae*).

Other families of fruits are abundant immunological and molecular data, but very little information on its possible clinical significance. Among vegetables, celery allergy is of particular interest for their ability to produce anaphylactic reactions (Ballmer-Weber et al., 2000).

The tomato, both raw and cooked is a regular feature in the diet. The awareness of this vegetable is particularly prevalent in the Mediterranean area, especially in children and adolescents, within is the most common clinical oral allergy syndrome. However, when there is an awareness associated latex, the most common manifestations are urticarial and anaphylaxis (Reche et al., 2001).

There are very few communications allergy to other vegetables. It is very rare lettuce allergy can cause allergic contact dermatitis, but not enough of allergic reactions upon ingestion data (Franck et al., 2000).

The allergens in fruits and vegetables are thermolabile, which facilitates tolerance sensitized individuals after specific treatments that inactivate their antigens.

f. **Nuts ("Nuts in Shell"):** Under the name of nuts, tree nuts, walnuts ("nuts") various seeds from different botanical families are included. It is a heterogeneous group of foods without Botanical related, but with great allergenic similarities and consumption patterns. Oleaginous fruits are consumed in dried form among which are: almonds, hazelnuts, cashews, walnuts, Brazil nuts, Pecan nut, pistachio, pine nuts, and sunflower seeds. Its stability against heat and digestive processes favor its high allergenicity, so often the reactions are intense and immediate. Allergy to nuts is one of the most common food allergies, although its prevalence varies according to age and geographic area.

They occur most often in children than in adults (Ewan, 1996) and, sometimes, may appear before the first known contact with the nut. It is likely that exposure to small amounts unnoticed or sensitization by other means explain these intense reactions. They can lead to severe clinical manifestations, even in small quantities, due to its presence as food ingredients or flavorings in various food products.

Allergy to nuts is often associated with allergies to various pollens. Most individuals with allergies to hazelnut are sensitized to pollens of birch and hazel (Ortolani et al., 2000) and confirmed that the major allergen in hazelnut is a 18 kDa protein homologous to Bet v 1 birch (Pastorello et al., 2002).

The major allergen of Brazil nuts (*Bertholletia excelsa*), Ber e 1 is a methionine-rich 2S protein composed of two subunits of 9 and 3 kDa. This protein has been used in transgenic studies to correct the deficit in methionine levels having soybeans. However, the commercial development of this GM soy has been abandoned, and that gene transfer of allergen (Ber e 1), of the Brazil nut, also transfers its allergenicity of soybean (Nordlee et al, 1996).

g. **Sesame:** The *Sesamum indicum* is native to tropical Africa, whose cultivation is widespread, for the use of plant seeds. Allergenic importance is great in those places where consumption is common. It is an ingredient that should be clearly identified and separated from nuts and peanuts, which can also contaminate. The prevalence and severity of allergy seed sesame has increased in recent years in Europe (Gangur et al., 2005) due to its introduction from Asian countries in the diet as food ingredient or oil, especially in bakery products, fast food, new foods and vegetarian products. Given its characteristics, sesame must be identified when used as ingredient in packaged foods, as indicated by Directive 2003/89 of the European Union (EU, 2003). However, many products and ready meals containing sesame are sold at fast food places, bakeries, restaurants, etc., whose ingredients are not easily identifiable and where cross contamination is more likely.

h. **Mustard:** Mustard is one of the most allergenic of spices on record to date, therefore its prevalence as allergenic potency. As for other food allergens, sensitization depends on the eating habits of the population. Allergens have been isolated from the seed of yellow mustard (*Sinapis alba*) and Eastern (*Brassica juncea*) and their primary structures have been studied in great detail (González de la Pena et al., 1993) (Monsalve et al., 1993). No all allergens of yellow mustard seed is a 15 kDa protein. Structural homology of an occupational allergen, Ric c 1, *Ricinus communis*, is known and is probably related to other 2S albumin present in soybean, cottonseed and pea.

3. **Other:** Latex, Anisakis, Mites, etc.: They are sometimes cause of serious clinical pictures, plus unexpected. Besides food used as additives, other conveyed by foods that can act as allergens. As most important, the following can be considered:
    a. **Latex:** Or natural rubber latex is a processed plant product obtained from the milky sap of many plants, though the only one who has been commercially exploited is from *Hevea brasiliensis* tree. Due to its elastic properties is used to make multiple everyday items such as gloves, condoms, pacifiers, baby bottle nipples, balloons, stickers, etc. .; and more specific as medical supplies, catheters, tourniquets, gloves, masks, etc. It is estimated consumption worldwide of 5.5 million tons per year. Latex allergy occurs by type I or immediate hypersensitivity mediated by IgE antibodies to latex proteins.

        The relationship between latex allergy and food allergy has two aspects to consider. On the one hand, it acts as a contaminant, in their contact with food proteins, handled with latex gloves. In this situation, there may be apparent signs of food allergy in patients allergic to latex. Furthermore, it is often an association of latex allergy and various fruits and vegetables allergens such as kiwi, chestnut, avocado, banana, papaya, figs, potatoes, peach, pineapple, grapes, celery, plum, tomato, etc…, which is known as "latex-fruit syndrome" (Wakelin & White, 1999), which is related to the existence in latex similar to those found in these plant antigens.
    b. **Anisakis:** The anisakiosis is a parasitic disease that is caused by parasitized fish larvae of Anisakis spp., consumed rare or undercooked. It is particularly important as health problem, in countries with high fish consumption. The adult parasite is found in the digestive tract of a variety of marine mammals, which act as definitive hosts (wales, dolphins, etc.) The larvae mature in the water and are eaten by small crustaceans that feed on various species of fish and cephalopods, which reached the stage of L3. The cycle is completed when the definitive hosts acquire carriers L3 intermediaries. Humans are an occasional host a result of eating contaminated fish larvae and he cannot complete its life cycle.

Clinical signs and symptoms develop as a result of inflammatory reaction caused by the penetration of larvae in the mucosa of the gastric wall. It can also cause manifestations of allergic reaction (hypersensitivity) immediate type ranging from urticarial or angioedema to anaphylactic shock and mixed frameworks with gastrointestinal and allergic clinic symptoms. In patients IgE antibodies primarily directed against antigens of the various structures of Anisakis larvae are detected. To the consumer, it should not consume rare fish that has not been previously frozen under 24 h, or fresh fish cooked to no more than 60 ° C for at least 5-10 minutes. The cooked on the grill or microwave are less secure than cooking or frying (AESAN, 2005) procedures.

c. **Mites (Dermatophagoides):** There are several publications of asthmatic patients sensitized to mites, *Dermatophagoides farinae* mainly no history of food allergy, anaphylactic reactions have presented different intensity by ingesting contaminated products made from flour mite. This contamination is common in places with warm, moist environment that favors growth of these mites. In Spain is described on inhabitants of the Canary Islands (Garcia-Robaina et al., 1997).
d. **Residues of Veterinary Drugs:** Sometimes animal foods may contain residues from veterinary treatment. Depending on the nature and risk of the same to human health, mandating absence or maximum limits in foodstuffs is regulated. Specifically, allergic reactions have been reported after ingestion of foods with residues of antibiotics such as ß-lactams and macrolides for which there are maximum permitted residues (Dewdney et al., 1991). Long such allergic reactions have been associated with the presence of penicillin in milk (Wicher and Reisman, 1980). Surveillance studies show a low incidence of detectable residues in most products (Figure 1).

Toxics in Foods

Although an agent causes food poisoning may be chemical or physical, in food toxicology it refers exclusively to chemicals. A term widely used in the drug area to define any foreign substance to the body in question is that of xenobiotic agent. However as Paracelsus said: "dosis sola facit venenum" even oxygen, that is essential to maintain the life of any aerobic organism, an atmosphere of pure oxygen is harmful to any mammal, as it is quickly consumed aminobutyric acid, moderator cerebral and nerve transmission, decrease and consequently serious nervous disorders occurs that end to convulsions and death (Repetto, 1981) occur. One could mention many examples which show the dictum of Paracelsus, indicating that the beneficial

Figure 1. Top eight allergies distribution, in children around the world
Extracted from Prevalence of allergies around the world: the big eight (ten, thirteen?). M. Fernandez-Rivas, Symposium on Sensitizing Properties of Proteins, Prague, 11-13 April 2012 (http:www.hesiglobal.org/files/public/Committee%20Presentations/PATC/Fernandez%20Rivasfor%20websiteAPPROVED.pdf)

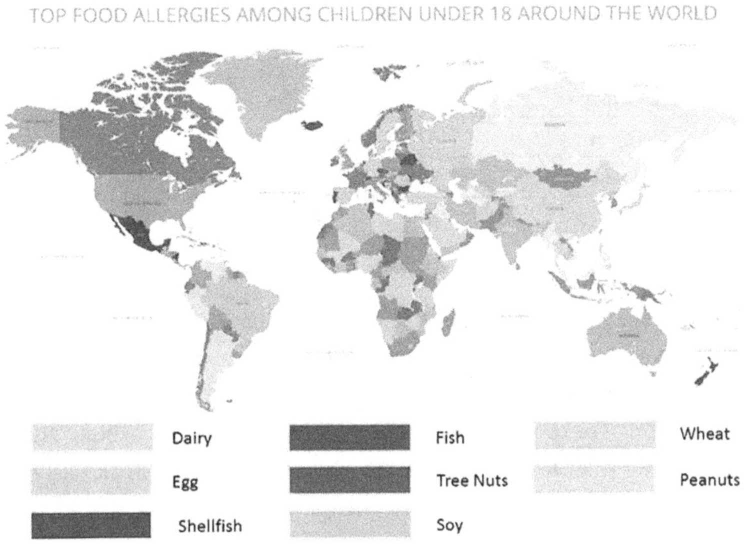

and harmful effect, of a substance depends on the dose. However, for each chemical there is a certain degree of toxicity.

Currently it is managing the concept of "potential toxicity," which has been proposed by Luckey and Venugopal, in an attempt to have a parameter to assess the toxicity of substances more accurately. This potential toxicity (pT) depends among other factors, the experienced animal species and route of administration. By definition, pT is the intake of base 10 logarithm of the inverse of the dose of a substance expressed in mol / kg, given produces a toxic effect. (Luckey & Venugopal, 1977; Repetto, 1981).

$$pT = -\log T$$

where,

T = toxic dose molar base.

Knowing the molecular weight (MW) of xenobiotic compound or agent is easy to calculate the pT, as shown in Table 5.

Table 5. Acute toxicity of some representative substances

Substance	DL 50 (mg/K)
Ethylic Alcohol	10.000
Sodic Phenobarbital	150
Strychnine	2
Nicotine	1
Tetrodotoxine	0,1
Dioxin	0,001
Botox	0,00001

From Klaassen et al., 1986.

Fungal toxins are probably the main cause of chronic toxicity in foods. Since the discovery of protein synthesis inhibitory fungal toxins (Fando et al, 1985), many fungi species has shown dangerous toxins able to appear in foods (Varga et al, 2003, Abarca et al, 2000). These fungi and their spores are sprayed around human environment in building (Cooley et al, 1998, Shelton B.G. et al, 2002), air (Zukiewicz-Sobczak 2013), water (Gonçalves et al, 2006) and food making places (Simeray et al, 1995).

Aspergillus species are probably the most extended fungi and play a key role in fungal toxicity. *Aspergillus oryzae* is used, in much classical Asian fermentations like, soy sauce,

sake and miso. Unfortunately is very difficult to distinguish at lance, between *Aspergillus oryzae,* and *A.flavus, A.restrictus, A.fumigatus* etc… species producers of fungal toxins.(EPA 1997).

Biological Factors that Influence Toxicity

The biological system which acts on the toxic agent is critical, because the effect will vary considerably according to the agency. This factor should be taken into account, since it is well known that among the different species of animals and humans there is great variation in sensitivity to toxic agents. The knowledge of the origin, development and course of poisoning in a particular animal should be established to scientifically based, extrapolate to humans. Precisely in toxicology, a specific branch known as Comparative Toxicology, which indicates on the basis of substantiated studies, animal model can be used to extrapolate experimental results to man. About the above, are some examples of animal models (Melby & Altman, 1976; Hodgson & Gutherie, 1980).

The effect of a toxic agent on a biological system results in an alteration of physiological equilibrium (homeostasis), so that poisoning is an illness and as such should be considered under pathos- chronic criterion, or must observe the developments in line time and we can classify it as acute poisoning, chronic or subacute.

Acute poisoning is defined as exposure to a xenobiotic agent that produces an almost immediate manifestation (sometimes in minutes), with a single administration of the poison, which can lead to poisoned to death, or total or partial recovery, which they may be or not sequels or nagging injuries.

In many cases of acute poisoning phenomenon, it happen reversibility except death. Overall subacute poisoning does not imply a lesser degree of severity of acute intoxication, but an evolution of subclinical disorders poisoning will appear.

Although this type of poisoning requires repetitive administration of toxic, not visible at the start conditions are present; however, the short term can present evidence of intoxication and some toxicologists believe that it is present, be exposed to the toxic biological system over a period that can range from one month to three months. Chronic poisoning occurs due to repeated exposure to the toxic agent.

This absorption occurs with relatively small toxic, which by itself does not produce visible amounts disorders initially, but the accumulation of xenobiotic agents in the body (typically in a specific organ or tissue) and over time are presented pathological conditions, and in most cases are irreversible. In this type of poisoning, initial conditions remain latent (subclinical) and are usually reversible; until for some reason, as it could be a decrease in normal physiological conditions (illness), you can highlight the poisoning. A classic chronic intoxication example, is the effect of carcinogenic substances, since in sub lethal doses, these compounds are not evident in the short term.

Poisoning requires three months to one or more years and when it manifests itself in clinical form, is very difficult to reverse the damage produced (Fabre & Truhaut, 1976; Repetto, 1981; Klaassen et al, 1986).

The concept of acceptable daily intake (ADI) or also called Acceptable Daily Intake (ADI), refers to the reduced expression of all available toxicological data for a given xenobiotic agent. DDA itself corresponds to the amount of a substance that can be ingested daily by an individual throughout his life, without as to cause damage to health. This level or dose is generally set by animal experimentation on acute and chronic toxicity (currently investigating mutagenic, teratogenic and carcinogenic) and preferably taking the value of the dose without observable effect (NOEL) for the most sensitive species. The maximum amount of xenobiotic that the most sensitive animal can ingest daily without adverse effect sought. However, it can be extrapolated to the human you have to take the safety factor (FS), which should generally consider interspecies or intra-species variation and the value of 100 (Pennington., 1998; Larry et al, 1990; Derache, 1990; Kotsonis et al, 1994).

Therefore the DDA is generally hundredth of NOEL for the most sensitive animal and expressed in mg / kg body weight. This DDA allows a high degree of probability, ensure a low risk of xenobiotic in question, but you will never say with absolute certainty safety.

Getting the DDA from NOEL: Acceptable Daily Intake or ADI

DDA = NOEL / FS

where,

NOEL = no-observed-effect dose (mg / kg pc- day)
SF = Safety factor (10 when the NOEL is of the same species; 100 for another)

Naturally Toxic Agents in Foods

Natural toxins found inherently in plant or animal foods, can be harmful when consumed in sufficient quantities. Natural toxins serve specific functions in ecosystems as chemical signals or as chemical defenses against predators, parasites or infectious microorganism. Obviously the molecules used have a wide range of chemical structures and toxicity levels.

The most common intoxications are those produced by toxic fungi. Every year inexpert people around the world die by toxic fungi ingestion. Although only a few of the 70-80 species of poisonous mushrooms are actually fatal when ingested, many of these deadly fungi bear an unfortunate resemblance to edible species and are thus especially dangerous. (Karlson-Stiber., Perssons, 2003)

They are near 2.000 species of poisonous plants in the world. Many times more than those considered as food (few hundred). Even many of this “nutritious” plants can become toxic if they are taken in excess or if they are not cooked in the right way. In addition, the toxicity of poisonous plants will change in dependence of sub-specie, as well as the geographical and climate conditions.

In culinary sciences are usual some plants that are very dangerous if they are ingested untreated: Potatoes (Solanine and glycoalkaloids), manioc, bamboo (Cyanide generating compounds and saponines), green beans (enzyme inhibitors). (Wink et al, 2008).

In animals, toxins may come from their proper metabolism or a chemical passed along the food chain. Is more frequent, that poisoning happens, eating marine animals than terrestrial ones. Marine toxins generated by toxic microalgae (Dinoflagellates) are accumulated in shellfish, fish and crustaceans and at end consumed by humans. Also microorganism and coral will produce neurotoxins (Tetrodotoxin) that may cause lethality after ingested (Chun-Fai Yu et al, 2004).

Culinary technics are very important in decrease or annulation of heat-labile toxins. One of most relevant examples is squid ink, used in Spanish and Italian gastronomy. The squid ink, contains toxic microorganism, melanin, melanin related products and L-Dopa. A single thermic treatment of 20 min. at 80° C is enough to neutralize toxicity of squid ink, and let it ready for food use (Fiore et al, 2004).

Food Additives and Toxicity

Food additives are natural or artificial substances, which are added to food in order to preserve or enhance its qualities, either preserving them from microorganisms, enhancing its taste, color or improving its texture. Safety or toxicity of additives it's depends on the substance itself and the amount used in final food. Both natural and synthetic products can be potentially mutagenic or cause allergic reactions (flour improvers, etc.) Another danger is the possibility to be used as cover, tampering or alterations of food, causing poisoning. (FAO/OMS, expert committee, 1965).

Pollutants Toxicity

During the past two hundred years humanity, has been discharging industrial waste in natural environment. Many of this industrial waste are chemically organic and may introduce itself inside food chain.

Persistent organic pollutants (POPs), are chemicals of global concern due to their potential for long-range transport, persistence in the environment, ability to bio-magnify and bio-accumulate in ecosystems, as well as their significant negative effects on human health and the environment. Humans are exposed to these chemicals in a variety of ways: mainly through the food we eat, but also through the air we breathe, in the outdoors, indoors and at the workplace. Many products used in our daily lives may contain POPs, which have been added to improve product characteristics, such as flame retardants or surfactants. As a result, POPs can be found virtually everywhere on our planet in measurable concentrations.

The most commonly encountered POPs are organic-chlorine pesticides, such as DDT, industrial chemicals, most notably polychlorinated biphenyls (PCB), as well as unintentional by-products of many industrial processes, especially polychlorinated di-benzo-p-dioxins (PCDD) and dibenzofurans (PCDF), commonly known as 'dioxins'.

However, an overall dietary risk assessment would require inclusion of other dietary sources of dioxins and dioxin-like PCBs. In many countries, an inadequate use of newspapers as starting of fire in home grills will produce the excess of POP needed, to appear a disease.

In order to address these risks, several steps have been taken to reduce or eliminate emissions of dioxins, dioxin-like PCBs and other related persistent organic pollutants (often referred to as POPs). Many countries have now implemented the Stockholm Convention on POPs (2001), which suggests ending commercial use of 12 POPs and reducing or eliminating their emission into the environment. To monitor reduction in human exposure WHO and UNEP run a monitoring program for POPs in breastmilk. A steady decline in levels has been observed since 1980 for most countries. (ONU, UNEP/POPS/POPRC.10/10, 2014)

In regard to food contamination, the FAO/WHO Codex Alimentarius Commission, which is a risk management body comprised of 169 member countries, is developing a draft code of practice for dioxins and dioxin-like PCBs in food, which identifies source-directed measures to reduce their presence in food, including fish, as well as a position paper, which provides an evaluation of the need for possible regulatory measures, such as limits in food and feed. (WHO, Food Safety Program updates, 2015)

Toxic Agents Generated in Food Processing

1. **Ethil-Carbamate/Urethane:** Ethyl carbamate (EC, urethane), is a naturally occurring component of all fermented foods and beverages. Because EC has shown a potential for carcinogenetic when administered in high doses in animal tests, production of EC is tried to be reduced during food production. The winemaker industry is interested in reducing EC levels in their products (Butzke & Bisson 1997).
2. **Allyl-Isothiocyanate:** Onion derived substances (Allyl-isocianates) has been used as bio-protective gas additives, to increase self-live of packed foods. Their use is not extended inside industry and exist some controversial opinions, about the advantages of their use. In a hand, there are natural biocides in the other hand may change the natural flavor of the product by adsorption.
3. **Pyrrolizidine Alkaloids:** Thirteen plant families are well known to contain pyrrolizidine alkaloid (PA) (IPCS, 1988). PA's are hepatotoxic, carcinogenic, genotoxic, teratogenic and sometimes pneumo-toxic. World-wide many episodes of PA intoxications have been reported involving ruminants as well as humans. Ruminants may eat the PA-plants directly as part of the forager, humans in an unconscious way taking contaminated grain or through ruminant's products (milk, meat, etc...). Also the microflora of the rumen and the origin specie of plant PA may vary the intensity of poisoning (Wiedenfeld & Edgar 2011).
4. **Alkenyl Benzenes and Derivatives:** Eugenol and methyleugenol, are aromatic compounds present in many natural herbs and plants used in culinary (Miele et al, 2001). Also may be presents in packaging of foods (Aurela et al, 2001),

as pollutants of non-vegetable foods. In both cases the presence of these molecules, at high concentratios may increase the risk of cellular mutagenicity and finally cancer (Dean 1978).

5. **Tannins:** Tannins are in all plants as part of the metabolism of cellulosic structures and have potential antioxidant activity (Hagerman, et al, 2015) and biocidal and antibiotic activity (Scalbert, 1991). These biological activities give to tannins relative toxic activities at high concentrations in animal feeds (Makkar 2003)
6. **Ethanol and Coffee:** Both may be qualified as "social drugs" and need to be ingested in baste quantities to become deadly toxic for humans. Many foods and food additives that are safe for human consumption can be extremely toxic to pets (Gugler et al, 2013). Even chronic ingestion of ethanol causes digestive mucosa irritation and changes in pets' intestine adsorption patterns (Bell et al, 1985).
7. **Diacetyl from Adverse Fermentations:** Diacetyl, is an important component in the flavor of food and it is known to be the chief component of the aroma of butter. It has been found in adverse fermentations of *Sacharomices Cerevisae* and has long been known. (Suomalainen & Ronkainen, 1968). Recently some strain of *Enterobacter Aerogenes*, are found to be able produce high levels of diacetyl during fermentation. (Zhao Ling et al, 2007). The absorption of diacetyl by air in mice shows relationship with obliterative bronchiolitis (OB) disease. This relation it has been observed also by Centers for Disease Control and Prevention (USA), in flavor-manufacturing industry workers. (CDC, 2007).
8. **Flavonoids:** Flavonoids are phenolic compounds that represent substantial constituents of the non-energetic part of the human diet. A group of metabolites of increasing interest are the phytoestrogens and phytosteroids, which are agonist or antagonist to the action of human endogen steroids. There are many chemical characterization and several biological studies of these compounds and many of them indicate the various possible medical applications, for example, in the decrease of symptomatology of menopause and the prevention and treatment of related diseases, in the prevention and treatment of cardiovascular diseases and in some types of cancer (Leyva et al, 2011). The studies about the toxicity of this natural compounds show a protective effect more than toxic one. (Fotsis et al, 1998) (Mishra et al, 2008).
9. **Maillard Reactions:** The Maillard reaction, is fundamental in culinary sciences for the production of aroma, taste, and color during the cooking of many foods (meat, bread, etc..). Recently it has been shown that these reactions may be accompanied by a reduction in nutritive value and the formation of toxic compounds (Ledl, & Schleicher, 2003). The increase of Strecker degradation reactions (Van Boekel M.A.J.S, 2006) larger the amount of toxic by-products

found. Mutagenic compounds like acrylamide are the final result of this decomposition reaction (Mottram et al, 2002).

10. **Lipid Thermodegradation:** When we heat food in contact with oil, a lot off physicochemical reactions happen at same time. To heat the frying oil to cooking, we have to raise the temperature above 100 ° C, trying not rise above the smoke point (which depends on the type of oil we use), normally in our houses, 120ºC. At this temperature, begins to realize the Maillard reaction. The sugars and amino acids from food react to give candy type products and finally decompose it into aldehyde compounds and pyrazines (Strecker degradation reaction) that are unhealthy enough.
Simultaneously, fatty acids (all oils are fatty acids, more or less purified), are degraded in a real chain of chemical reactions. Fatty acid of our oil, bind with oxygen from air to give hydro-peroxide molecules. Food fat decomposition give more (generally saturated, climbing of cholesterol) free fatty acids and semi-decomposed fats (mono-glycerides, di-glycerides and glycerin). Finally, with increasing temperature, we obtain dimers, trimers, epoxides, alcohols, simple acids, hydrocarbons and ketones. That is, all a wide variety of organic compounds, more or less toxic.
Regarding the type of oil oxidation by heat, always increases the acidity, so if we start heating an oil of lower acidity, it will take longer to upload this to levels that makes it disgusting sensory. Special oils, which sell for fryers are almost pure fatty acids (high oleic, etc. ...), this means they can be used longer without degradation, but its organoleptic characteristics are very low. In the market are also sold anti-oxidant compounds to add to the frying oil that make it longer shelf-life, but usually is cheaper to optimize the use of standard oil in the kitchen.
11. **Sucrose and Tooth Decay:** Relationship between sucrose, bacterial adhesion and tooth decay are well stablishing. Glycoprotein and plaque formation is a fast process that fixes anaerobic bacteria like *Streptococcus mutans*, in teeth surface. Lactic acid generated by bacterial metabolism causes teeth cavity.
In modern cuisine, use of polysaccharides based, food additives (thickening and gel-forming agents), modulate the effect of bacterial adhesion to tooth (Steinberg et al, 2005).

FUTURE RESEARCH DIRECTIONS

The main matter is the difficulty to obtain data about ADIS and NOEL, fine referenced, that may be used in food or culinary process. In the other hand, to understand this data is mandatory a minimum level of toxicology knowledge. Basic food toxicology and culinary sciences should be a basic knowledge to be study in food technology, food production and culinary sciences careers. Day by day, allergen and toxin detection thresholds are increasing in the same ratio than technology, but some answer remains unresolved (Taylor S.L. et al, 2004). Protective measures are running, but their real effect on population is unknown at time (Moneret-Vautrin, & Kanny 2004). Many review on food allergens thresholds, have try to clarify this questions, but the relationships between allergen presence and toxic/immune-reaction remain unclear (Kirsch et al, 2009) (Green et al, 2002) (Crevel et al, 2008) (Morisset, et al, 2003) (Nowak-Wegrzyn et al, 2009) (Fernandez 2012)

CONCLUSION

Adverse reactions to foods produced by allergies, food intolerances and toxins, are an emerging health problem. The incidence of these diseases presents a continued increase in recent years. The most effective way to avoid the adverse food reactions is eliminated from the diet of susceptible people components that trigger the adverse effect, making an exclusion diet. For consumers with allergies, exposure to a small amount of food that is sensitive can provoke severe reactions, including anaphylactic shock which can compromise their life. There is great variation in sensitivity of different food allergens among the population, and there is currently no consensus on allergen levels, with the exception of gluten, which may lead to an allergic reaction in susceptible people. That is why they have to have all the necessary information about the composition of foods to make a right choice according to the needs and becomes an essential element of food safety.

REFERENCES

Abarca, M. L., Bragulat, M. R., Castellá, G., & Cabañes, F. J. (n.d.). Ochratoxin A production by strains of Aspergillus niger var. niger. *Applied and Environmental Microbiology*, *60*, 2650–2652. PMID:8074536

Agencia Española de Seguridad Alimentaria y Nutrición. (2012). *Guía para la aplicación del sistema de trazabilidad en la empresa agroalimentaria. Alcalá, 56 - 28071 Madrid. Artes Gráficas Palermo, S.L, Alcalá E. B., Agencia Española de Seguridad Alimentaria y Nutrición*. AESAN.

Alimentarius, C. (2006). *Anteproyecto de Norma Revisada para Alimentos Exentos de Gluten*. Retrieved October 5, 2006, from ftp://ftp.fao.org/Codex/ccnfsdu28/cl06_05s.pdf

Añíbarro, B., Garcia-Ara, M. C., Martin Esteban, M., Boyano, T., Diaz Pena, J. M., & Ojeda, J. A. (1997). Peculiarities of egg allergy in children with bird protein sensitization. *Annals of Allergy, Asthma & Immunology*, *78*(2), 213–216. doi:10.1016/S1081-1206(10)63389-3 PMID:9048530

Aurela, B., Ohra-Aho, & Söderhjelm, L. (n.d.). Migration of alkylbenzenes from packaging into food and Tenax®. *Packaging Technology and Science, 14*(2), 71–77.

Ballmer-Weber, B. K., Vieths, S., Luttkopf, D., Heuschmann, P., & Wüthrich, B. (2000). Celery allergy confirmed by double-blind, placebo-controlled food challenge: A clinical study in 32 subjects with a history of adverse reactions to celery root. *The Journal of Allergy and Clinical Immunology*, *106*(2), 373–378. doi:10.1067/mai.2000.107196 PMID:10932083

Bell, A.E., Sellers, L.A., Allen, A., Cunliffe, W.J., Morris, E.R., & Ross-Murphy, S.B. (1985). Properties of Gastric and Duodenal Mucus: Effect of Proteolysis, Disulfide Reduction, Bile, Acid, Ethanol, and Hypertonicity on Mucus Gel structure. *Gastroenterology, 88*(1), 269–280.

Bellanti, J. A., Sabra, A., & Zeligs, B. J. (2004). Gastrointestinal immunopathology and food allergy. *Annals of Allergy, Asthma & Immunology*, *93*(5Suppl 3), S26–S32. doi:10.1016/S1081-1206(10)61729-2 PMID:15562871

Berjia, F. L., Poulsen, M., & Nauta, M. (2014). Burden of diseases estimates associated to different red meat cooking practices. *Food and Chemical Toxicology*, *66*, 237–244. doi:10.1016/j.fct.2014.01.045 PMID:24491261

Bernhisel-Broadbent, J., Dintzis, H. M., Dintzis, R. Z., & Sampson, H. A. (1994). Allergenicity and antigenicity of chicken egg ovomucoid (Gal dIII) compared with ovalbumin (Gal d I) in children with egg allergy and in mice. *The Journal of Allergy and Clinical Immunology*, *93*(6), 1047–1059. doi:10.1016/S0091-6749(94)70054-0 PMID:8006309

Beyer, K., Morrow, E., Li, X. M., Bardina, L., Bannon, G. A., Burks, A. W., & Sampson, H. A. (2001). Effects of cooking methods on peanut allergenicity. *The Journal of Allergy and Clinical Immunology*, *107*(6), 1077–1081. doi:10.1067/mai.2001.115480 PMID:11398088

Bock, S. A. (1987). Prospective appraisal of complaints of adverse reactions to foods in children during the first 3 years of life. *Pediatrics*, *79*, 683–688. PMID:3575022

Bock, S. A., & Atkins, F. M. (1989). The natural history of peanut allergy. *The Journal of Allergy and Clinical Immunology*, *83*(5), 900–904. doi:10.1016/0091-6749(89)90103-6 PMID:2715549

Butzke, C. E., & Bisson, L. F. (1997). *Ethyl Carbamate Preventative Action Manual*. Retrieved from http://www.cfsan.fda.gov/~frf/ecaction.html

Centers for Disease Control and Prevention (CDC). (2007). Fixed obstructive lung disease among workers in the flavor-manufacturing industry--California, 2004-2007. *MMWR Morb Mortal Wkly Rep.*, *56*(16), 389-93.

Chun-Fai, Yu., Yu, P. H., Chan, P., Yan, Q., & Wong, P.-K. (2004). Two novel species of tetrodotoxin-producing bacteria isolated from toxic marine puffer fishes. *Toxicon*, *44*(6), 641–647. doi:10.1016/j.toxicon.2004.07.021 PMID:15501290

Cooley, J. D., Wong, W. C., Jumper, C. A., & Straus, D. C. (1998). Correlation between the prevalence of certain fungi and sick building syndrome. *Occupational and Environmental Medicine*, *55*(9), 579–584. doi:10.1136/oem.55.9.579 PMID:9861178

Cordle, C. T. (2004). Soy protein allergy: Incidence and relative severity. *The Journal of Nutrition*, *134*(5), 1213S–1219S. PMID:15113974

Crespo, J. F., Pascual, C., Burks, A. W., Helm, R. M., & Martín Esteban, M. (1995a). Frequency of food allergy in a pediatric population from Spain. *Pediatric Allergy and Immunology*, *6*(1), 39–43. doi:10.1111/j.1399-3038.1995.tb00256.x PMID:7550764

Crespo, J. F., Pascual, C., Domínguez, C., Ojeda, I., Martín Muñoz, F., & Martín Esteban, M. (1995b). Allergic reactions associated with airborne fish particles in IgE-mediated fish hypersensitive patients. *Allergy*, *50*(3), 257–261. doi:10.1111/j.1398-9995.1995.tb01143.x PMID:7677242

Crevel, R. W. R., Ballmer-Weber, B. K., Holzhauser, T., Hourihane, J., Knulst, A. C., Mackie, A. R., & Taylor, S. L. et al. (2008). Thresholds for allergens and their value to different stakeholders. *Allergy*, *63*(5), 597–609. doi:10.1111/j.1398-9995.2008.01636.x PMID:18394134

Dean, B. J. (1978). Genetic toxicology of benzene, toluene, xylenes and phenols. *Mutation Research: Reviews in Genetic Toxicology*, *47*(2), 75–97. doi:10.1016/0165-1110(78)90014-3 PMID:415231

Derache, R. (1990). *Toxicología y seguridad de los alimentos*. Barcelona, Spain: Ed. Omega.

Dewdney, J. M., Maes, L., Raynaud, J. P., Blanc, F., Scheid, J. P., Jackson, T., & Verschueren, C. et al. (1991). Risk Assessment of antibiotic residues of ß–lactams and macrolides in food products with regard to their immunoallergic potential. *Food and Chemical Toxicology*, *29*(7), 477–483. doi:10.1016/0278-6915(91)90095-O PMID:1894215

Directive of the European Union 1169/2011. (2011). *Regulation (EU) No 1169/2011 of the European Parliament and of the Council of 25 October 2011 on the provision of food information to consumers.*

Directive of the European Union 2003/89. (2003). *Directive 2003/89/EC of the European Parliament and of the Council of 10 November 2003 amending Directive 2000/13/EC as regards indication of the ingredients present in foodstuffs.*

Dolan, L. C., Matulka, R. A., & Burdock, G. A. (2010). Naturally Occurring Food Toxins. *Toxins*, *2*(9), 2289–2332. doi:10.3390/toxins2092289 PMID:22069686

EPA-Attachment. (1997). *I-Final Risk Assessment of* Aspergillus oryzae. EPA.

Ewan, P. W. (1996). Clinical study of peanut and nut allergy in 62 consecutive patients: New features and associations. *British Medical Journal*, *312*(7038), 1074–1078. doi:10.1136/bmj.312.7038.1074 PMID:8616415

Fabre, R., & Truhaut, R. (1976). Toxicología. Ed. Paraninfo.

FAO-WHO. (1965). *Food and Agriculture Organization of the United Nations*. World Health Organization.

Fernandez, M. (2012). *Prevalence of allergies around the world: the big eight (ten, thirteen?).* Symposium on sensitizing properties of proteins, Prague, Czech Republic.

Fiore, G., Poli, A., Cosmo, A. D., D'ischia, M., & Palumbo, A. (2004). Dopamine in the ink defence system of *Sepia officinalis*: Biosynthesis, vesicular compartmentation in mature ink gland cells, nitric oxide (NO)/cGMP-induced depletion and fate in secreted ink. *The Biochemical Journal*, *378*(3), 785–791. doi:10.1042/bj20031864 PMID:14670074

Fotsis, T., Pepper, M. S., Montesano, R., Aktas, E., Breit, S., Schweigerer, L., & Adlercreutz, H. et al. (1998). 7Phytoestrogens and inhibition of angiogenesis. *Bailliere's Clinical Endocrinology and Metabolism*, *12*(4), 649–666. doi:10.1016/S0950-351X(98)80009-8

Franck, P., Kanny, G., Dousset, B., Nabet, P., & Moneret-Vautrin, D. A. (2000). Lettuce allergy. *Allergy*, *55*(2), 201–202. doi:10.1034/j.1398-9995.2000.00373.x PMID:10726743

Gangur, V., Kelly, C., & Navuluri, L. (2005). Sesame allergy: A growing food allergy of global proportions? *Annals of Allergy, Asthma & Immunology*, *95*(1), 4–11. doi:10.1016/S1081-1206(10)61181-7 PMID:16095135

García Ara, M. C., Boyano, M. T., Díaz Pena, J. M., Martín Muñoz, F., Pascual, C., García, G., & Martín Esteban, M. (2003). Incidencia de alergia a proteínas de leche de vaca en el primer año de vida y su repercusión en el consumo de hidrolizados. *Anales de Pediatria (Barcelona, Spain)*, *58*(2), 100–105. doi:10.1016/S1695-4033(03)78012-6

Garcia-Robaina, J. C., Eraso, E., Martinez, J., Martinez, A., De la Torre Morin, F., Hernandez-Nieto, L., & Guisantes, J. et al. (1997). Sensitization to *Blomia kulagini* in a general population of a subtropical region of Spain (Canary Islands). *Allergy*, *52*(7), 727–731. doi:10.1111/j.1398-9995.1997.tb01229.x PMID:9265987

Gonçalves, A. B., Russell, R., & Paterson, M. (2006). Survey and significance of filamentous fungi from tap water. *International Journal of Hygiene and Environmental Health*, *209*(3), 257–264. doi:10.1016/j.ijheh.2005.12.001 PMID:16459143

González, R., Varela, J., Carreira, J., & Polo, F. (1995). Soybean hydrophobic protein and soybean hull allergy. *Lancet*, *346*(8966), 48–49. doi:10.1016/S0140-6736(95)92676-3 PMID:7603155

González de la Pena, M. A., Villalba, M., Garcia-Lopez, J. L., & Rodriguez, R. (1993). Cloning and expression of the major allergen from yellow mustard seeds Sen a1. *Biochemical and Biophysical Research Communications*, *190*(2), 648–653. doi:10.1006/bbrc.1993.1097 PMID:8093997

Green, B. J., Mitakakis, T. Z., & Tovey, E. R. (2002). Allergen detection from 11 fungal species before and after germination. *The Journal of Allergy and Clinical Immunology*, *111*(2), 285–289. doi:10.1067/mai.2003.57 PMID:12589346

Gugler, K., Piscitelli, C., & Dennis, J. (2013). Hidden dangers in the kitchen: Common foods toxic to dogs and cats. *Compend Contin Educ Vet*, *35*(7), E2. PMID:23677840

Hagerman, A. E., Riedl, K. M., Jones, G. A., Sovik, K. N., Ritchard, N. T., Hartzfeld, P. W., & Riechel, T. L. (2015). High Molecular Weight Plant Polyphenolics (Tannins) as Biological Antioxidants. *Journal of Agricultural and Food Chemistry*, *46*(5), 1887–1892. doi:10.1021/jf970975b

Hodgson, E., & Gutherie, F. E. (Eds.). (1980). Introduction to Biochemical Toxicity. New York: Academic Press.

Houba, R., Doekes, G., & Heederik, D. (1998). Occupational respiratory allergy in bakery workers: A review of the literature. *American Journal of Industrial Medicine*, *34*(6), 529–546. doi:10.1002/(SICI)1097-0274(199812)34:6<529::AID-AJIM1>3.0.CO;2-I PMID:9816411

International Programme on Chemical Safety (IPCS). (1988). *Environmental health criteria 80 - pyrrolizidine alkaloids*. Geneva, Switzerland: World Health Organization.

Jansen, J. J. N., Kardinaal, A. F. M., Huijbers, G., Viieg-Boerstra, B. J., Martens, B. P. M., & Ockhuizen, T. (1994). Prevalence of food allergy and intolerance in the adult Dutch population. *The Journal of Allergy and Clinical Immunology*, *93*(2), 446–456. doi:10.1016/0091-6749(94)90353-0 PMID:8120272

Kanny, G., Moneret-Vautrin, D. A., Flabbee, J., Beaudouin, E., Morisset, M., & Thevenin, F. (2001). Population study of food allergy in France. *The Journal of Allergy and Clinical Immunology*, *108*(1), 133–140. doi:10.1067/mai.2001.116427 PMID:11447395

Karlson-Stiber C., Perssons H. (2003). Cytotoxic fungi--an overview. *Toxicon.*, *42*(4), 339-49.

Kima, C. (2015). *The Psychology of Overeating. Food and the Culture of Consumerism. Bloomsbury Academic*. New York: Bloomsbury Publishing.

Kirsh, S., Fourdrilis, S., Dobson, R., Scippo, M.-L., Rogister, G. M., & De Pauw, E. (2009). Quantitative methods for food allergens, a review. *Analytical and Bioanalytical Chemistry*, *395*(1), 57–67. doi:10.1007/s00216-009-2869-7 PMID:19543718

Klaassen, C. D., Casarett, L. J., & Amdur, M. O. (1986). *Toxicology: the basic science of poisons*. Ed Macmillan.

Kotsonis, F. N., Tschanz, C., Butchko, H. H., & Stargel, W. W. (1996). The Clinical Evaluation of a Food Additive: Assessment of Aspartame. CRC Press.

Larry Branen, A., Davidson, P. M., Salminen, S., & Thorngate, J. H. III, (Eds.). (2002). *Food Additives*. New York: Marcel Dekker, Inc.

Ledl, F., & Schleicher, E. (2003). New Aspects of the Maillard Reaction in Foods and in the Human Body. *Angewandte Chemie International Edition in English*, *29*(6), 565–594. doi:10.1002/anie.199005653

Leung, P. S., Chow, W. K., Duffey, S., Kwan, H. S., Gershwin, M. E., & Chu, K. H. (1996). IgE reactivity against a crossreactive allergen in crustacea and mollusca: Evidence for tropomyosin as the common allergen. *The Journal of Allergy and Clinical Immunology*, *98*(5), 954–961. doi:10.1016/S0091-6749(96)80012-1 PMID:8939159

Leyva, E., Navarro-Tovar, G., Loredo-Carrillo, S.E., & Santos Díaz, M.D.S. (2011). Biosíntesis y actividad biológica de fitoestrógenos y fitoesteroides. *Bol. Soc. Quím. Méx.*, *5*(2-3), 35-43.

Ling, Z., Wang, J., Bao, Y., Fuy, Y., Liu, B., & An, L. (2007). Selection of Enterobacter aerogenes mutant with High Productivity of Diacetyl and Analysis of Fermentation Kinetics. Biotechnology.

Lopez-Torrejon, G., Salcedo, G., Martin-Esteban, M., Diaz-Perales, A., Pascual, C. Y., & Sanchez-Monge, R. (2003). Lenc 1, a major allergen and vicilin from lentil seeds: Protein isolation and cDNA cloning. *The Journal of Allergy and Clinical Immunology*, *112*, 1208–1215. doi:10.1016/j.jaci.2003.08.035 PMID:14657885

Luckey, T. D., & Venugopal, B. (1977). Metal Toxicity in Mammals. *Human Ecology*, *7*(1), 99–101.

MacDonald, T. T., & Di Sabatino, A. (2009). The Immunologic Basis for Gastrointestinal Food Allergy. *Current Opinion in Gastroenterology*, *25*(6), 521–526. doi:10.1097/MOG.0b013e3283306236 PMID:19654542

Makkar, H. P. S. (2003). Effects and fate of tannins in ruminant animals, adaptation to tannins, and strategies to overcome detrimental effects of feeding tannin-rich feeds. *Small Ruminant Research*, *49*(3), 241–256. doi:10.1016/S0921-4488(03)00142-1

Mandallaz, M. M., de Weck, A. L., & Dahinden, C. A. (1988). Bird-egg syndrome. Cross-reactivity between bird antigens and egg-yolk livetins in IgE-mediated hypersensitivity. *International Archives of Allergy and Immunology*, *87*(2), 143–150. doi:10.1159/000234664 PMID:3192303

Martín Esteban, M. (2006). Alergia a fórmulas de sustitución en alérgicos a proteínas de leche de vaca. *Pediátrika*, *1*, 12–15.

Melby, E. C., & Altman, N. H. (Eds.). (1976). *Handbook of Laboratory Animal Science* (Vol. 2). Cleveland, Ohio, USA: IIICRC Press.

Metcalfe, D. (1984). Food hypersensitivity. *The Journal of Allergy and Clinical Immunology*, *73*(6), 749–762. doi:10.1016/0091-6749(84)90442-1 PMID:6609945

Miele, M., Dondero, R., Ciarallo, G., & Mazzei, M. (2001). Methyleugenol in Ocimum basilicum L. Cv. Genovese Gigante. *Journal of Agricultural and Food Chemistry*, *49*(1), 517–521. doi:10.1021/jf000865w PMID:11170620

Mishra, P., Kale, R. K., & Kar, A. (2008). Chemoprevention of mammary tumorigenesis and chemomodulation of the antioxidative enzymes and peroxidative damage in prepubertal Sprague Dawley rats by Biochanin A. *Molecular and Cellular Biochemistry*, *312*(1-2), 1–9. doi:10.1007/s11010-008-9714-8 PMID:18273562

Moneret-Vautrin, D. A., & Kanny, G. (2004). Update on threshold doses of food allergens: Implications for patients and the food industry. *Current Opinion in Allergy and Clinical Immunology*, *4*(3), 215–219. doi:10.1097/00130832-200406000-00014 PMID:15126945

Monsalve, R. I., González de la Peña, M. A., Menéndez-Arias, L., López-Otín, C., Villalba, M., & Rodríguez, R. (1993). Characterization of a new oriental-mustard (Brassica juncea) allergen, Bra j IE: Detection of an allergenic epitope. *The Biochemical Journal*, *293*(3), 625–632. doi:10.1042/bj2930625 PMID:7688955

Morisset, M., Moneret-Vautrin, D. A., Kanny, G., Guénard, L., Beaudouin, E., Flabbée, J., & Hatahet, R. (2003). Thresholds of clinical reactivity to milk, egg, peanut and sesame in immunoglobulin E-dependent allergies: Evaluation by double-blind or single blind placebo-controlled oral challenges. *Clinical and Experimental Allergy*, *33*(8), 1046–1051. doi:10.1046/j.1365-2222.2003.01734.x PMID:12911777

Mottram, D. S., Bronislaw, L. W., & Dodson, A. T. (2002). Food chemistry: Acrylamide is formed in the Maillard reaction. *Nature*, *419*(6906), 448–449. doi:10.1038/419448a PMID:12368844

Nordlee, J. A., Taylor, S. L., Townsend, J. A., Thomas, L. A., & Bush, R. K. (1996). Identification of a Brazil-nut allergen in transgenic soybeans. *The New England Journal of Medicine*, *334*(11), 688–692. doi:10.1056/NEJM199603143341103 PMID:8594427

Nowak-Wegrzyn, A., Assa'ad, A. H., Bahna, S. L., Bock, S. A., Sicherer, S. H., & Teuber, S. S. (2009). Work Group report: Oral food challenge testing. *The Journal of Allergy and Clinical Immunology*, *123*(6), S365–S383. doi:10.1016/j.jaci.2009.03.042 PMID:19500710

ONU/UNEP/POPS. (2014). *Tenth meeting of the Persistent Organic Pollutants Review Committee (POPRC.10)*. FAO Headquarters. Retrieved from http://chm.pops.int/TheConvention/POPsReviewCommittee/Meetings/POPRC10/Overview/tabid/3779/mctl/ViewDetails/EventModID/871/EventID/514/xmid/11873/Default.aspx

Ortolani, C., Ballmer-Weber, B. K., Hansen, K. S., Ispano, M., Wüthrich, B., Bindslev-Jensen, C., & Pastorello, E. A. et al. (2000). Hazelnut allergy: A double-blind, placebo-controlled food challenge multicenter study. *The Journal of Allergy and Clinical Immunology*, *105*(3), 577–581. doi:10.1067/mai.2000.103052 PMID:10719310

Palosuo, K. (2003). Update on wheat hypersensitivity. *Current Opinion in Allergy and Clinical Immunology*, *3*(3), 205–209. doi:10.1097/00130832-200306000-00009 PMID:12840704

Pascual, C., Martín Esteban, M., & Fernández Crespo, J. (1992). Fish allergy: Evaluation of the importance of cross-reactivity. *The Journal of Pediatrics*, *121*(5), S29–S34. doi:10.1016/S0022-3476(05)81403-9 PMID:1447631

Pastorello, E. A., Farioli, L., Pravettoni, V., Ispano, M., Scibola, E., Trambaioli, C., & Ortolani, C. et al. (2000). The maize major allergen, which is responsible for food-induced allergic reactions, is a lipid transfer protein. *The Journal of Allergy and Clinical Immunology*, *106*(4), 744–751. doi:10.1067/mai.2000.108712 PMID:11031346

Pastorello, E. A., Vieths, S., Pravettoni, V., Farioli, L., Trambaioli, C., Fortunato, D., & Conti, A. et al. (2002). Identification of hazel-nut major allergens in sensitive patients with positive double-blind, placebo- controlled food challenge results. *The Journal of Allergy and Clinical Immunology*, *109*(3), 563–570. doi:10.1067/mai.2002.121946 PMID:11898007

Pennington, J. A. T. (1998). Dietary exposure models for nitrates and nitrites. *Food Control*, *9*(6), 385–395. doi:10.1016/S0956-7135(98)00019-X

Pereira, M. J., Belver, M. T., Pascual, C. Y., & Martin Esteban, M. (2002). The allergenic significance of legumes. *Allergologia et Immunopathologia*, *30*, 346–353. doi:10.1016/S0301-0546(02)79152-0 PMID:12464170

Reche, M., Pascual, C. Y., Vicente, J., Caballero, T., Martín Muñoz, F., Sánchez, S., & Martín Esteban, M. (2001). Tomato allergy in children and young adults: Cross-reactivity with latex and potato. *Allergy*, *56*(12), 1197–1201. doi:10.1034/j.1398-9995.2001.00279.x PMID:11736750

Repetto, M. (1981). *Toxicología Avanzada* (D. de Santos, Ed.). Madrid, Spain.

Rojas-Hijazo, B., Garces, M. M., Caballero, M. L., Alloza, P., & Moneo, I. (2006). Unsuspected lupin allergens hidden in food. *International Archives of Allergy and Immunology*, *141*(1), 47–50. doi:10.1159/000094181 PMID:16804325

Sampson, H. A. (2004). Update on Food allergy. *Current Reviews of Allergy and Clinical Immunology*, *113*(5), 805–819. doi:10.1016/j.jaci.2004.03.014 PMID:15131561

Sanz Ortega, J., Martorell Aragonés, A., & Michavila Gómez, A. (2001). Estudio de la incidencia de alergia mediada por IgE frente a la proteína de la leche de vaca en el primer año de vida. *Anales Espanoles de Pediatria*, *545*, 36–39.

Scalbert, A. (1991). Antimicrobial properties of tannins. *Phytochemistry*, *30*(12), 3875–3883. doi:10.1016/0031-9422(91)83426-L

Shelton, B. G., Kirkland, K. H., Flanders, W. D., & Morris, G. K. (2002). Profiles of Airborne Fungi in Buildings and Outdoor Environments in the United States. *Applied and Environmental Microbiology*, *68*(4), 1743–1753. doi:10.1128/AEM.68.4.1743-1753.2002 PMID:11916692

Simeray, J., Mandin, D., & Chaumont, J.-P.Impact on the Study of Allergies. (1995). Variations in the Distribution of Fungal Spores in the Atmosfere of Bakehouses. Impact on the Study of Allergies. *Grana*, *34*(4), 269–274. doi:10.1080/00173139509429056

Steinberg, D., Feldman, M., Ofek, I., & Weiss, E. I. (2005). Cranberry high molecular weight constituents promote *Streptococcus sobrinus* desorption from artificial biofilm. *International Journal of Antimicrobial Agents*, *25*(3), 247–251. doi:10.1016/j.ijantimicag.2004.10.014 PMID:15737520

Stockholm Convention on POPs. (2001). Available in: http://chm.pops.int/TheConvention/POPsReviewCommittee/ReportsandDecisions/tabid/3309/Default.aspx

Suomalainen, H., & Ronkainen, P. (1968). The production of aroma compounds by yeast. *J. Insl. Brew*, *85*, 149-156.

Tareke, E., Rydberg, P., Karlsson, P., Eriksson, S., & Törnqvist, M. (2000). Acrylamide: A Cooking Carcinogen? *Chemical Research in Toxicology*, *13*(6), 517–522. doi:10.1021/tx9901938 PMID:10858325

Taylor, S. L., Hefle, S. L., Bindslev-Jensen, C., Atkins, F. M., Andre, C., Bruijnzeel-Koomen, C., . . . Abbott, P. (2004). *A consensus protocol for the determination of the threshold doses for allergenic foods: how much is too much?* Faculty Publications in Food Science and Technology. Retrieved from http://digitalcommons.unl.edu/foodsciefacpub/36

Taylor, S. L., Straton, J. E., & Nordlee, J. A. (1989). Histamine poisoning (scombroid fish poisoning): An allergy-like intoxication. *Journal of Toxicology. Clinical Toxicology*, *27*(4-5), 225–240. doi:10.3109/15563658908994420 PMID:2689658

Van Boekel, M.A.J.S. (2006). *Formation of flavour compounds in the Maillard reaction*. Academic Press.

Varga, J., Rigó, K., Tóth, B., Téren, J., & Kozakiewicz, Z. (2003). Evolutionary Relationships among Aspergillus Species Producing Economically Important Mycotoxins. *Food Technology and Biotechnology*, *41*(1), 29–36.

Wakelin, , & White, . (1999). Natural rubber latex allergy. *Clinical and Experimental Dermatology*, *24*(4), 245–248. doi:10.1046/j.1365-2230.1999.00470.x PMID:10457121

WHO. (2015). *Food Safety Program updates*. Retrieved from. http://www.who.int/mediacentre/factsheets/fs225/en/

Wicher, K., & Reisman, R. (1980). Anaphylactic reaction to penicilin (or penicilin-like substantce) in soft drink. *The Journal of Allergy and Clinical Immunology*, *66*(2), 640. doi:10.1016/0091-6749(80)90063-9 PMID:6967496

Wiedenfeld, H., & Edgar, J. (2011). Toxicity of pyrrolizidine alkaloids to humans and ruminants. *Phytochemistry Reviews*, *10*(1), 137–151. doi:10.1007/s11101-010-9174-0

Wink, M., & Van Wyk, B. E. (2008). Mind-altering and poisonous plants of the world. Timber Press.

Young, E., & Stoneham, M. D. (1994). A population study of food intolerance. *Lancet*, *343*(8906), 1127–1130. doi:10.1016/S0140-6736(94)90234-8 PMID:7910231

Zukiewicz-Sobczak, W. (2013). The role of fungi in allergic diseases. *Postep Derm Alergol*, *1*, 42–45. doi:10.5114/pdia.2013.33377 PMID:24278044

Chapter 10
Perspective Uses of Essential Oils in Functional Foods and Antimicrobial Packaging Material

Tripti Malik
Dolphin (P.G.) Institute of Biomedical and Natural Sciences, India

ABSTRACT

Functional foods are recently introduced to assure superior nutritional quality; contain biologically active compounds in defined amounts. These foods have to be effectively packaged and stored in order to prevent microbial spoilage and risk of food borne infections. Recently, food technologists and scientists are formulating the Essential Oil (EOs) containing functional foods. The antibacterial, antifungal, antioxidant and anti-carcinogenic properties of EOs have been proved by a number of researchers. Health conscious consumers prefer natural additives, hence these volatile oils due to their green image can be safely used as a replacement of synthetic preservatives. The shelf life of functional foods can be improved by antimicrobial packaging incorporating EOs and their derivatives in the edible films and coatings. EOs can be easily fabricated as microencapsules and nanoparticles, which increases their stability and solubility. Hence EOs are considered as the most usable additives in future functional foods.

DOI: 10.4018/978-1-5225-0607-2.ch010

INTRODUCTION

The 'food' has been traditionally defined as the nutritious substances required for the maintenance of life and growth. As the food consumption habits have been changed globally, so there is lot of concern on the health consequences. Especially in the developing countries nutritional status of an individual faces the challenges of ageing, globalization and urbanization (Kearney, 2010). As diet and health are closely related, nutritional deficiencies can result into number of diseases (Burkert, 2014; Levine & Labuza, 1990). In addition to the nutritional and sensory implications, the food items have also been proven to improve the psycho-physical well-being and associated with prevention of certain diseases (Menrad, 2003). Hence in the present context, the food is not only intended to satisfy the hunger but it should also have additional nutritional and sensory properties, which can play an important role in physical and mental health of the consumers. Due to modernized life style, in urban regions a large portion of daily diet comprises of ready-to-eat and novel food types, which are highly prone to microbial spoilage and pose risk to the consumers. The traditional food items are replaced with the fast food due to their easy availability and quick processing (Ashakiran & Deepthi, 2012). There has been increasing interest in developing novel types of effective and non-toxic antimicrobial compounds to protect the food against contamination and the consumer against infection. Essential oils (EOs) due to their unique combinative properties of aroma, flavour and fragrance have been preferably used in food items since ancient times. This chapter offers an insight into exhaustive applications of EOs for development of future functional foods for the additional health benefits.

FUNCTIONAL FOODS

Newer food products such as nutraceuticals, medifoods and vitafoods; collectively termed as functional foods have now been designed and been included in the diet regimens of health conscious consumers (Azzurra & Paola, 2009). Functional foods are the foods and food components that provide allied health benefits in addition to the basic nutrition. It also includes conventional foods, fortified, enriched or enhanced foods and dietary supplements (Clydesdale, 2004). A plethora of these foods are available in the market; their consumption is not only required for the maintenance of health. In addition to the benefits to health, these foods have gained popularity because of their convenience (Frewer *et al.,* 2003).

The consumption of functional foods has enormously increased worldwide and is highly preferred over with the treatment of diseases (Castro *et al.,* 2005). Functional foods which contain probiotics and prebiotics can be used in the prevention and treatment of several diseases such as cardiovascular diseases, cancer, diabetes, hypertension (Alissa and Ferns, 2012) as well as infectious diseases (Singh & Bhatia, 2011).

Health benefits of these beneficial foods have been attributed to biologically active components which impart health benefits or desirable physiological effects (Hasler, 2002). These physiologically active compounds which are derived from plants are refereed as "phytochemicals" or in general also called botanicals (Rodriguez *et al.*, 2006; Bloch, 2003; Bruulsema, 2000). Significant health potential of various phytochemicals such as carotenoids, phenolic compounds (flavonoids, phytoestrogens, phenolic acids), phytosterols and phytostanols, tocotrienols, organosulfur compounds (allium compounds and glucosinolates), and nondigestible carbohydrates (dietary fiber and prebiotics) have been already proved by clinical and experimental studies (Rodriguez *et al.*, 2006). Research is also enduring on the beneficial effects of other phytochemicals such as glucosinolates, isothiocyanates (Dinkova-Kostova &d Kostov, 2012), terpenes, terpenoids, phytoestrogens and saponins (Dillard & German, 2000). The consumer acceptability of functional foods chiefly depends on their appearance and taste; hence should be incorporated with good flavouring agents.

ESSENTIAL OILS AS FOOD FLAVOURING AGENTS IN FUNCTIONAL FOODS

An EO is a concentrated hydrophobic liquid containing volatile aroma compounds derived from 'quinta-essentia' of plants (Cowan, 1999; Singh & Malik, 2008; Lee *et al.*, 2004). According to ISO, EOs are defined as the products obtained from different parts of plants through distillation by steam distillation, hydro distillation and pressing the citrus fruit pericarp techniques (UNIDO & FAO, 2005). EOs are actually secondary metabolites present in special cells or groups of cells or in glandular hair in non-woody parts (stem, leaves, flowers and fruits) of aromatic plants (Pasqua *et al.*, 2005). Chemically EOs are enriched in terpenes $[(C_5H_8)_n]$. Additionally may also contain terpenoids, phenylpropanes and specific compounds containing nitrogen and sulphur (Bassole & Juliani, 2012; Smadja, 2009; Dorman & Deans, 2000). EOs have been traditionally used for their pleasing aroma. These aromatic oils have a great usage in cosmetics, flavouring, folk medicine, perfumery and pharmaceuticals. EOs are known to soothe the body and soul, have physical and psychological healing effects and bring an euphoria to the body. The applications of EOs for therapeutic purposes is termed as 'aromatherapy', which was first introduced by Rene Maurice Gattefose (1937), and was later rediscovered by Dr. Jean Valnet (Singh & Maurya, 2005). In India, applications of EOs has been mentioned in the

Vedic literature of India. The use of aromatics as flavours and fragrances has also been compiled in Ayurveda "Gandhshastra"(NIIR Board; Singh and Malik, 2008). Remarkable antibacterial, antifungal, antioxidant, anti-carcinogenic and biological properties of EOs have also been proved (Malik *et al.*, 2015a; Malik *et al.*, 2011; Malik & Singh, 2010).

The enormous application of flavours in food items is also supported by the fact that the global trade of flavouring products accounts to 7 billion US Dollars, out of which 16% is due to natural products and essential oils (Dubal *et al.* 2008). EOs or extracts from common culinary herbs and spices are also valued by Europe Union as the world's biggest importer (UNIDO & FAO, 2005). Flavour enhancement properties and medicinal properties of various culinary herbs and spices have been historically known. Some of the spices which are used in Indian cuisine are black pepper, chillies, cardamom, cinnamon, clove, curcuma, dried ginger, fennel, garlic and mustard seeds. Indian food is also seasoned and flavoured with herbs such as basil, coriander, dill, fenugreek, green onions, lemongrass, thyme, wintergreen etc. Not only Indian cuisines but in many other cuisines of different countries herbs and spices are also added (Kaefer & Milner, 2008; Tapsell *et al.*, 2006). It is well recognized that the addition of dietary EOs improves the digestive processes which is the actual reason behind adding the herbs and spices in the food items. Due to aroma and culinary properties, EOs extracted from some of the carminative herbs are also used in bakery products, meat and fish dishes, icecream and alcoholic beverages (Kordsardouei *et al.*, 2013; Sahib *et al.*, 2012; Rather *et al.*, 2012; Bajaj and Urooj, 2006; Diaaz-Maroto *et al.,* 2005; Badei *et al.* 2000).

The addition of EOs is not only anticipated for a pleasing aroma but these also improve the digestion; encourages the consumer to bite and chew. When ingested these oils stimulates production of saliva in mouth, enhances digestion of food in the intestine. The immune system may also get strengthened, as EOs also stimulates antibody production and toxin removal (Nam *et al.*, 2008). Ingestion of EOs enhances the secretion of bile, mucus and digestive enzymes have been found to increase (Jang *et al.*, 2007; Manzanilla *et al.*, 2004; Platel, 2001). An essential oil derived from *Mentha longifolia* ssp. *Hymalaiensis,* rich in cis and trans-Piperitone Oxide and Piperitenone Oxide, has been formulated as candy, hard sugar, sugar-Free, toffee and hard-boiled candy. It provides a physical warming sensation when administered to the oral cavity; has been developed as a method for achieving a physical warming sensation (http://patents.justia.com/patent/20140010768). *Citrus sinensis* essential oil (orange sweet oil) is mostly used as flavouring agents of soft drinks, baked goods and confectioneries, soaps, other cleansing products and aerosols. Its health benefits includes anti-inflammatory, antidepressant, antispasmodic, antiseptic, aphrodisiac, carminative, diuretic, tonic, sedative and cholagoguitic activities. (Health Benefits n.d).

Tagetes EO (80 to 120 ppm) emulsified with propylene glycol has been added to a beverage made from the pulp of mango (variety totapuri) to achieve a distinct enhancement in fresh mango. A higher perception of beverage added with EO was judged by a trained sensory panel and it also scored better in consumer acceptability test[1].

In addition to flavour EOs also increase feed intake (Deyoe *et al.,*1962). Flavour and Extract Manufacturers Association (FEMA) Expert Panel has evaluated each EO on a case by case basis and have also applied their scientific judgment (Smith *et al.*, 2005). FEMA has also laid the lower limit, upper limit and mean value of each EO to be used as a flavouring agent (FAO/WHO, 2009).

ANTIOXIDANT ACTIVITY OF ESSENTIAL OILS IN HUMAN BODY AND THEIR ROLE IN THE PREVENTION OF DISEASES

In the human body, cell death and tissue damage results due to exogenous chemical and endogenous metabolic processes which produce highly reactive free radicals (Saleh *et al.*, 2010). Oxidative stress in humans results due to generation of active oxygen molecules which are an underlying cause of various inflammatory diseases such as cancer, cardiovascular diseases, atheroesclerosis, cataract, Alzheimer's and Parkinson's diseases (Parejo *et al.*, 2002). In healthy individuals, the production of free radicals is balanced by the antioxidative defense system. Oxidative stress may also result in liver dysfunction disorders such as subclinical hepatitis without jaundice, inflammatory necrotic hepatitis, liver cirrhosis and hepatocellular carcinoma in which reactive oxygen species are generated (Zhu *et al.*, 2012; Tanikawa & Torimura, 2006). These volatile oils as antioxidants may play an important role in prevention of brain dysfunction, cancer, cardiovascular diseases, disorders of immune system, heart diseases, type 2 diabetes, and neurodegenerative diseases (Maen & Cock, 2015; Opara *et al.,* 2014; Kamatou *et al.*, 2010; Kaefer & Milner, 2008; Aruoma *et al.*, 1998).

In addition to this, EOs as additives are effective in retarding the process of lipid peroxidation in oils and fatty foods. They also act by free radical scavenging, by termination of peroxides and also prevent lipid oxidation (Amorati *et al.*, 2013; Miguel, 2010). Due to the hepatoprotective properties the consumption of *Rosmarinus officinalis* (Rosemary) EO has been recommended by European Medicines Agency (EMA) for treatment of certain clinical disorders such as dyspepsia and mild spasmodic disorders of the gastrointestinal tract. Its clinical application as an adjuvant in the relief of minor muscular and articular pain and use in minor peripheral circulatory disorders is also permitted (Raskovic *et al.*, 2014). *Trachyspermum ammi* (Ajwain) EO has also been used for the treatment of digestive and inflammatory diseases also possess strong anti-oxidant properties (Kamaljeet *et al.*, 2012). The principle active constituents of *T.ammi* EO which are phenols, mainly thymol (35-60%) are considered to be responsible for its free radical scavenging properties (Chatterjee *et al.*, 2013).

EOs of some of the culinary herbs also possess antioxidant (Miguel, 2010; Tanabe *et al.,* 2002), antimicrobial (Thompson *et al.*, 2013; Pittman *et al.,* 2011; O' Bryan *et al.*, 2008; Škrinjar & Nemet, 2009), antithrombotic (Ballabeni *et al.*, 2007; Ballabeni *et al.*, 2004), anti-inflammatory (Miguel, 2010) and pharmacological properties (deSousa, 2011). Some EOs have a role in lowering the cholesterol; the hypocholestero-lemic effect of lemongrass oil is due to the inhibition of 3-hydroxy-3-methylglutaryl-coenzyme A (HMG-CoA) reductase activity which is a key regulatory enzyme in the cholesterol synthesis process (Krishan & Narang, 2014; Elson 1989). EOs from coriander seed, lemon balm, peppermint, pine and tea tree oils have exhibited strong antibacterial activity, can be used in the formulations of herbal medicines against gastrointestinal disorders such as irritable bowel syndrome (Thompson *et al.*, 2013).

EOs have also shown anti-cancerous properties. *Origanum dictamnus*(dittany) EO and its active component has shown anti-proliferative activity and cytotoxicity against HepG2cells (a human experimental model of hepatocellular carcinoma), can be applied as a promising chemopreventiveagent (Mitropoulo *et al.*, 2015). However, the quantity of EOs and their components to be added in food and confectionery products at such as low concentrations which shouldn't alter the organoleptic qualities. EOs extracted from spices and herbs can also be used as flavouring agents in medicines, which excites reflux flow of saliva and many psycosomatic and psychological diseases which are associated with loss of appetite (Mohiuddin *et al.*, 2012).

IMMUNOMODULATORY AND ANTI-INFLAMMATORY ACTIVITY OF EOs

Essential oils and their components have showed promising immunostimulant activity on both specific and non-specific immune mechanisms, proved by *in vitro* as well as *in vivo* animal studies. In an *in vivo* study, immunomodulatory effect of geranial, geranial acetate, gingerol, and eugenol oils was evaluated by studying humoral and cell-mediated immune responses using rats as the animal model. The essential oils were tested for hypersensitivity and hemagglutination reactions, using sheep red blood cells (SRBC) as the antigen; haemagglutinating antibody titre (HAT) and delayed type hypersensitivity (DTH) response were the test parameters studied after the oral ingestion. An increase was reported for both the parameters and the foot pad thickness response was also higher; indicated significant immunostimulant activity on both the specific and non-specific immune mechanisms (Farhath *et al.*, 2012).

In another study, potentiation of antigen-specific T cell-mediated immunity and macrophage activity was observed for EO of Niaouli (Melaleuca quinquenervia). However, the humoral response was not enhanced (Nam *et al.*, 2008). The immunomodulatory effect of garlic EO was explained due to its ability to enhance the production of interleukins, tumor necrosis factor (TNF-α), interferon (INF-γ). Garlic EO also increases phagocytosis of peritoneal macrophages, and secretary metabolism of macrophages. The antioxidant function and number of antigen presenting cells (APC) was also increased (Hanieh *et al.*, 2010). Garlic EO in diets also improved antibody response against Newcastle disease virus, increased weight of spleen and bursa of Fabricious, and augmented hypersensitivity cutaneous basophilic response (Krishan & Narang, 2014; Rahimi *et al.*, 2011).

Cinnamaldehyde, a major constituent of cinnamon EO inhibits the cyclo-oxygenase (COX-2) activity, which is responsible for its anti-inflammatory activity (Guo *et al.*, 2005). Phenylpropanoids, active constituents of EOs has shown potent inflammatory activity by various mechanisms (Silveira *et al.*, 2014). The traditional use of Phenethyl alcohol has been supported *in vitro* on the contraction of isolated tracheal smooth muscle in guinea pig, prevented histamine-induced bronchoconstriction, which indicates anti-asthmatic effect (Chi *et al.*, 2009). The phenolic compounds of EOs possess suppress the metabolism of inflammatory prostaglandins such as TNF-α, IL-1β and IL-6; the precursors arachidonic acid and thromboxane A_2 (Silveira *et al.*, 2014). *Nigella sativa* EO sold under the trade name, 'dNigellone' is advised orally to patients suffering from bronchial asthma. In clinical studies on the patients of allergic diseases, including allergic rhinitis, bronchial asthma, atopic eczema administration of dNigellone, decreased the IgE, and eosinophil count, endogenous cortisol in plasma and urine; can be effectively used as an adjuvant for the treatment of allergic diseases (Salem *et al.*, 2005).

ESSENTIAL OILS AS PRESERVATIVES IN FOOD ITEMS

Packaging through the traditional methods is associated with loss of nutrients. The use of synthetic preservatives constitutes another approach for food preservation. Chemical preservatives such as calcium propionate, sodium nitrate, sodium nitrite, sulfites (sulfur dioxide, sodium bisulfite, potassium hydrogen sulfite) and disodium EDTA are usually added in the packaged food products to extend their shelf-life (Abdulmumeen *et al.*, 2012; Noel *et al.*, 1990). These chemicals are found to be associated with serious health problems like cancer, allergies, asthma, hyperactivity, and hormonal problems. Moreover, the addition of chemical food preservatives may result in adverse changes in organoleptic properties and loss of nutrients; may also be incompatible with some components of food items (Doyle, 2007; Rasooli, 2007). The consumers have a negative perception of synthetic food additives, which has spurred an interest for search of natural alternatives. Hence, the use of these synthetic preservatives for food items has to be restricted. The conception that EOs can substitute food preservatives has been supported by their antioxidant and antimicrobial properties. Incorporation of essential oils and their derivatives into food items and in packaging constitutes an option in 'Hurdle technology', which is a latest approach in food technology, also called combined Methods/processes or barrier technology. Different food items which can be preserved with EOs as preservatives include meat and meat products, sea foods, vegetables, cereals based products and dairy products (Perricone, 2005).

ANTIMICROBIAL PROPERTIES OF ESSENTIAL OILS

Antimicrobial potential of number of volatile oils has been well documented by various researchers. EOs of *Ocimum basilicum* (basil), *Cymbopogon flexosus* (lemongrass), *Pelargonium graveolens* (geranium), *Mentha arvensis* (mentha) have been shown to be highly effective against both bacterial (*Bacillus cereus*, *Salmonella enteritidis* and *Salmonella typhimurium)* and fungal (*Aspergillus flavus* and *Aspergillus niger*) pathogens associated with food borne infections. The lowest value of MIC was observed for basil and lemongrass oil for *Bacillus cereus* and *Salmonella enteritidis* respectively (Malik *et al*., 2008). A spice used in Turkish cuisine, *Satureja cuneifolia* has shown considerable antibacterial activity against *P.aeruginosa*, *B.cereus*, *Sarcina lutea*, *E. coli* and *S. aureus* (Kan *et al.,* 2006). Oregano spice which is used as flavouring in tea, salads and meat dishes, in the form of water extract or hydrosol, showed significant bactericidal effect against *E. coli* 0157: H7, *Listeria monocytogens* 4b, *S. aureus* and *Yersinia enterocolitica* (Gulmez *et al.*, 2006). High preservative potential for food and cosmetic industries were attributed to *Artemisia afra,* and *Rosmarinus offcinalis* essential oil which displayed high antimicrobial activity against 41 microbial strains causing food spoilage and/or poisoning (Mangena & Muyima, 1999). The preservation of meat products was found to be improved by application of volatile oils in the study of Aureli *et al.* (1992), as shelf life was found to increase because of reduction of microbial load. 32 plant essential oils commonly used in food industry were tested against four strains of *L. monocytogenes* and one strain of *L. innocua* by paper disc diffusion and inhibition curve method. Five EOs, namely cinnamon, clove, origanum, prevents and thyme showed antibacterial activity even at lower concentration (1:50 v/v). Pimento oil showed most remarkable and rapid activity. In a minced pork meat food matrix, thyme oil reduced *L. monocytogenes* population by 100 fold over the first week of storage. The shelf life of seafoods can be increased by dipping them in solutions of garlic oil and its constituents; carvacrol and thymol. *Moraxella, Flavobacteruim* and *vibrioniaceae* were more sensitive to compounds whereas *Alcaligenes* strains were resistant. The "dipping" treatment followed by storage at low temperature extended the shelf life by reducing both the total microbial load by about 100 fold and the volatile bases nitrogen (VB-N). Antimicrobial activities of allspice, garlic and oregano essential oils were investigated against *Salmonella enterica* and *Listeria monocytogenes* in tomato puree film-forming solutions. The results indicated that the antimicrobial activities against the three pathogens were in the following order: oregano oil > allspice oil > garlic oil (Du *et al.*, 2009). EOs of *Lavandula angustifolia, Eucalyptus globulus* and *Satureja hortensis* inhibited *Salmonella enterica* at different concentrations added to whole liquid eggs stored at 7°C (Djenane *et al.*, 2013). Not only antibacterial but prominent antifungal activity of *Citrus lemon, Cymbopogon citrates, Lippia alba, Lippia microphbylla* and *Peumus boldus* EOs against mould strains (*Aspergillus flavus, A. niger, Fusarium* spp., *Penicillium* spp. and *Rhizopus* spp.) has been reported. The phytochemicals citral, eugenol and myrcene have also shown prominent antimould activity (deSouza *et al.,* 2005). *O. dictamnus* essentialoil and its main components namely, carvacrol, γ-terpinene, p-cymene and linalool were effective against *Staphylococcus aureus, Staphylococcus epidermidis, Escherichia coli, Listeria monocytogenes, Salmonella Enteritidis, Salmonella typhimurium, Saccharomyces cerevisiae*, and *Aspergillus niger* (Mitropoulo *et al.* 2015).

Some components of EOs derived from spices and condiments selectively inhibits pathogenic intestinal bacteria, hence may have a pharmacological role in balancing the microflora of intestine, can be added used as the probiotic alternative to the antibiotics. For example, Cinnamaldehyde and eugenol have broad spectrum activity against many pathogenic bacteria, fungi and viruses. These have also determined to be effective against *Helicobacter pylori,* the causative agent of peptic ulcers and gastric malignancy. *H. pylori* was significantly inhibited at 2μg/ml; were also active at low pH (Ali *et al.*, 2005).

In an *in vivo* study, EO has been found to bind to the fimbriae of pathogenic bacteria and reduce the adherence of pathogens (for example, *E. coli* and *Cl. perfringens*) with intestinal wall (Jamroz *et al.*, 2006). The inhibitory activity of some EOs can also be explained to the deregulation of virulence factors of certain pathogenic microorganisms. *Ocimum gratissimum* EO has shown remarkable antioxidant and inhibitory activity against *E. coli* protease, a virulence factor which plays a crucial role in numerous pathologic processes. Proteolytic enzymes are involved in arthritis, tumor invasion and metastasis, infections and a number of degenerative diseases (Adesegun, 2013). Some EOs have also exhibited anti-viral activity in experimental studies. *Nigella sativa* EO has shown a remarkable antiviral effect against murine cytomegalovirus infection. In addition, elevation of IFN-γ in serum for a prolonged time was also observed (Salem and Hussain, 2000). Wu *et al.* (2010) have advocated that the oral administration of a commercial essential oil blend, On Guard™ *(wild orange, clove, cinnamon, eucalyptus and rosemary EO) for protection against H1N1 influenza virus. The potential antiviral activity was observed as the virus was incubated with essential oil in Madin-Darby canine kidney (MDCK) cells. The antiviral effect was proposed to be due to inhibition of viral protein translation. In order to optomize their use as preservatives in food items the antimicrobial efficacy of a number of EOs their antimicrobial efficacy against microorganisms has been studied in different food models (Table 1).

MECHANISM OF ANTIMICROBIAL ACTION OF ESSENTIAL OILS

The antimicrobial activity of essential oils is related to the respective composition of the volatile oils, the structural configuration of the constituent components of the volatile oils and their functional groups. As EOs are a complex mixture of diverse constituents hence the antimicrobial action can't be explained due to a single molecule. Additionally, each microbial cell has different target sites. Cell wall, cell membrane, cell proteins and specific enzymes includes some of the target sites. Quorum sensing, cell division and production of micobial toxins can also be altered by EOs and their constituents (Table 2). The susceptibility of different microorganisms differs; the difference may also be observed between different strains. In addition, intrinsic and extrinsic conditions are also responsible for susceptibility and resistance of pathogens towards EOs (Singh and Malik, 2008).

Some active constituents have been associated with the antimicrobial activity (Prabuseenivasan *et al.*, 2006). Terpenes, the backbone of EO structure have either low or nil antimicrobial activity (Hyldgard, 2012; Rao *et al.*, 2010). The hydroxyl group was found to be important in the antibacterial activity and swarming inhibition of *P.mirabilis* (Malik *et al.*, 2015b). Mostly alcohols, phenols and aldehydes are considered to be responsible for the cytotoxicity of essential oils (Bruni *et al.*, 2003). Alcohols are known to possess bactericidal rather than bacteriostatic activity against vegetative cells (Malik *et al.* 2015a). Phenolic compounds, such as thymol and carvacrol, cause structural and functional damages to the cytoplasmic membrane (Sikkema *et al.*, 1995). Thymol causes the disruption of both outer- and inner membranes, interacts with membrane proteins and intracellular targets of microbial cell (Hyldgard, 2012). Eugenol inhibits various enzymes such as ATPase,

Table 1. Studies on antimicrobial efficacy of EOs in food models

Food Items	Chemical Constituent/ Essential Oil	Microorganisms Tested	References
Meat and Meat Products	Eugenol and coriander, clove, oregano, and thyme oils	wide range of microorganisms, including bacteria, yeasts and moulds	Speranza and Corbo (2010)
	Thyme oil	*L. monocytogenes*	Lemay *et al.*, (2002); Singh *et al.* (2004)
Seafood Products	oregano oil	*Photobacterium phosphoreum*	Speranza and Corbo(2010)
	thymol	Total bacterial count	Del Nobile *et al.* (2009)
	oregano, thyme, basil, marjoram, lemongrass, ginger, and clove	Foodborne Pathogens and Spoilage Bacteria	Barbosa *et al.* (2009)
Vegetables and Fruits	Lemongrass and geraniol	*Salmonella enteritidis, Escherichia coli,* and *Listeria innocua*	Raybaudi-Massilia *et al.* (2006)
	cinnamon, palmarosa, and lemongrass	*Salmonella enteritidis, Escherichia coli,* and *Listeria innocua*	Raybaudi-Massilia *et al.* (2009)
	lemongrass, oregano oil, and vanillin	Total bacterial count	Rojas-Graü *et al.* (2007)
	Clove, eucalyptus, orange rind	*Aspergillus, Mucor* and *Rhizopus*	Lakshmi and Naidu, 2010
	Chiliadenus & Origanum	*Bacillus cereus, Staphylococcus aureus, Escherichia coli* and *Pseudomonas aeruginosa*	Al-fawwaz and Alsohaili, 2015
Dairy Products	Terpineol	Total microbial count	Fisher and Phillips, 2008
	Chiliadenus & Origanum	*Bacillus cereus, Staphylococcus aureus, Escherichia coli* and *Pseudomonas aeruginosa*	Al-fawwaz and Alsohaili, 2015
	Basil, Caraway, Coriander, Dill, lemonbalm	*Bacillus cereus, Escherichia coli, Lactobacillus delbrueckii, Listeria monocytogenes, Streptococcus thermophilus*	Mohamed *et al.*, 2013
	Thyme	Total bacterial count, coliforms, enterococci	Dostálová *et al.*, 2013
Cereal-Based Products	thymol		Del Nobile *et al.* (2009)
	lemon balm, garden sage, coriander, thyme, peppermint, cinnamon	*Fusarium, Aspergillus, Pichia, Saccharomyces* and *Hyphopichia*	Sulaman *et al.*, 2013

Table 2. Different targets in a bacterial cell on which EO and their constituents act

Targets in Microbial Cell	Essential Oil/Chemical Component	Tested Microorganisms	References
ATP and ATPases	Eugenol & Carvacrol	*Escherichia coli, Listeria monocytogenes* and *Lactobacillus sakei*	Gill and Holley 2006;
	Oregano	*Listeria monocytogenes*	Caillet and Lacroix, 2006
	Cinnamaldehyde	*Escherichia coli, Listeria monocytogenes* and *Lactobacillus sakei*	Gill & Holley, 2006
	Cinnamaldehyde	*Bacillus cereus*	Kwon *et al.*, 2003
Cell wall	Oregano	*E. coli*	Gaunt *et al.*, 2005
	Eugenol or carvacrol	*E. coli, Listeria monocytogenes* and *Lactobacillus sakei*	Gill and Holley, 2006
Increase in permeability of Cell Membrane, cell lysis, leakage of cell contents	African basil	*E. coli, Klebsiella sp., L. innocua, L. monocytogenes,Proteus mirabilis, Pseudomonas aeruginosa, Salmonella enteritidis, Shigella flexneri, Staphylococcus aureus*	Nakamura et al.(1999), Cimanga et al.(2002), Nguefack et al.(2004)
	Bishop's weed (carom,ajwain)	Gram-positive strains Gram-negative strains	Paul (2011)
	Vanillin	*E. coli*	Fitzgerald *et al.*, 2004
	Carvacrol, Thymol, and trans-cinnamaldehyde	*E. coli* and *S. typhimurium*	Helander et al.,1998
	Carvacrol	*Bacillus cereus*	Ultee *et al.*, 2002
	Thymol and carvacrol, Oregano	*Pseudomonas aeruginosa* and *Staphylococcus aureus*	Lambert *et al.*, 2001
Inhibition of cell division	Cinnamaldehyde	*E. coli*	Domadia *et al.*, 2007
Inhibition of microbial toxin	Carvacrol	*B. cereus* (diarrheal toxin)	Ultee and Smid, 2001
	Oregano	*S. aureus* (enterotoxin)	De Souza *et al.*, 2010
Specific enzymes	Cinnamon	*Pseudomonas aeruginosa* and *Staphylococcus aureus*	Bouhdid *et al.*, 2010
Quorum sensing	Cinnamaldehyde	*Vibrio harveyi*	Niu et al.,2006; Gilbert,2006; Brackman *et al.*, 2008
	Clove oil	*Chromobacterium violaceum* and *Pseudomonas aeruginosa.*	Khan *et al.*, 2009
	Rose, geranium, lavender and rosemary, eucalyptus and citrus oils	*Chromobacterium violaceum* and *Escherichia coli*	Szabo *et al.*, 2010

continued on following page

Table 2. Continued

Targets in Microbial Cell	Essential Oil/Chemical Component	Tested Microorganisms	References
ATP and ATPases	Eugenol & Carvacrol	*Escherichia coli, Listeria monocytogenes* and *Lactobacillus sakei*	Gill and Holley 2006;
	Oregano	*Listeria monocytogenes*	Caillet and Lacroix, 2006
	Cinnamaldehyde	*Escherichia coli, Listeria monocytogenes* and *Lactobacillus sakei*	Gill & Holley, 2006
	Cinnamaldehyde	*Bacillus cereus*	Kwon *et al.,* 2003
Cell wall	Oregano	*E. coli*	Gaunt *et al.,* 2005
	Eugenol or carvacrol	*E. coli, Listeria monocytogenes* and *Lactobacillus sakei*	Gill and Holley, 2006
Increase in permeability of Cell Membrane, cell lysis, leakage of cell contents	African basil	*E. coli, Klebsiella sp., L. innocua, L. monocytogenes,Proteus mirabilis, Pseudomonas aeruginosa, Salmonella enteritidis, Shigella flexneri, Staphylococcus aureus*	Nakamura et al.(1999), Cimanga et al.(2002), Nguefack et al.(2004)
	Bishop's weed (carom,ajwain)	Gram-positive strains Gram-negative strains	Paul(2011)
	Vanillin	*E. coli*	Fitzgerald *et al.,* 2004
	Carvacrol, Thymol, and trans-cinnamaldehyde	*E. coli* and *S. typhimurium*	Helander et al.,1998
	Carvacrol	*Bacillus cereus*	Ultee *et al.,* 2002
	Thymol and carvacrol, Oregano	*Pseudomonas aeruginosa* and *Staphylococcus aureus*	Lambert *et al.,* 2001
Inhibition of cell division	Cinnamaldehyde	*E. coli*	Domadia *et al.,* 2007
Inhibition of microbial toxin	Carvacrol	*B. cereus* (diarrheal toxin)	Ultee and Smid, 2001
	Oregano	*S. aureus (*enterotoxin)	De Souza *et al.,* 2010
Specific enzymes	Cinnamon	*Pseudomonas aeruginosa* and *Staphylococcus aureus*	Bouhdid *et al.,* 2010
Quorum sensing	Cinnamaldehyde	*Vibrio harveyi*	Niu et al.,2006; Gilbert,2006; Brackman *et al.,* 2008
	Clove oil	*Chromobacterium violaceum* and *Pseudomonas aeruginosa.*	Khan *et al.,* 2009
	Rose, geranium, lavender and rosemary, eucalyptus and citrus oils	*Chromobacterium violaceum* and *Escherichia coli*	Szabo *et al.,* 2010

histidine decarboxylase, amylase, and protease recovery is impaired (Gill & Holley, 2006).

The primary mode of action of yeast cells is proposed to be the inhibition of cell division. The other antifungal mechanisms include the disruption of membranes, mitochondrial enzymes and sterol biosynthesis (Hyldgard, 2012).

Pronounced antimicrobial activity is also explained due to higher number of unsaturated bonds in the structure of EO constituents. The presence of formate moiety in the structure appeared to increase the activity of parent compound. The formate group acts like a hetero atom which increases the antimicrobial activity because of presence of lone pairs of electrons (Malik *et al.* 2015b; Dorman and Deans, 2000). Several antimicrobial studies have shown that Gram- negative bacteria are usually less susceptible than Gram-positive bacteria. Lesser susceptibility can be explained due to the outer membrane of Gram- negative bacteria in which hydrophilic lipopolysaccharides (LPS), acts as a barrier toward macromolecules and hydrophobic compounds (Perricone, 2015; Trombetta *et al.*, 2005). Among the Gram-positive bacteria, Lactic acid bacteria are observed to be the most resistant; can be attributed to ATP generation by substrate level phosphorylation (Perricone, 2015) (Table 2).

ESSENTIAL OILS IN MOOD FOODS AND BEVERAGES

The mechanism of physiological relaxation due to aroma is explained as the stimulation of the olfactory system and production of signals that project to the olfactory bulb, where smell images are produced. These images are then analyzed and are recognized by the brain (Buck, 2000). Hence EO containing functional foods can also be developed as 'mood foods and beverages', which may be designed to enhance mental performance, brain function and cognitive ability. Among the other substances such as chocolate, caffeine etc, EOs also bring about transient mood changes (Hammersley & Reid, 2009). EOs such as Lavender, Hiba and Vanilla have been tested and validiated experimentally for their anti-anxiety properties (Moss *et al.*, 2008; Martin, 1996).

The olfactory impact of EOs of Lavender (*Lavandula angustifolia*) and Rosemary (*Rosmarinus officinalis*) on cognition and mood has been evaluated. Rosemary EO has shown significant enhancement of performance for overall quality of memory and secondary memory factors (Moss *et al.*, 2003). Aroma of *Salvia officinalis* has resulted in significant enhancement effect in the quality of memory factor (Fu *et al.*, 2013). Hence, their oral consumption may also prove to be beneficial in improving the physiological processes of human body. The effect of an experimental drink containing milk casein flavoured with eucalyptus oil has been found to be positive in physiological relaxation. Milk casein is an important ingredient in health assisting foods but has got a bitter taste hence has to be mixed with various flavours, most commonly used is grapefruit-orange flavor. Eucalyptus EO added with casein has shown a beneficial effect on stress control as salivary cortisol levels decreased in the human study subjects (Park *et al.*, 2007). The oral consumption of *Salvia lavandulaefolia* EO (50µl) was proved to be a potent inhibitor of human acetylcholine sterase (AChE), lead to improved performance of secondary memory and attention tasks at 1h post dose in human participants (Kennedy *et al.*, 2011).

Some EOs can be used as aphrodisiac, for example Nutmeg (*Myristica fragrans)* has been used to improve sexual function and enhances the sex drive, may be used as a safe and effective herbal remedy in treating sexual disorders. Eugenol, a constituent of number of EOs including has also been used as an aphrodisiac because of its vasolidatory and smooth muscle relaxant properties (Okonkwo & Ogu, 2014; Tajuddin *et al.*, 2005; Tajuddin *et al.*, 2003).

The consumption of peppermint EO (in the form of decaffeinated tea) has been observed to improve performance of individuals in a memory task and physiological measures. Peppermint intake produces calming effects, reduces both the heart rate and blood pressure, increases EEG activity (Fox *et al.*, 2012). Peppermint aroma causes an improvement in tasks related to attentional processes, virtual recognition memory, working memory, and visual-motor response. Ingestion of peppermint EO also improves atheletic activity as it has significant effects on the spirometric measurements (FVC_1, PIF, and PEF), visual reaction time, audio reaction time, systolic blood pressure, diastolic blood pressure, heart rate, breath rate, grip force, vertical jump test, and long jump test (Meamarbashi,2014).

The fragrances of EOs and their main components affect the autonomic nerves, lipolysis and appetite in experimental animals. For example in study grapefruit oil and its major component, limonene enhanced the renal sympathetic activity (RSNA) and suppressed gastric vagal (parasympathetic) nervous activity (GVNA). The plasma glycerol concentration was increased while the appetite was decreased. Opposite effects on the autonomic nerves, the plasma glycerol concentration and appetite were observed with stimulation by the aroma of lavender oil and its major component, linalool (Shen *et al.*, 2005a; Shen *et al.*, 2005b).

The shelf life of unpasteurized fruit juices can be increased with the addition of EOs. Apple, pear,and melon juices when added with Lemongrass and geraniol, were found effective against *E. coli*, *Salmonella* sp., and *Listeria* spp. (Raybaudi-Massilia *et al.*,2006). Eucalyptus EO has been found to be a potent inhibitor of spoilage yeasts in mixed fruit juice (Tyagi *et al.*, 2014).

To further enhance the health benefits EOs are also proposed to be used as additives in fermented drinks. EOs flavoured fermented milk products such as flavoured curd beverages or flavoured yogurt will not only provide protection against the gut pathogens, but will also curb the antibiotic resistant microorganisms and are also

Figure 1. Combinatorial properties of essential oils because of which they can be used as constituents in functional foods

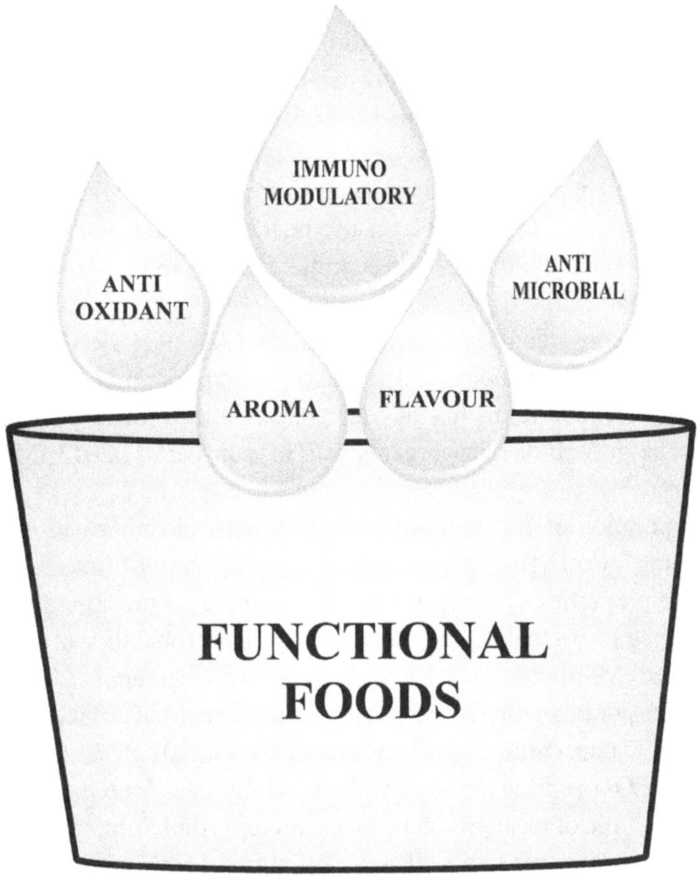

proposed to increase their shelf life. These beverages will function as both probiotic health product and preventive antimicrobial product against enteric pathogens (Hitoshi, 2012; Shipradeep *et al.*, 2012). EOs are also deveolped in solid dosage forms as chewable tablets or orally disintegrating tablet consisting of eucalyptus oil, peppermint and clove essential oil releases essential oil in the oral cavity or in gastrointestinal cavity. These essential oils when ingested prior to bed will improve the quality of sleep. Sodium chloride added to it would further increase its antimicrobial activity (US 20110150995 A1).

This extensive review depicts the remarkable antibacterial, antifungal, antioxidant, anti-carcinogenic and biological properties of EOs. Hence the unique combinative properties of essential oils will not only impart a pleasing aroma but will also enhance the health benefits of functional foods (Figure 1).

ESSENTIAL OILS IN EDIBLE FILMS AND PACKAGING

The use of edible films and coatings (EFC) is a new alternative to extend the shelf life of food items. Edible films and coatings are made from food-grade proteins and carbohydrates, are also compostable and biodegradable (Falguera *et al.*, 2011; Debeaufort *et al.*, 1998). These can also be consumed with the food product ; functions as barriers to water vapour, oxygen, and carbon dioxide and may also carry substances to inhibit pathogenic and spoilage microorganisms (Miksusanti & Masril, 2013) . Natural antimicrobial agents can also be incorporated, leads to the development of antimicrobial edible films and coatings (AEFC) (Sánchez-González *et al.*, 2011; Maftoonazad & Badii, 2009).

Since EOs are considered as Generally Regarded As Safe (GRAS) by US – FDA (Kim *et al.*, 1995), these could be added into the food packaging as antimicrobials. Their addition into food items not only enhances the flavour of packed food, but also inhibits the growth of microorganisms (Hosseinii *et al.*, 2013; Maftoonazad & Badii, 2009).

The incorporation of EO is multifunctional, hence it is termed as "active or smart packaging". Packaging of EOs modifies the matrix of films improves water vapour barrier properties of protein-based films, increase the strength of the film and its resistance to stretching, the transparency, and probability of food spoilage are also reduced (Maftoonazad & Badii, 2009; Perez-Gago *et al.*, 2006;). A starch edible film incorporated with Ginger EO showed best antibacterial and antioxidant activity at 3% EO concentration (Miksusanti & Masril, 2013).

Addition of EOs to edible films is an advanced approach for the preservation and extension of shelf life of meat products. Whey protein edible film incorporated with essential oils (cinnamon oil, clove oil, anise oil, turmeric oil, guava leaf oil, nutmeg oil and lime oil) in different concentration were found to be inhibitory against major molds (*Aspergillus flavus*, *Penicillium* sp.) and bacteria (*Staphylococcus aureus*) which are usually found on dried fish (*Decapterus maruadsi*) (Matan, 2012). Soy protein edible films incorporated with different concentration of oregano (OR) or thyme (TH) essential oils were found to be highly inhibitory for *Escherichia coli*, *E. coli* O157:H7 and *Staphylococcus aureus.* The inhibitory effects were also observed on fresh ground beef during refrigerated storage at 4 °C (Emiroglu *et al.*, 2010).

In the past some essential oils have been reported as anti-quorum sensing in bacteria ((Szabo *et al.*, 2010); which inhibits the cell to cell communication, an important step in pathogenesis of virulent microorganisms. Oregano EO was formulation as a pectin edible film. Pectin-Oregano EO inhibited the quorum sensing not only in *Chromobacterium violaceum*, the model bacteria. But significant inhibitory results were also reported against *Escherichia coli* O157:H7, *Salmonella Choleraesuis*, *Staphylococcus aureus*, and *Listeria monocytogenes* (Alvarez et al., 2014).

Edible coatings enriched with EOs have also proved to be beneficial for fresh cut fruits/vegetables improves the antioxidant protection, prevents the browning reactions and hence the consequent quality loss in fruits and vegetables is managed without any adverse effect on their sensory acceptability (Espitia *et al.*, 2014; Ponce *et al.* 2008; Rojas-Grau *et al.*, 2006).

An edible film was constituted with apple puree solution (APEF) and incorporated with oregano, cinnamon, and lemongrass EOs; was investigated for mechanical, physical and bactericidal properties. Bactericidal activities of APFFS, expressed as BA50 values; defined as the percentage of antimicrobial that killed 50% of the bacteria under the test conditions. BA50 values ranged from 0.019% for oregano oil to 0.094% for cinnamon oil. The addition of EOs also decreased water vapor permeability and increased oxygen permeability of the film (Rojas-Grau *et al.*, 2006). In another study, Thyme EO and apple skin polyphenols (ASP) were added to prepare açaí edible films, showed adequate physical-mechanical properties and antimicrobial activity against *Listeria monocytogenes* (Espitia *et al.*, 2014). Moreover, the antioxidant activity of edible films prepared from biopolymers of several sources such as fish skin gelatin and chitosan incorporated with different EOs were also found to be higher (Perdones *et al.*,2011; Tongnuanchan *et al.*,2014).

Otoni *et al.* (2014) have developed coarse emulsions and nano-emulsions of different edible films with clove bud *(Syzgium aromaticum)* EO and oregano (*Origanum vulgare*) EOs and then edible film was prepared by adding methylcellulose. The resulting film had higher rigidity and flexibility for packing of bread slices. Even after the storage of 10 days, calcium propionate lost its effectiveness, whereas the edible films carrying EOs droplets delayed the growth of bread mold. The edible films fabricated for the preservation of fruits and vegetables are incorporated with EOs, which acts both as anti-oxidant as well as anti-browning agent. Hence the natural color of the fruits and vegetables are maintained and loss of their bioactive compounds is also minimized (Sitonio & Menegalli, 2014).

LIMITATIONS IN APPLICATIONS OF EOs AS FUNCTIONAL FOODS

This comprehensive review has revealed that EOs have enormous health benefits, however the information on their mode of action, as well as the exact supplementation level and their interaction with food ingredients for desired effects in literature is inadequate. As EOs are marked by an intense aroma, may cause a negative organoleptic impact upon addition in food items even at low concentrations. A threshold concentration has to be worked out which should be effective and also acceptable for the consumers. The variation in organoleptic properties of the final product due to the addition of EO can be managed by a mild temperature treatment. Additionally a mild thermal treatment also enhances the antimicrobial efficacy of the essential oil by influencing the vapour pressure of the molecules (Belleti *et al.*, 2007; Gardini *et al.*, 2001).

Sometimes it is speculated to increase the concentration of EOs to overcome the loss in effectiveness due to food matrix components; can only be applied to the spicy food items, in others it will result turn food non-palatable and consumers tend to avert due to strong odour (Lv *et al.*, 2011). The low yield of EO indicates to these are highly concentrated and hence are not equivalent to the whole plant; should be preferably diluted before application (Balchin, 1996). As these compounds are photosensitive, light may degrade the active compound during storage and deteriorate optical properties like luminosity; hence measures should be taken to eliminate their photo-deterioration (Singh & Malik, 2008).

The interaction of EOs with food matrix is also a matter of concern, as these may interact with fat, protein and starch components, due to which efficacy is lost. High fat content of food reduces the action of EOs in meat products. High amount of fat and/or protein in foodstuffs protect the bacteria from the action of the EO as hydrophobicity of oil increases it dissolves more in the lipid phase of the food, due to which less is available to act on bacterial cells which are present in the aqueous phase (Mejlholm & Dalgaard, 2002). For example, mint oil has lower antibacterial effect on *Listeria monocytogenes* in high fat food (Tassou *et al.*, 1996). The low water activity of food also reduces the action of EO on e target bacterial cell (Smith-Palmer *et al.*, 2001). The physical structure of food item also determines the efficacy. Antimicrobial effect of EO in broth medium was determined to be higher as compared with the gel against *Salmonella typhimurium* (Speranza & Corbo, 2010).

The random and inappropriate use of EOs in food items may pose certain risks to human health due to mutational events, carcinogenic effects and genetic damages. A bioassay method has been developed for testing the toxicity of essential oils in which the hatching rate of the eggs and different stages in their life cycle has been used as a criterion for toxicity (Svoboda and Hampson, 1998). In animals EOs are administered by stomach tube and chronic feeding studies and their toxicological effects have been determined (Lee *et al.*, 2004). Cytotoxicity and genotoxicity tests of these substances on different human cells are evaluated by trypan blue dye exclusion test, MTT assay, single cell gel electrophoresis and DNA diffusion assay; higher concentrations of EOs and their components have shown toxicity (Sinha, 2014). In order to elude the hypersensitivity concerns these have been tested for allergic contact dermatitis and photosensitization (Pednelar *et al.*, 2013). Although these have been classified under GRAS by US-FDA; their incorporation in food items should be critically analyzed by the regulatory bodies of different countries so as to evaluate EOs and impose proper regulations for their usage (Sinha, 2014).

FUTURE PERSPECTIVES

As the bioactivity of EOs is altered by food components, pH, temperature and gaseous environments; hence, in order to ensure their safe and effective application, future studies regarding the mode of action of EOs, contraindications, synergistic effects are further required (Hyldgard, 2012). Development of edible films and packaging is an initiative in the preservation of food items. Experts from diverse fields such as nutrition, medical sciences immunology, chemistry, food technology and engineering have to come altogether for pragmatic production of edible films and coating.

EOs and their additive components as phytochemicals can be easily fabricated as microcapsules or nanoparticles, and then can be suitably added to the food items. Microencapsulation includes formation of a robust shell around the EO emulsion droplets, which will be effective for increasing their solubility and stability (Otoni *et al.*, 2014; Maftoonazad & Badii, 2009). There should be a release system for EO from packaging or a fuming system inside the packaging to ensure maximum activity of their active compounds (Tongunacha *et al.*, 2014).

The future of EOs containing functional foods depends on their practical efficacy in promoting human health. Their efficacy need to be confirmed by large investigating teams of researchers from different areas. Animal model and cell/tissue studies can authenticate the *in-vitro* studies, but the results need to be validated in humans. EOs and antibiotics when administered together have shown synergistic antimicrobial effects (Malik *et al.*, 2011; Choi *et al.*, 2009). Hence the application of combinations of antibiotics/preservatives/EO components and essential oils can be a futuristic approach in the food preservation (Boire *et al.*, 2013).

CONCLUSION

EOs have been traditionally used as ingredients in food items because of their flavour and fragrance. Recently, the addition use of EOs is gaining momentum in dietary industry due to their unique amalgamating properties of aroma and flavour. Functional foods consisting of EOs and their active constituents are now being developed which serves the rationale of anti-oxidant and antimicrobial agent. EOs are associated with additional properties viz. anti-anxiety, mood alleviating, anti-inflammatory and immuno-modulatory, properties; which further enhances the market value of functional foods. Hence, functional foods formulated using EOs have versatile applications; if included in daily diet regimens will potentially reduce the disease burden. Hence these should essentially be included in the diet. Moreover, EOs are now being incorporated into edible films and coatings which constitutes a novel approach for food preservation.

REFERENCES

Abdulmumeen, H.A., Risikat, A.N. & Sururah, A.R. (2012). Food: Its preservatives, additives and applications. *International Journal of Chemical and Biochemical Sciences,* 36-47.

Adesegun, A. S., Samuel, F. O., Anthony, O. B., & Nurudeen, O. A. (2013). Antioxidant and Inhibitory Properties of Essential Oil of *Ocimum Gratissimum* Against Extracellular Protease of *Escherichia coli. IOSR Journal Of Pharmacy., 3*(1), 50–55. doi:10.9790/3013-31305055

Al-fawwaz, A. T., & Alsohaili, S. A. (2015). Antimicrobial Activity of *Varthemia iphinoides* and *Majorana syriaca* Essential Oils from Jordan and Their Potential Use as Natural Food Preservatives. *Journal of Natural Sciences Research., 5*(22), 155.

Albarracín, H., Alfonso, A., & Sánchez, B. (2012). Application of essential oils as a preservative to improve the shelf life of *Nile tilapia* (Oreochoromisniloticus). *Revista de la facultad de química farmacéutica, 19*(1), 34-40.

Ali, S. K., Khan, A. A., Ahmed, I., Musaddiq, M., Ahmed, K. S., Polasa, H., & Ahmed, N. et al. (2005). Antimicrobial activities of eugenol and cinnamaldehyde against human gastric pathogen *Helicobacter pylori. Annals of Clinical Microbiology and Antimicrobials, 4*(1), 20. doi:10.1186/1476-0711-4-20 PMID:16371157

Alissa, E. M., & Ferns, G. A. (2012). Functional Foods and Nutraceuticals in the Primary Prevention of Cardiovascular Diseases. *Journal of Nutrition and Metabolism, 2012*, 1–16. doi:10.1155/2012/569486 PMID:22570771

Alvarez, M. V., Luis, A., Ortega-Ramirez, M., Gutierrez-Pacheco, M., Bernal-Mercado, A. T., Rodriguez-Garcia, I., & Ayala-Zavala, J. F. (2014). Oregano essential oil-pectin edible films as anti-quorum sensing and food antimicrobial agents. *Frontiers in Microbiology., 5*, 699. doi:10.3389/fmicb.2014.00699 PMID:25566215

Amorati, R., Foti, M. C., & Valgimigli, L. (2013). Antioxidant Activity of Essential Oils. *Journal of Agricultural and Food Chemistry, 61*(46), 10835–10847. doi:10.1021/jf403496k PMID:24156356

Aruoma, O. I. (1998). Free radicals, oxidative stress, and antioxidants in human health and disease. *Journal of the American Oil Chemists' Society, 75*(2), 199–212. doi:10.1007/s11746-998-0032-9

Ashakiran & Deepthi, R. (2012). Fast Foods and their Impact on Health. *Journal of Krishna Institute of Medical Sciences University., 2*, 7–15.

Aureli, P., Costantini, A., & Zolea, S. (1992). Antimicrobial activity of some plant essential oils against *Listeria monocytogenes*. *Journal of Food Protection*, *55*, 344–348.

Azzura, A., & Paola, P. (2009). *Consumers' behaviours and attitudes toward healthy food products: The case of Organic and Functional foods*. Paper presented at 113th EAAE Seminar "A resilient European food industry and food chain in a challenging world", Chania, Crete, Greece.

Badei, A. Z., Hemeda, H. H., Hafez, S. A., & Hassanen, N. H. (2000). Effect of baking and storage on the essential oil components of anise and cumin biscuits. *Egyptian Journal of Agricultural Research.*, *78*, 321–334.

Bajaj, S., Urooj, A., & Prabhasankar, P. (2006). Effect of incorporation of mint on texture, colour and sensory parameters of biscuits. *International Journal of Food Properties.*, *9*(4), 691–700. doi:10.1080/10942910600547632

Balchin, M. L. (2006). Aromatherapy Science. In *A Guide for Healthcare Professionals* (1st ed.). USA: Pharmaceutical Press.

Ballabeni, V., Tognolini, M., Chiavarini, M., Impicciatore, M., Bruni, R., Bianchi, A., & Barocelli, E. (2004). Novel antiplatelet and antithrombotic activities of essential oil from Lavandula hybrida Reverchon "grosso". *Phytomedicine*, *11*(7-8), 596–601. doi:10.1016/j.phymed.2004.01.002 PMID:15636172

Ballabeni, V., Tognolinia, M., Bertonia, S., Brunib, R., Guerrinibm, A., Ruedac, G. M., & Barocellia, E. (2007). Antiplatelet and antithrombotic activities of essential oil from wild Ocotea quixos (Lam.) Kosterm. (Lauraceae) calices from Amazonian Ecuador. *Pharmacological Research*, *55*(1), 23–30. doi:10.1016/j.phrs.2006.09.009 PMID:17079160

Ballard, C., O'Brien, J., Reichelt, K., & Perry, E. (2002). Aromatherapy as a safe and effective treatment for the management of agitation in severe dementia: The results of a double blind, placebo controlled trial. *The Journal of Clinical Psychiatry*, *63*(7), 553–558. doi:10.4088/JCP.v63n0703 PMID:12143909

Barbosa, L. N., Rall, V. L. M., Fernandes, A. A. F., Ushimaru, P. I., Probst, I. S., & Fernandes, A. (2009). Essential oils against foodborne pathogens and spoilage bacteria in minced meat. *Foodborne Pathogens and Disease*, *6*(6), 725–728. doi:10.1089/fpd.2009.0282 PMID:19580445

Baron, R. A. (1990). Environmentally-induced positive affect: Its impact on self efficacy, task performance, negotiation and conflict. *Journal of Applied Social Psychology*, *20*(5), 368–384. doi:10.1111/j.1559-1816.1990.tb00417.x

Baron, R. A., & Thomley, J. (1994). A whiff of reality. *Environment and Behavior*, *26*(6), 766–784. doi:10.1177/0013916594266003

Bartram, T. (1995). *Encyclopaedia of herbal medicines*. Dorset, UK: Grace publishers.

Bassole, I. H., & Juliani, H. R. (2012). Essential oils in combination and their antimicrobial properties. *Molecules (Basel, Switzerland)*, *17*(4), 3989–4006. doi:10.3390/molecules17043989 PMID:22469594

Belletti, N., Kamdem, S.S., Patrignani, F., Lanciotti, R.., Covelli, A., & Gardini, F. (2007). *Antimicrobial activity of aroma compounds against* Saccharomyces cerevisiae *and improvement ofmicrobiological stability of soft drinks as assessed by logistic regression*. Academic Press.

Bloch, A. S. (2003). Nutrition for health promotion: Phytochemicals, functional foods, and alternative approaches to combat obesity. *Dental Clinics of North America*, *47*(2), 411–423. doi:10.1016/S0011-8532(02)00109-X PMID:12699239

Boire, N. A., Riedel, S., & Parrish, N. M. (2013). Essential Oils and Future Antibiotics: New Weapons against Emerging‘ Superbugs’? *Journal of Ancient Diseases & Preventive Remedies.*, *1*(2), 1–5. doi:10.4172/2329-8731.1000105

Bond, A., & Lader, M. (1974). The use of analogue scales in rating subjective feelings. *The British Journal of Medical Psychology*, *47*(3), 211–218. doi:10.1111/j.2044-8341.1974.tb02285.x

Bouhdid, S., Abrini, J., Amensour, M., Zhiri, A., Espuny, M. J., & Manresa, A. (2010). Functional and ultrastructural changes in *Pseudomonas aeruginosa* and *Staphylococcus aureus* cells induced by *Cinnamomum verum* essential oil. *Journal of Applied Microbiology*, *109*(4), 1139–1149. doi:10.1111/j.1365-2672.2010.04740.x PMID:20456525

Brackman, G., Defoirdt, T., Miyamoto, C., Bossier, P., Calenbergh, S. V., Nelis, H., & Coenye, T. (2008). Cinnamaldehyde and cinnamaldehyde derivatives reduce virulence in *Vibrio* spp. by decreasing the DNA-binding activity of the quorum sensing response regulator LuxR. *BMC Microbiology*, *8*(1), 149. doi:10.1186/1471-2180-8-149 PMID:18793453

Brewer, M. S. (2006). Natural Antioxidants: Sources, Compounds, Mechanisms of Action, and Potential Applications. *Comprehensive Reviews in Food Science and Food Safety*, *10*(4), 221–247. doi:10.1111/j.1541-4337.2011.00156.x

Bruni, R., Medici, A., Andreotti, E., Fantin, C., Muzzoli, M., Dehesa, M., & Sacchetti, G. et al. (2003). Chemical composition and biological activities of *Isphingo* essential oil, a traditional *Ecuadorian* spice from *Ocotea quixus* (Lam.) Kosterm. (Lauraceae) flower calices. *Food Chemistry*, *85*(3), 415–421. doi:10.1016/j.foodchem.2003.07.019

Bruulsema, T. W. (2000). Functional Food Components: A Role for Mineral Nutrients? *Better Crops.*, *84*(2), 4–5.

Buck, L. B. (2000). The molecular architecture of odor and pheromone sensing in mammals. *Cell*, *100*(6), 611–618. doi:10.1016/S0092-8674(00)80698-4 PMID:10761927

Burkert, N.T., & Muckenhuber, J., Großscha, Ra´sky & Freidl, W. (2014). Nutrition and Health – The Association between Eating Behavior and Various Health Parameters: A Matched Sample Study. *PLoS ONE*, *9*(2), e88278. PMID:24516625

Caillet, S., & Lacroix, M. (2006). Effect of gamma radiation and oregano essential oil on murein and ATP concentration of *Listeria monocytogenes. Journal of Food Protection*, *69*, 2961–2969. PMID:17186665

Castro, I. A., Barroso, L. P., & Sinnecker, P. (2005). Functional foods for coronary heart disease risk reduction: A meta-analysis using a multivariate approach. *The American Journal of Clinical Nutrition*, *82*(1), 32–40. PMID:16002797

Chatterjee, S., Goswami, N., & Kothari, N. (2013). Evaluation of antioxidant activity of essential oil from Ajwain (Trachyspermum ammi) seeds. *International Journal of Green Pharmacy.*, *7*(2), 140–144. doi:10.4103/0973-8258.116396

Chi, T., Ji, X., Xia, M., Rong, Y., Qiu, F., & Zou, L. (2009). Effect of six extractions from Wuhu decoction on isolated tracheal smoothe muscle in Guinea pig. *Zhongguo Shiyan Fangjixue Zazhi*, *15*, 52–55.

Choi, J., Kang, O., Lee, Y., Oh, Y.-C., Chae, H.-S., Jang, H.-J., & Kwon, D.-Y. et al. (2009). Antibacterial activity of methylgallate isolated from Galla Rhois or carvacrol combined with nalidixic acid against nalidixic acid resistant bacteria. *Molecules (Basel, Switzerland)*, *14*(5), 1773–1780. doi:10.3390/molecules14051773 PMID:19471197

Cimanga, K., Kambu, K., Tona, L., Apers, S., DeBruyne, T., Hermans, N., & Tott, Ã. (2002). Correlation between chemical composition and antibacterial activity of essential oils of some aromatic medicinal plants growing in the Democratic Republic of Congo. *Journal of Ethnopharmacology*, *79*(2), 213–220. doi:10.1016/S0378-8741(01)00384-1 PMID:11801384

Clydesdale, F. (2004). Functional foods: Opportunities and challenges. IFT Expert Panel Report. *Food Technology*, *58*, 35–40.

Cowan, M. M. (1999). Plant products as antimicrobial agents. *Clinical Microbiology Reviews*, *12*, 564–582. PMID:10515903

De Souza, E. L., Barros, J. C., Oliveira, C. E. V., & Conceição, M. L. (2010). Influence of *Origanum vulgare* L. essential oil on enterotoxin production, membrane permeabliltiy and surface characteristics of *Staphylococcus aureus*. *International Journal of Food Microbiology*, *137*(2-3), 308–311. doi:10.1016/j.ijfoodmicro.2009.11.025 PMID:20015563

Debeaufort, F., Quezada-Gallo, J., & Voilley, A. (1998). Edible films and coatings: Tomorrow's packaging: A review. *Critical Reviews in Food Science and Nutrition*, *38*(4), 299–313. doi:10.1080/10408699891274219 PMID:9626488

Del Nobile, M. A., Corbo, M. R., Speranza, B., Sinigaglia, M., Conte, A., & Caroprese, M. (2009). Combined effect of MAP and active compounds on fresh blue fish burgher. *International Journal of Food Microbiology*, *135*(3), 281–287. doi:10.1016/j.ijfoodmicro.2009.07.024 PMID:19755204

deSouza, E. L., Lima, E. O., Freire, K. R. L., & Sousa, C. P. (2005). Inhibitory action of some essential oils and phytochemicals on the growth of moulds isolated from foods. *Brazilian Archives of Biology and Technology.*, *48*(2), 245–250. doi:10.1590/S1516-89132005000200011

Deyoe, C. W., Davies, R. E., Krishnan, R., Khaund, R., & Couch, J. R. (1962). Studies on the taste performance of chick. *Poultry Science*, *47*(3), 781–784. doi:10.3382/ps.0410781

Diaaz-Maroto, M. C., & Hidalgo, I. J. D. (2005). Saa nchez-Palomo, E. & Peä rez-Coello, M.S. (2005).Volatile components and key odorants of fennel (*Foeniculum vulgare* Mill.) and thyme (*Thymus vulgaris* L.) Oil extracts obtained by simultaneous distillation–extraction and supercritical fluid extraction. *Journal of Agricultural and Food Chemistry*, *53*(13), 5385–5389. doi:10.1021/jf050340+ PMID:15969523

Dillard, C. J., & Bruce German, J. (2000). Phytochemicals: Nutraceuticals and human health. *Journal of the Science of Food and Agriculture*, *80*(12), 744–1756. doi:10.1002/1097-0010(20000915)80:12<1744::AID-JSFA725>3.0.CO;2-W

Dinkova-Kostova, A. T., & Kostov, R. V. (2012). Glucosinolates and isothiocyanates in health and disease. *Trends in Molecular Medicine*, *18*(6), 337–347. doi:10.1016/j.molmed.2012.04.003 PMID:22578879

Djenane, D., Yangüela, J., Roncalés, P., & Aider, M. (2013). Use of essential oils as natural food preservatives: Effect on the growth of *Salmonella Enteritidis* in liquid whole eggs stored under abuse refrigerated conditions. *Journal of Food Research.*, *2*(3), 65–78. doi:10.5539/jfr.v2n3p65

Domadia, P., Swarup, S., Bhunia, A., Sivaraman, J., & Dasgupta, D. (2013). Inhibition of bacterial cell division protein FtsZ by cinnamaldehyde. *Biochemical Pharmacology*, *74*(6), 831–840. doi:10.1016/j.bcp.2007.06.029 PMID:17662960

Dorman, H., & Deans, S. G. (2000). Antimicrobial agents from plants: Antibacterial activity of plant volatile oils. *Journal of Applied Microbiology*, *88*(2), 308–316. doi:10.1046/j.1365-2672.2000.00969.x PMID:10736000

Dorman, H., & Deans, S. G. (2000). Antimicrobial agents from plants: Antibacterial activity of plant volatile oils. *Journal of Applied Microbiology*, *88*(2), 308–316. doi:10.1046/j.1365-2672.2000.00969.x PMID:10736000

Doyle, M. E. (2007). *Microbial food spoilage — losses and control strategies: a brief review of the literature*. FRI Briefings. Retrieved from www.wisc.edu/fri/

Du, W.-X., Olsen, C. W., Avena-Bustillo, R. J., McHugh, T. H., Levin, C. E., Mandrell, R., & Friedman, M. (2009). Antibacterial effects of allspice, garlic and oregano essential oil in tomato films determined by overlay and vapour phase methods. *Journal of Food Science*, *74*(7), M390–M397. doi:10.1111/j.1750-3841.2009.01289.x PMID:19895486

Dubal, S.A., Tilkari, Y.P., Momin, S.A. & Indrakant, V.B. (2008). Biotechnological routes in flavour industries. *Advanced Biotechnology*. 20-31.

Edris, A. (2007). Pharmaceutical and Therapeutic Potentials of Essential Oils and Their Individual Volatile Constituents. *Phytotherapy Research*, *21*(4), 308–323. doi:10.1002/ptr.2072 PMID:17199238

Elson, C. E., Underbakke, G. L., Hanson, P., Shrago, E., Wainberg, R. H., & Qureshi, A. A. (1989). Impact of lemongrass oil, an essential oil, on serum cholesterol. *Lipids*, *24*(8), 677–679. doi:10.1007/BF02535203 PMID:2586227

Emiroğlu, Z. K., Yemiş, G. P., Coşkun, B. K., & Andoğan, K. (2010). Antimicrobial activity of soy edible films incorporated with thyme and oregano essential oils on fresh ground beef patties. *Meat Science*, *86*(2), 283–288. doi:10.1016/j.meatsci.2010.04.016 PMID:20580990

Espitia, P. J. P., Avena-Bustillos, R. J., Du, W. X., Chiou, B. S., Williams, T. G., Wood, D., & Soares, N. F. F. et al. (2014). Physical and Antibacterial Properties of Açaí Edible Films Formulated with Thyme Essential Oil and Apple Skin Polyphenols. *Journal of Food Science*, *79*(5), M903–M910. doi:10.1111/1750-3841.12432 PMID:24749789

Falguera, V., Quintero, J. P., Jiménez, A., Muñoz, J. A., & Ibarz, A. (2011). Edible films and coatings: Structures, active functions and trends in their use. *Trends in Food Science & Technology*, *22*(6), 292–303. doi:10.1016/j.tifs.2011.02.004

Farhath, S., Vijaya, P. P., & Manivannan, V. (2013). Immunomodulatory activity of geranial, geranial acetate, gingerol, and eugenol essential oils: Evidence for humoral and cell-mediated responses. *Avicenna Journal of Phytomedicine.*, *3*(3), 1–5. PMID:25050278

Fisher, K., & Phillips, C. (2008). Potential antimicrobial uses of essential oils in food:is citrus the answer? *Trends in Food Science & Technology*, *19*(3), 156–164. doi:10.1016/j.tifs.2007.11.006

Fitzgerald, D. J., Stratford, M., Gasson, M. J., & Narbad, A. (2005). Structure-function analysis of the vanillin molecule and its antifungal properties. *Journal of Agricultural and Food Chemistry*, *53*(5), 1769–1775. doi:10.1021/jf048575t PMID:15740072

Fox, M., Krueger, E., Putterman, L., & Schroeder, R. (2012). The Effect of Peppermint on Memory Performance. *Journal of Advanced Student Science.*, *01*, 1–7.

Frewer, L., Scholderer, J., & Lambert, N. (2003). Consumer acceptance of functional foods: Issues for the future. *British Food Journal*, *105*(10), 714–731. doi:10.1108/00070700310506263

Fu, Z., Wang, H., Hu, X., Sun, Z., & Han, C. (2013). The Pharmacological Properties of *Salvia* Essential Oils. *Journal of Applied Pharmaceutical Science*, *3*(07), 122–127.

Gardini, F., Lanciotti, R., & Guerzoni, M. E. (2001). Effect of trans-2-hexenal on the growth of *Aspergillus flavus* in relation to its concentration, temperature and water activity. *Letters in Applied Microbiology*, *33*(1), 50–55. doi:10.1046/j.1472-765X.2001.00956.x PMID:11442815

Gaunt, L., Higgins, S., & Hughes, J. (2005). Decontamination of surface borne bacteria by ionized antimicrobial vapours. *Journal of Electrostatics*, *63*(6-10), 809–814. doi:10.1016/j.elstat.2005.03.076

Gill, A. O., & Holley, R. A. (2006). Inhibition of membrane bound ATPases of *Escherichia coli* and *Listeria monocytogenes* by plant oil aromatics. *International Journal of Food Microbiology, 111*(2), 170–174. doi:10.1016/j.ijfoodmicro.2006.04.046 PMID:16828188

Gu, X., & Manautou, J. E. (2012). Molecular mechanisms underlying chemical liver injury. *Expert Reviews in Molecular Medicine, 14*, e4. doi:10.1017/S1462399411002110 PMID:22306029

Gulmez, M., Oral, N., Guven, A., Vatansever, L., & Baz, E. (2006). Antibacterial activity of oregano tea and a commercial oregano water against *Escherichia coli* O157/:H7, *Listeria monocytogenes* 4b, *Staphylococcus aureus* and *Yersinia enterocolitica* O3. *Internet Journal of Food Safety, 8*, 7–13.

Guo, J., Huo, H., Zhao, B., Liu, H., Li, L., Ma, Y., & Jiang, T. et al. (2005). Cinnamaldehyde reduces IL-1β-induced cyclooxygenase-2 activity in rat cerebral microvascular endothelial cells. *European Journal of Pharmacology, 537*(1-3), 174–180. doi:10.1016/j.ejphar.2006.03.002 PMID:16624280

Hammersley, R., & Reid, M. (2009). Theorising transient mood after ingestion. *Neuroscience and Biobehavioral Reviews, 33*(3), 213–222. doi:10.1016/j.neubiorev.2008.07.010 PMID:18775746

Hanieh, H., Narabara, K., Piao, M., Gerile, C., Abe, A., & Kondo, Y. (2010). Modulatory effects of two levels of dietary Alliums on immune response and certain immunological variables, following immunization, in White Leghorn chickens. *Animal Science Journal, 81*(6), 673–680. doi:10.1111/j.1740-0929.2010.00798.x PMID:21108687

Hasler, C. M. (2002). Functional Foods: Benefits, Concerns and Challenges—A Position Paper from the American Council on Science and Health. *The Journal of Nutrition, 132*(12), 3772–3781. PMID:12468622

Health Benefits of Orange Essential Oil. (n.d.). Retrieved from: https://www.organicfacts.net/health-benefits/essential-oils/orange-essential-oil.html

Helander, I. M., Alakomi, H. L., Latva-Kala, K., Mattila-Sandholm, T., Pol, I., Smid, E. J., & von Wright, A. et al. (1998). Characterization of the action of selected essential oil components on Gram-negative bacteria. *Journal of Agricultural and Food Chemistry, 46*(9), 3590–3595. doi:10.1021/jf980154m

Hinneberg, I., Dorman, D. H. J., & Hiltunen, R. (2006). Antioxidant activities of extracts from selected culinary herbs and spices. *Food Chemistry, 97*(1), 122–129. doi:10.1016/j.foodchem.2005.03.028

Hitoshi, A. (2012). Beneficial Effects of Fragrances. In *Beverages on Human Health, Nutrition, Well-Being and Health*. Retrieved from http://www.intechopen.com/books/nutrition-well-being-and-health/beneficial-effects-of-fragrances-in-beverages-on-human-health

Hosseini, M. S., Nasari, M., Zarai, A., Lotfollahian, H., Riyazi, S. R., & Meimandipour, A. (2013). Effects of lemon essential oil on gastrointestinal tract, blood parameter and immune responses in broilers. *Annals of Biological Research*, *4*(10), 47–51. Retrieved from http://patents.justia.com/patent/20140010768

Hyldgard, M., Mygind, T., & Meyer, R. L. (2012). Essential oils in food preservation: Mode of action, synergies, and interactions with food matrix components. *Frontiers in Microbiology*, *2*(12), 1–24.

Islam, S. N., Begum, P., Ahsan, T., Huque, S., & Ahsan, M. (2004). Immunosuppressive and cytotoxic properties of *Nigella sativa. Phytotherapy Research*, *18*(5), 395–398. doi:10.1002/ptr.1449 PMID:15174000

Jamroz, D., Wertelecki, T., Houszka, M., & Kamel, C. (2006). Influence of diet type on the inclusion of plant origin active substances on morphological and histochemical characteristics of the stomach and jejunum walls in chicken. *Journal of Animal Physiology and Animal Nutrition*, *90*(5-6), 255–268. doi:10.1111/j.1439-0396.2005.00603.x PMID:16684147

Jang, I. S., Ko, Y. H., Kang, S. Y., & Lee, C. Y. (2007). Effect of a commercial essential oil on growth performance, digestive enzyme activity and intestinal microflora population in broiler chickens. *Animal Feed Science and Technology*, *134*(3-4), 304–315. doi:10.1016/j.anifeedsci.2006.06.009

Joint FAO/WHO Expert Committee on Food Additives. Meeting. (2009). *Safety evaluation of certain food additives*. Author.

Kaefer, C. M., & Milner, J. A. (2008). The Role of Herbs and Spices in Cancer Prevention. *The Journal of Nutritional Biochemistry*, *19*(6), 347–361. doi:10.1016/j.jnutbio.2007.11.003 PMID:18499033

Kamaljeet, D. N., Thakur, N., Tomar, S., Lalit, S., & Thakur, R. (2012). *Trachyspermum ammi* (Ajwain): A comprehensive Review. *International Research Journal of Pharmacy.*, *3*(5), 133–138.

Kamatou, G. P. P., & Viljoen, A. M. (2010). A review of the application and pharmacological properties of α-bisabolol and α-bisabolol-rich oils. *Journal of the American Oil Chemists' Society*, *87*(1), 1–7. doi:10.1007/s11746-009-1483-3

Kan, Y., Ucan, U. S., Kartal, M., Altun, M. L., Aslan, S., Sayar, E., & Ceyhan, T. (2006). GC-MS analysis and antibacterial activity of cultivated *Satureja cuneifolia* Ten. essential oil. Turkish. *Journal of Chemistry*, *30*, 253–259.

Kearney, J. (2010). Food consumption trends and drivers. *Philosophical Transitions of the Royal Society*, *365*(1554), 2793–2807. doi:10.1098/rstb.2010.0149 PMID:20713385

Kennedy, D. O., Dodd, F. L., Robertson, B. C., Okello, E. J., Reay, J. L., Scholey, A. B., & Haskell, C. F. (2011). Monoterpenoid extract of sage (*Salvia lavandulaefolioa*) with cholinesterase injhibiting properties improves cognitive performance and mood in healthy adults. *Journal de Pharmacologie*, *25*(8), 1088–1100. PMID:20937617

Khan, M. S. A., Zahin, M., Hasan, S., Husain, F. M., & Ahmad, I. (2009). Inhibition of quorum sensing regulated bacterial functions by plant essential oils with special reference to clove oil. *Letters in Applied Microbiology*, *49*(3), 354–360. doi:10.1111/j.1472-765X.2009.02666.x PMID:19627477

Kim, J., Maurice, R. M., & Wei, C. (1995). Antibacterial Activity of some essential oil components against five food borne pathogens. *Journal of Agricultural and Food Chemistry*, *43*(11), 2839–2845. doi:10.1021/jf00059a013

Kordsardouei, H., Barzegar, M., & Sahari, M. A. (2013). Application of *Zataria multiflora* Boiss. and *Cinnamon zeylanicum* essential oils as two natural preservatives in cake. *Avicenna Journal of Phytomedicine.*, *3*(3), 238–247. PMID:25050280

Krishan, G., & Narang, A. (2014). Use of essential oils in poultry nutrition: A new approach. *Journal of Advanced Veterinary and AnimalResearch.*, *1*(4), 156–162.

Kwon, J. A., Yu, C. B., & Park, H. D. (2003). Bacteriocidal effects and inhibition of cell separation of cinnamicaldehyde on *Bacillus cereus*. *Letters in Applied Microbiology*, *37*(1), 61–65. doi:10.1046/j.1472-765X.2003.01350.x PMID:12803558

Lakshmi, B. S., & Naidu, K. C. (2010). Antimicrobial efficacy of essential oil *Syzygium aromaticum* against common infectants of storage cereals and fruits. *Journal of Pharmacy Research*, *3*(10), 2544.

Lee, K. W., Everts, H., & Beynen, A. C. (2004). Essential oils in broiler nutrition. *International Journal of Poultry Science*, *3*(12), 738–752. doi:10.3923/ijps.2004.738.752

Lemay, M. J., Choquette, J., Delaquis, P. J., Gariépy, C., Rodrigue, N., & Saucier, L. (2002). Antimicrobial effect of natural preservatives in a cooked and acidified chicken meat model. *International Journal of Food Microbiology*, *78*(3), 217–226. doi:10.1016/S0168-1605(02)00014-4 PMID:12227640

Levine, A. S., & Labuza, T. P. (1990). Food systems: The relationship between health and food science/technology. *Environmental Health Perspectives*, *86*, 233–238. doi:10.1289/ehp.9086233 PMID:2401259

Lv, F., Liang, H., Yuan, Q., & Li, C. (2011). antimicrobial effects and mechanism of action of selected plant essential oil combinations against four food-related microorganisms. *Food Research International*, *44*(9), 3057–3064. doi:10.1016/j.foodres.2011.07.030

Maen, A., & Cock, I. E. (2015). Inhibitory activity of Australian culinary herb extracts against the bacterial triggers of selected autoimmune diseases. *Pharmacognosy Communications.*, *5*(2), 130–139. doi:10.5530/pc.2015.2.4

Maftoonazad, N., & Badii, F. (2009). Use of Edible Films and Coatings to Extend the Shelf Life of Food Products. *Recent Patents on Food. Nutrition & Agriculture.*, *1*(2), 162–170.

Malik, T., & Singh, P. (2010). Antimicrobial effects of essential oils against uropathogens with varying sensitivity to antibiotics. *Asian Journal of Biological Sciences.*, *3*(2), 92–98. doi:10.3923/ajbs.2010.92.98

Malik, T., & Singh, P. (2015a). Antimicrobial activity of aromachemicals against uropathogens. 2015. *Journal of Environmental and Applied Research.*, *03*(02), 86–91.

Malik, T., Singh, P., Pant, S., Chauhan, N., Kumar, V., & Swarup, S. (2015b). Inhibition of swarming behavior in P. mirabilis by Pelargonium graveolens L her Essential oil. *Bangladesh Journal of Medical Sciences*, *14*(4), 384. doi:10.3329/bjms.v14i4.20004

Malik, T., Singh, P., Pant, S., Kumar, N., Chauhan, N., & Lohani, H. (2008). Antimicrobial activity of essential oils on pathogens associated with food borne infections. *Journal of Medicinal and Aromatic Plant Sciences*, *30*, 314–319.

Malik, T., Singh, P. S., Pant, S., Chauhan, N., & Lohani, H. (2011). Potentiation of antimicrobial activity of ciprofloxacin by *Pelargonium graveolens* essential oil against selected uropathogens. *Phytotherapy Research*, *25*(8), 1225–1228. doi:10.1002/ptr.3479 PMID:21618302

Mangena, T., & Muyima, N. Y. O. (1999). Comparative evaluation of the antimicrobial activities of essential oils of *Artemisia afra, Pteronia incana* and *Rosamarinus officinalis* on selected bacteria and yeast strains. *Letters in Applied Microbiology*, *28*(4), 291–296. doi:10.1046/j.1365-2672.1999.00525.x PMID:10212442

Manzanilla, E. G., Perez, J. F., Martin, M., Kamel, C., Baucells, F., & Gasa, J. (2004). Effect of plant extracts and formic acid on the intestinal equilibrium of early-weaned pigs. *Journal of Animal Science*, *82*, 3210–3218. PMID:15542467

Martin, G. N. (1996). Olfactory remediation: Current evidence and possible applications. *Social Science & Medicine*, *43*(1), 63–70. doi:10.1016/0277-9536(95)00334-7 PMID:8816011

Matan, N. (2012). Antimicrobial activity of edible film incorporated with essential oils to preserve dried fish (*Decapterus maruadsi*). *International Food Research Journal.*, *19*(4), 1733–1738.

Meamarbashi, A. (2014). Instant effects of peppermint essential oil on the physiological parameters and exercise performance. *Avicenna Journal of Phytomedicine.*, *4*(1), 72–78. PMID:25050303

Mejlholm, O., & Dalgaard, P. (2002). Antimicrobial effect of essential oils on the seafood spoilage micro-organism *Photobacterium phosphoreum* in liquid media and fish products. *Letters in Applied Microbiology*, *34*(1), 27–31. doi:10.1046/j.1472-765x.2002.01033.x PMID:11849488

Menrad, K. (2003). Market and marketing of functional food in Europe. *Journal of Food Engineering*, *56*(2-3), 181–188. doi:10.1016/S0260-8774(02)00247-9

Miguel, M. G. (2010). Antioxidant and Anti-Inflammatory Activities of Essential Oils. *Molecules (Basel, Switzerland)*, *15*(12), 9252–9287. doi:10.3390/molecules15129252 PMID:21160452

Miksusanti, H., & Masril, K. I. (2013). Antibacterial and Antioxidant of Uwi (Dioscorea Alata L) Starch Edible Film Incorporated with Ginger Essential Oil. *International Journal of Bioscience. Biochemistry and Bioinformatics.*, *3*(4), 354–356.

Mitropoulou, G., Fitsiou, E., Stavropoulou, E., Papavassilopoulou, E., Vamvakias, M., Pappa, A., Oreopoulou, A., & Kourkoutas, Y. (2015).Composition, antimicrobial, antioxidant, and antiproliferative activity of *Origanum dictamnus*(dittany) essential oil. *Microbial Ecology in Health & Disease, 26*, 26543-26552.

Mohamed, S. H. S., Zaky, W. M., Kassem, J. M., Abbas, H. M., Salem, M. M. E., & Said-Al Ahl, H. A. H. (2013). Impact of antimicrobial properties of some essential oils on cheese yoghurt quality. *World Applied Sciences Journal*, *27*(4), 497–507.

Mohiuddin, M., & Chowdhry, M.J., Alam, & Hossain, M.K. (2012). Chemical composition of essential oils of four flavouring plants used by the tribal people of Bandarban hill district in Bangladesh. *International Journal of Medicinal & Aromatic Plants.*, *2*(1), 106–113.

Moss, M., Cook, J., Wesnes, K., & Duckett, P. (2003). Aromas of rosemary and lavender essential oils differentially affect cognition and mood in healthy adults. *The International Journal of Neuroscience*, *113*(1), 15–38. doi:10.1080/00207450390161903 PMID:12690999

Moss, M., Hewitt, S., Moss, L., & Wesnes, K. (2008). Modulation of cognitive performance and mood by aromas of peppermint and Ylang-Ylang. *The International Journal of Neuroscience*, *118*(1), 59–77. doi:10.1080/00207450601042094 PMID:18041606

Nakamura, C. V., Ueda-Nakamura, T., Bando, E., & Negr, Ã. (1999). Antibacterial activity of *Ocimum gratissimum* L. essential oil. *Memorias do Instituto Oswaldo Cruz*, *94*(5), 675–678. doi:10.1590/S0074-02761999000500022 PMID:10464416

Nam, S. Y., Chang, M. H., Don, Z. J. S., Seo, H. J., & Oh, H. K. (2008). Essential oil of niaoulipreferentially potentiates antigen-specific cellular immunity and cytokine production by macrophages. *Immunopharmacology and Immunotoxicology*, *30*(3), 459–474. doi:10.1080/08923970802135187 PMID:18668393

Nguefack, J., Tamgue, O., Dongmo, J. B. L., Dakole, C. D., Leth, V., Vis-mer, H. F., & Nkengfack, A. E. et al. (2012). Synergistic action between fractions of essential oils from *Cymbopogon citratus, Ocimum gratissimum* and *Thymus vulgaris* against *Penicillium expansum. Food Control*, *23*(2), 377–383. doi:10.1016/j.foodcont.2011.08.002

Niu, S., Afre, S., & Gilbert, E. S. (2006). Sub inhibitory concentrations of cinnamaldehyde interfere with quorum sensing. *Letters in Applied Microbiology*, *43*(5), 489–494. doi:10.1111/j.1472-765X.2006.02001.x PMID:17032221

Noel, P., Briand, E., & Dumont, J. P. (1990). Role of nitrite in flavour development in uncooked cured meat products: Sensory assessment. *Meat Science*, *28*(1), 1–8. doi:10.1016/0309-1740(90)90015-X PMID:22055434

O'Bryan, C. A., Crandall, P. G., Chalova, V. I., & Ricke, S. C. (2008). Orange essential oils antimicrobial activities against Salmonella spp. *Journal of Food Science*, *73*(6), M264–M267. doi:10.1111/j.1750-3841.2008.00790.x PMID:19241555

Okonkwo, C., & Assumpta, O. (2014). Nutritional Evaluation of Some Selected Spices Commonly Used in the South-Eastern Part of Nigeria. *Journal of Biology. Agriculture and Healthcare, 15*(4), 97–103.

Opara, E. I., Diaaz-Maroto, M. C., & Hidalgo, I. J. D. (2014). Culinary Herbs and Spices: Their Bioactive Properties, the Contribution of Polyphenols and the Challenges in Deducing Their True Health Benefits. *International Journal of Molecular Sciences, 15*(10), 19183–19202. doi:10.3390/ijms151019183 PMID:25340982

Otoni, C. G., Silvania, F. O. P., Medeiros, E.A.A., & Soares, N. de F. F. (2014). Edible Films from Methylcellulose and Nanoemulsions of Clove Bud art *Syzygium aromaticum* and Oregano (*Origanum vulgare*) Essential Oils as Shelf Life Extenders for Sliced Bread. *J. Agric. Food Chemistry, 62*(22), 5214–5219.

Parejo, I., Iadomat, V., Bastida, J., Rosas-romero, A., Flerlage, N., Burillo, J., & Codina, C. (2002). Comparison between the Radical Scavenging Activity and Antioxidant Activity of Six Distilled and Nondistilled Mediterranean Herbs and Aromatic Plants. *Journal of Agricultural and Food Chemistry, 50*(23), 6882–6890. doi:10.1021/jf020540a PMID:12405792

Parejo, I., Iadomat, V., Bastida, J., Rosas-romero, A., Flerlage, N., Burillo, J., & Codina, C. (2002). Comparison between the Radical Scavenging Activity and Antioxidant Activity of Six Distilled and Nondistilled Mediterranean Herbs and Aromatic Plants. *Journal of Agricultural and Food Chemistry, 50*(23), 6882–6890. doi:10.1021/jf020540a PMID:12405792

Park, B. J., Morikawa, T., Ogata, T., Washida, K., Iwamoto, M., Nakamura, H., & Miyazaki, Y. (2009). Physiological effects of ingesting eucalyptus EO with milk casein peptide. *Silva Fennica, 43*(1), 173–179. doi:10.14214/sf.223

Pasqua, R. D., Feo, V. D., Francesco, V., & Mauriello, G. (2005). *In vitro* antimicrobial activity of essential oils from Mediterranean Apiaceae, Verbenaceae and Lamiaceae food borne pathogens and spoilage bacteria. *Annals of Microbiology, 55*(2), 139–143.

Paul, S., Dubey, R. C., Maheswari, D. K., & Kang, S. C. (2011). *Trachyspermum ammi* (L.) fruit essential oil influencing on membrane permeability and surface characteristics in inhibiting food–borne pathogens. *Food Control, 22*(5), 725–731. doi:10.1016/j.foodcont.2010.11.003

Perdones, Á., Vargas, M., Atarés, L., & Chiralt, A. (2011). Physical, Antioxidant and Antimicrobial Properties of Chitosan-Cinnamon Leaf oil Films as Affected by Oleic Acid. *Food Hydrocolloids, 36*, 256–264. doi:10.1016/j.foodhyd.2013.10.003

Perez-Gago, M. B., Serra, M., & del R'ıo, M. A. (2006). Color change of fresh-cut apples coated with whey protein concentrate-based edible coatings. *Postharvest Biology and Technology*, *39*(1), 84–92. doi:10.1016/j.postharvbio.2005.08.002

Perricone, M., Arace, E., Corbo, M. R., Sinigaglia, M., & Bevilacqua, A. (2015). Bioactivity of essential oils:a review on their interaction with food components. *Frontiers in Micribiology.*, *6*(76), 1–7. PMID:25709605

Pittman, C. I., Pendleton, S., Bisha, B., O'Bryan, C. A., Belk, K. E., Goodridge, L., & Ricke, S. C. et al. (2011). Activity of citrus essential oils against *Escherichia coli* O157:H7 and *Salmonella* spp. and effects on beef subprimal cuts under refrigeration. *Journal of Food Science*, *76*(6), M433–M438. doi:10.1111/j.1750-3841.2011.02253.x PMID:22417514

Platel, K., & Srinivasan, K. (2001). Studies on the influence of dietary spices on food transit time in experimental rats. *Nutrition Research (New York, N.Y.)*, *21*(9), 1309–1314. doi:10.1016/S0271-5317(01)00331-1

Ponce, A. G., Roura, S. I., Del valle, C. E., & Moreira, M.R. (2008). Antimicrobial and Antioxidant Activities of Edible Coatings Enriched with Natural Plant Extracts: In Vitro and In Vivo Studies. Postharvest Biology and Technolog., 49(2), 294-300.

Prabuseenivasan, S., Jayakumar, M., & Ignacimuthu, S. (2006). *In vitro* antibacterial activity of some plant essential oil. *BMC Complementary and Alternative Medicine*, *6*(1), 1–8. doi:10.1186/1472-6882-6-39 PMID:16412227

Rahimi, S., Zadeh, T., Karimi, M. A., Omidbaigi, R., & Rokni, H. (2011). Effect of the three herbal extracts on growth performance, immune system, blood factors and intestinal selected bacterial population in broiler chickens. *Journal of Agriculture Science and Technology.*, *13*, 527–539.

Rao, A., Zhang, Y., Muend, S., & Rao, R. (2010). Mechanism of anti- fungal activity of terpenoid phenols resembles calcium stress and inhibition of the TOR pathway. *Antimicrobial Agents and Chemotherapy*, *54*(12), 5062–5069. doi:10.1128/AAC.01050-10 PMID:20921304

Rašković, A., Milanović, I., Pavlović, N., Ćebović, T., Vukmirović, S., & Mikov, M. (2014). Antioxidant activity of rosemary (*Rosmarinus officinalis* L.) essential oil and its hepatoprotective potential. *BMC Complementary and Alternative Medicine*, *14*(1), 225–234. doi:10.1186/1472-6882-14-225 PMID:25002023

Rasooli, I. (2007). Food Preservation – A Biopreservative Approach. *Food*, *1*(2), 111–136.

Rather, M. A., Dar, B. A., Sofi, S. N., Bhat, B. A., & Qurishi, M. A. (2012). Volatile components and key odorants of fennel (Foeniculum vulgare Mill.) and thyme (Thymus vulgaris L.) Oil extracts obtained by simultaneous distillation–extraction and supercritical fluid extraction. *Journal of Agricultural and Food Chemistry*, *53*, 5385–5389. PMID:15969523

Raybaudi-Massilia, R. M., Mosqueda-Melgar, J., & Martin-Belloso, O. (2006). Antimicrobial activity of essential oils on *Salmonella enteritidis, Escherichiacoli*, and *Listeriainnocua* in fruitjuices. *Journal of Food Protection*, *69*, 1579–1586. PMID:16865889

Raybaudi-Massilia, R. M., Mosqueda-Melgar, J., Sobrino-Lopez, A., Soliva-Fortuny, R., & Martín-Belloso, O. (2009). Use of malic acid and other quality stabilizing compounds to assure the safety of freshcut"fuji" apples by inactivation of *Listeria monocytogenes, Salmonella Enteridis*, and *Escherichia coli* O157:H7. *Journal of Food Safety*, *29*(2), 236–252. doi:10.1111/j.1745-4565.2009.00153.x

Rodriguez, E. B., Flavier, M. E., Rodriguez-Amaya, D. B., & Amaya-Farfán, J. (2006). Phytochemicals and functional foods. Current situation and prospect for developing countries. *Segurança Alimentar e Nutricional, Campinas*, *13*(1), 1–22.

Rojas-Grau¨, M. A., & Roberto, J. (2006). Mechanical, Barrier, and Antimicrobial Properties of Apple Puree Edible Films Containing Plant. *Journal of Agricultural and Food Chemistry*, *54*(24), 9262–9267. doi:10.1021/jf061717u PMID:17117819

Sahib, N. J., Anwar, F., Gilani, A. H., Hamid, A. A., Saari, A., & Khalid, M. (2012). Coriander (Coriandrum sativum L.): A PotentialSource of High-Value Components for Functional Foods and Nutraceuticals- A Review. *Phytotherapy Research*, *27*(10), 1439–1456. PMID:23281145

Saleh, M. O., Clark, S., Woodward, B., & Deolo-Sobogun, S. A. (2010). Antioxidant and free radical scavenging of essential oils. *Ethnicity & Disease*, *20*, 78–82. PMID:20521390

Salem, M. L. (2005). Immunomodulatory and therapeutic properties of the *Nigella sativa* L. seed. *International Immunopharmacology*, *5*(13-14), 1749–1770. doi:10.1016/j.intimp.2005.06.008 PMID:16275613

Salem, M. L., & Hossain, M. S. (2000). Protective effect of black seed oil from *Nigella sativa* against murine cytomegalovirus infection. *International Journal of Immunopharmacology*, *22*(9), 729–740. doi:10.1016/S0192-0561(00)00036-9 PMID:10884593

Sánchez-González, L., Pastor, C., Vargas, M., Chiralt, A., González-Martínez, C., & Cháfer, M. (2011). Effect of Hydroxypropylmethylcellulose and Chitosan Coatings with and Without Bergamot Essential Oil on Quality and Safety of Cold-Stored Grapes. *Postharvest Biology and Technology*, *60*(1), 57–63. doi:10.1016/j.postharvbio.2010.11.004

Shen, J., Niijima, A., Tanida, M., Horii, Y., Maeda, K., & Kastuya, N. (2005a). Olfactory stimulation with scent of grapefruitoil affects autonomic nerves, lipolysis and appetite in rats. *Neuroscience Letters*, *380*(3), 289–294. doi:10.1016/j.neulet.2005.01.058 PMID:15862904

Shen, J., Niijima, A., Tanida, M., Horii, Y., Maeda, K., & Nagai, K. (2005b). Olfactory stimulation with scent of lavender oil affects autonomic nerves, lipolysis and appetite in rats. *Neuroscience Letters*, *383*(1-2), 188–193. doi:10.1016/j.neulet.2005.04.010 PMID:15878236

Shipradeep, K. S., Khare, R.S., Ojha, S., Kundu, K., & Kundu, S. (2012). Development of Probiotic Candidate in Combination with Essential Oils from Medicinal Plant and Their Effect on Enteric Pathogens: A Review. Gastroenterology Research and Practice.

Sikkema, J., DeBont, J. A. M., & Poolman, B. (1995). Mechanisms of membrane toxicity of hydrocarbons. *Microbiological Reviews*, *59*, 201–222. PMID:7603409

Silveira e Sá, R. C., Andrade, L. N., Oliveira, R. R. B., & Sousa, D. P. (2014). A Review on Anti-Inflammatory Activity of Phenylpropanoids Found in Essential Oils. *Molecules (Basel, Switzerland)*, *19*(2), 1459–1480. doi:10.3390/molecules19021459 PMID:24473208

Singh, A., Singh, R. K., Bhunia, A. K., & Singh, N. (2004). Efficacy of plant essential oils as antimicrobial agents against *Listeria monocytogenes* in hot-dogs. *LWT-Food Science & Technology*, *36*(8), 787–794. doi:10.1016/S0023-6438(03)00112-9

Singh, G., & Maurya, S. (2005). Antimicrobial, antifungal and insecticidal investigations on essential oils – an overview. *Natural Product Radiance*, *4*(3), 179–192.

Singh, M. P., & Bhatia, A. (2011). Role of functional foods in periodontal health and disease. *Indian Journal of Dental Advancements*, *3*(3), 587–592. doi:10.5866/3.3.587

Singh, P., & Malik, T. (2008). Essence of plants: essential oils as antimicrobials. In P. Parihar & L. Parihar (Eds.), *Advances in Applied Microbiology* (pp. 137–148). Bikaner, India: Agrobios Publishers.

Singh, P., & Malik, T. (2008). Essence of plants: essential oils as antimicrobials. In P. Parihar & L. Parihar (Eds.), *Advances in Applied Microbiology* (pp. 137–148). Bikaner, India: Agrobios Publishers.

Sinha, S., Jothiramajayam, M., Ghosh, M., & Mukherjee, A. (2014). Evaluation of toxicity of essential oils palmarosa, citronella, lemongrass and vetiver in human lymphocytes. *Food and Chemical Toxicology*, *68*, 71–77. doi:10.1016/j.fct.2014.02.036 PMID:24650756

Škrinjar, M. M., & Neme, N. T. (2009). Antimicrobial effects of spices and herbs essential oils. *Acta Periodica Technologica.*, *40*(40), 195–209. doi:10.2298/APT0940195S

Smadja, J. (2009). Essential oils: chemical composition and localization. In Essential oils and green extractions and applications (pp. 194-213). Har Krishan Bhalla and Sons.

Smith, R.L., Cohen, S.M., Doull, J., Feron, V.J., Goodman, J.I., & Marnett, L.J, Porto Ghese, P.S., & Adams, T.B. (2005). A procedure for the safety evaluation of natural flavor complexes used as ingredients in food: Essential oils. *Food and Chemical Toxicology*, *43*(3), 345–363. PMID:15680674

Smith-Palmer, A., Stewart, J., & Fyfe, L. (2001). The potential application of plant essential oils as natural food preservatives in soft cheese. *Food Microbiology*, *18*(4), 463–470. doi:10.1006/fmic.2001.0415

Speranza, B., & Corbo, M. R. (2010). Essential oils for preserving perishable foods: possibilities and limitations. In Application of Alternative Food Preservation Technologies to Enhance Food Safety and Stability, (pp. 35-57). Sharjah, UAE: Bentham Publisher.

Sumalan, R. M., Alexa, E., & Poiana, M. A. (2013). Assessment of inhibitory potential of essential oils on natural mycoflora and *Fusarium* mycotoxins production in wheat. *Chemistry Central Journal*, *7*(32), 1–12. PMID:23409841

Svoboda, K. P., Ingli, A., Hampson, J., Galambosi, B., & Asakawa, Y. (1998). Biomass production, essential oil yield and composition of *Myrica gale* L. harvested from wild populations in Scotland and Finland. *Flavour and Fragrance Journal*, *13*(6), 367–372. doi:10.1002/(SICI)1099-1026(199811/12)13:6<367::AID-FFJ724>3.0.CO;2-M

Szabo, M. A., Vagra, G. J., Hohmann, J., Schelz, Z., Szegedi, E. E., Amaral, L., & Molnar, J. (2012). Inhibition of quorum sensing signals by essential oils. *Phytotherapy Research*, *24*(5), 782–786. doi:10.1002/ptr.3010 PMID:19827025

Tajuddin, A. S., & Latif, A. (2005). An experimental study of sexual function improving effect of *Myristica fragrans* Houtt. *BMC Complementary and Alternative Medicine*, *5*(1), 16. doi:10.1186/1472-6882-5-16 PMID:16033651

Tajuddin, S., Ahmed, S., & Latif, A. (2003). Aphrodisiac activity of 50% ethanolic extracts of *Myristica fragrans* houtt and *Syzygium aromatican* (L) Merr. And Perry (clove) in male mice. A comparative study. *BMC Complementary and Alternative Medicine*, *3*(1), 6. doi:10.1186/1472-6882-3-6 PMID:14567759

Tanabe, H., Yoshida, M., & Tomita, N. (2002). Comparison of the antioxidant activities of 22 commonly used culinary herbs and spices on the lipid oxidation of pork meat. *Animal Science Journal*, *73*(5), 389–393. doi:10.1046/j.1344-3941.2002.00054.x

Tanikawa, K., & Torimura, T. (2006). Studies on oxidative stress in liver diseases: Important future trends in liver research. *Medical Molecular Morphology*, *39*(1), 22–27. doi:10.1007/s00795-006-0313-z PMID:16575511

Tapsell, L.C., Hemphill, I., Cobiac, L., Sullivan, D.R., Fenech, M., & Patch, C.S., Roodenrys, ... Inge, K.E. (2006). Health benefits of herbs and spices: The past, the present, the future. *The Medical Journal of Australia*, *185*, S1–S24. PMID:17022438

Tassou, C., Drosinos, E. H., & Nychas, G. J. E. (1996). Inhibition of resident microbial flora and pathogen inocula on cold fresh fish fillets in olive oil, oregano, and lemon juice under modified atmosphere or air. *Journal of Food Protection*, *59*, 31–34.

Thompson, A., Meah, D., Ahmed, N., Conniff-Jenkins, R., Chileshe, E., Phillips, C. O., & Row, P. E. et al. (2013). Comparison of the antibacterial activity of essential oils and extracts of medicinal and culinary herbs to investigate potential new treatments for irritable bowel syndrome. *BMC Complementary and Alternative Medicine*, *13*(1), 338–350. doi:10.1186/1472-6882-13-338 PMID:24283351

Tongnuanchan, P., Benjakul, S., & Prodpran, T. (2014). Physico Chemical Properties, Morphology and Antioxidant Activity of Film from Fish Skin Gelatin Incorporated with Root Essential Oils. *Journal of Food Engineering*, *117*(3), 350–360. doi:10.1016/j.jfoodeng.2013.03.005

Trombetta, D., Castelli, F., Sarpietro, M. G., Venuti, V., Cristani, M., Daniele, C., & Bisignano, G. et al. (2005). Mechanisms of antibacterial action of three monoterpenes. *Antimicrobial Agents and Chemotherapy*, *49*(6), 2474–2478. doi:10.1128/AAC.49.6.2474-2478.2005 PMID:15917549

Tyagi, A. K., Bukvicki, D., Gottardi, D., Tabanelli, G., Montanari, C., Malik, A., & Guerzoni, M. E. (2014). Eucalyptus Essential Oil as a Natural Food Preservative In Vivo and In Vitro Antiyeast Potential. BioMed Research International.

Ultee, A., Bennik, M. H., & Moezelaar, R. (2002). The phenolic hydroxyl group of carvacrol is essential for action against the food-borne pathogen *Bacillus cereus*. *Applied and Environmental Microbiology*, *68*(4), 1561–1568. doi:10.1128/AEM.68.4.1561-1568.2002 PMID:11916669

Ultee, E., & Smid, J. (2001). Influence of carvacrol on growth and toxin production by *Bacillus cereus*. *International Journal of Food Microbiology*, *4*(3), 373–378. doi:10.1016/S0168-1605(00)00480-3 PMID:11294360

UNIDO & FAO. (2005). *Herbs, spices and essential oils:post-harvest operations in developing countries*. Vienna: United Nations Industrial development Organization & Food and Agriculture organization of United Nations (UNIDO).

Wu, S., Patel, K.B., Booth, L.J. Metcalfb, J.P., Lin, H.K., & Wu, W. (2010). *Protective essential oil attenuates influenza virus infection: An in vitro study in MDCK cells*. Academic Press.

Xiao, Z., Liu, W., Zhu, G., Zhou, R., & Niu, Y. (2014). A review of the preparation and application of flavour and essential oils microcapsules based on complex coacervation technology. *Journal of the Science of Food and Agriculture*, *94*(8), 1482–1494. doi:10.1002/jsfa.6491 PMID:24282124

Zhu, R., Wang, Y., Zhang, L., & Guo, Q. (2012). Oxidative stress and liver disease. *Hepatology Research*, *42*(8), 741–749. doi:10.1111/j.1872-034X.2012.00996.x PMID:22489668

KEY TERMS AND DEFINITIONS

Aphrodisiac: A food, drink or other thing that stimulates sexual desire.

Carminative: An agent that prevents or relieves flatulence and in infants, may help in treatment of colic.

Cognitive Ability: The mental process of knowing, including aspects such as awareness, perception, reasoning and judgement.

Generally Recognized As Safe: A state label assigned by the FDA (US Food and Drug Administration) to a listing of substances not known to be hazardous to health.

Genotoxicity: Destructive effect on cell's DNA material, thereby causing cancer or mutation.

Immunomodulatory: Capability of modifying or regulating one or more immune functions.

Microencapsulation: The process of enclosing chemical substances in microcapsules.

Nanoparticle: A microscopic particle of matter that is measured on the nanoscale, usually that measures less than 100nanometers.

Phytochemical: A nonnutritive bioactive plant substance, such as flavonoid or carotenoid, considered to have a beneficial effect on human health.

ENDNOTE

1 http://www.allindianpatents.com/patents/238344-a-process-and-formulation-for-the-preparation-of-enhanced-mango-flavor-beverage.

Compilation of References

Abarca, M. L., Bragulat, M. R., Castellá, G., & Cabañes, F. J. (n.d.). Ochratoxin A production by strains of Aspergillus niger var. niger. *Applied and Environmental Microbiology*, *60*, 2650–2652. PMID:8074536

Abass, E. H., Zair, S. K., Mohammud, T. K., & Nagem, S. A. (2014). Recovery of pure Hesperidin from Iraqi Sweet Oranges Peel and study the effect in some bacteria. *Baghdad Science Journal*, *11*(2), 455–460.

Abbeddou, S., Rischkowsky, B., Richter, E. K., Hess, H. D., & Kreuzer, M. (2011). Modification of milk fatty acid composition by feeding forages and agro-industrial byproducts from dry areas to Awassi sheep. *Journal of Dairy Science*, *94*(9), 4657–4668. doi:10.3168/jds.2011-4154 PMID:21854938

Abdulmumeen, H.A., Risikat, A.N. & Sururah, A.R. (2012). Food: Its preservatives, additives and applications. *International Journal of Chemical and Biochemical Sciences,* 36-47.

Abuelsaad, A. S., Mohamed, I., Allam, G., & Al-Solumani, A. A. (2013). Antimicrobial and immunomodulating activities of hesperidin and ellagic acid against diarrheic *Aeromonas hydrophila* in a murine model. *Life Sciences*, *93*(20), 714–722. doi:10.1016/j.lfs.2013.09.019 PMID:24090709

AbuGhazaleh, A. A., Riley, M. B., Thies, E. E., & Jenkins, T. C. (2005). Dilution rate and pH effects on the conversion of oleic acid to trans C 18: 1 positional isomers in continuous culture. *Journal of Dairy Science*, *88*(12), 4334–4341. doi:10.3168/jds.S0022-0302(05)73120-9 PMID:16291625

Adesegun, A. S., Samuel, F. O., Anthony, O. B., & Nurudeen, O. A. (2013). Antioxidant and Inhibitory Properties of Essential Oil of *Ocimum Gratissimum* Against Extracellular Protease of *Escherichia coli. IOSR Journal Of Pharmacy.*, *3*(1), 50–55. doi:10.9790/3013-31305055

Agencia Española de Seguridad Alimentaria y Nutrición. (2012). *Guía para la aplicación del sistema de trazabilidad en la empresa agroalimentaria. Alcalá, 56 - 28071 Madrid. Artes Gráficas Palermo, S.L, Alcalá E. B., Agencia Española de Seguridad Alimentaria y Nutrición.* AESAN.

Ahmadi, S., & McKenna, K. (2003). Keratitis-ichthyosis-deafness syndrome and carotenaemia. *Clinical and Experimental Dermatology*, *28*(4), 394–396. doi:10.1046/j.1365-2230.2003.01316.x PMID:12823302

Aii, T., Tamaki, M., Shimabukuro, H., Hayasawa, H., Shimizu, T., & Ishida, S. (1999). Conjugated linoleic acid content in milk fat of the cows fed a large amount of linseed. *Animal Science Journal*, *70*(6), 535–541.

Akroum, S., Bendjeddou, D., Satta, D., & Lalaoui, K. (2010). Antibacterial, antioxidant and acute toxicity tests on flavonoids extracted from some medicinal plants. *International Journal of Green Pharmacy*, *4*(3), 165–169. doi:10.4103/0973-8258.69174

Alastruey-Izquierdo, A., Cuenca-Estrella, M., Monzon, A., Mellado, E., & Rodriguez-Tudela, J. L. (2008). Antifungal susceptibility profile of clinical Fusarium spp. isolates identified by molecular methods. *The Journal of Antimicrobial Chemotherapy*, *61*(4), 805–809. doi:10.1093/jac/dkn022 PMID:18263569

Albarracín, H., Alfonso, A., & Sánchez, B. (2012). Application of essential oils as a preservative to improve the shelf life of *Nile tilapia* (Oreochoromisniloticus). *Revista de la facultad de química farmacéutica, 19*(1), 34-40.

Alberti, K. G. M., Zimmet, P., Shaw, J., & Group, I. E. T. F. C. (2005). The metabolic syndrome—a new worldwide definition. *Lancet*, *366*(9491), 1059–1062. doi:10.1016/S0140-6736(05)67402-8 PMID:16182882

Alexandrakis, G., Alfonso, E. C., & Miller, D. (2000). Shifting trends in bacterial keratitis in south Florida and emerging resistance to fluoroquinolones. *Ophthalmology*, *107*(8), 1497–1502. doi:10.1016/S0161-6420(00)00179-2 PMID:10919897

Al-fawwaz, A. T., & Alsohaili, S. A. (2015). Antimicrobial Activity of *Varthemia iphinoides* and *Majorana syriaca* Essential Oils from Jordan and Their Potential Use as Natural Food Preservatives. *Journal of Natural Sciences Research.*, *5*(22), 155.

Alfonso, E. C., Mandelbaum, S., Fox, M. J., & Forster, R. K. (1986). Ulcerative keratitis associated with contact lens wear. *American Journal of Ophthalmology*, *101*(4), 429–433. doi:10.1016/0002-9394(86)90641-0 PMID:3963102

Alimentarius, C. (2006). *Anteproyecto de Norma Revisada para Alimentos Exentos de Gluten*. Retrieved October 5, 2006, from ftp://ftp.fao.org/Codex/ccnfsdu28/cl06_05s.pdf

Ali, S. K., Khan, A. A., Ahmed, I., Musaddiq, M., Ahmed, K. S., Polasa, H., & Ahmed, N. et al. (2005). Antimicrobial activities of eugenol and cinnamaldehyde against human gastric pathogen *Helicobacter pylori. Annals of Clinical Microbiology and Antimicrobials*, *4*(1), 20. doi:10.1186/1476-0711-4-20 PMID:16371157

Alissa, E. M., & Ferns, G. A. (2012). Functional Foods and Nutraceuticals in the Primary Prevention of Cardiovascular Diseases. *Journal of Nutrition and Metabolism*, *2012*, 1–16. doi:10.1155/2012/569486 PMID:22570771

Alonso, L., Cuesta, E. P., & Gilliland, S. E. (2003). Production of free conjugated linoleic acid by Lactobacillus acidophilus and Lactobacillus casei of human intestinal origin. *Journal of Dairy Science*, *86*(6), 1941–1946. doi:10.3168/jds.S0022-0302(03)73781-3 PMID:12836928

Alvarez, M. V., Luis, A., Ortega-Ramirez, M., Gutierrez-Pacheco, M., Bernal-Mercado, A. T., Rodriguez-Garcia, I., & Ayala-Zavala, J. F. (2014). Oregano essential oil-pectin edible films as anti-quorum sensing and food antimicrobial agents. *Frontiers in Microbiology.*, *5*, 699. doi:10.3389/fmicb.2014.00699 PMID:25566215

Alvarez-Suarez, J. M., Giampieri, F., Tulipani, S., Casoli, T., Di Stefano, G., Gonzalez-Paramas, A. M., & Battino, M. (2014). One-month strawberry-rich anthocyanin supplementation ameliorates cardiovascular risk, oxidative stress markers and platelet activation in humans. *The Journal of Nutritional Biochemistry*, *25*(3), 289–294. doi:10.1016/j.jnutbio.2013.11.002 PMID:24406274

Alves, M. J., Ferreira, I. C., Froufe, H. J., Abreu, R. M., Martins, A., & Pintado, M. (2013). Antimicrobial activity of phenolic compounds identified in wild mushrooms, SAR analysis and docking studies. *Journal of Applied Microbiology*, *115*(2), 346–357. doi:10.1111/jam.12196 PMID:23510516

Amadou, , Gounga, & Le. (2013). Millets: Nutritional composition, some health benefits and processing – A Review.Emir. *Journal of Food & Agriculture*, *25*(7), 501–508. doi:10.9755/ejfa.v25i7.12045

Amorati, R., Foti, M. C., & Valgimigli, L. (2013). Antioxidant Activity of Essential Oils. *Journal of Agricultural and Food Chemistry*, *61*(46), 10835–10847. doi:10.1021/jf403496k PMID:24156356

Anand, P., Kunnumakkara, A. B., Newman, R. A., & Aggarwal, B. B. (2007). Bioavailability of Curcumin: Problems and Promises. *Molecular Pharmaceutics*, *4*(6), 807–818. doi:10.1021/mp700113r PMID:17999464

Anderson, N. E., & Clydesdale, F. M. (1980). Effects of processing on the dietary fiber content of wheat bran, pureed green beans and carrots. *Journal of Food Science*, *45*(6), 1533–1537. doi:10.1111/j.1365-2621.1980.tb07556.x

Ando, A., Ogawa, J., Kishino, S., & Shimizu, S. (2003). CLA production from ricinoleic acid by lactic acid bacteria. *Journal of the American Oil Chemists' Society*, *80*(9), 889–894. doi:10.1007/s11746-003-0790-1

Ando, A., Ogawa, J., Sugimoto, S., Kishino, S., Sakuradani, E., Yokozeki, K., & Shimizu, S. (2009). Selective production of cis-9, trans-11 isomer of conjugated linoleic acid from trans-vaccenic acid methyl ester by Delacroixia coronata. *Journal of Applied Microbiology*, *106*(5), 1697–1704. doi:10.1111/j.1365-2672.2008.04139.x PMID:19226396

Añíbarro, B., Garcia-Ara, M. C., Martin Esteban, M., Boyano, T., Diaz Pena, J. M., & Ojeda, J. A. (1997). Peculiarities of egg allergy in children with bird protein sensitization. *Annals of Allergy, Asthma & Immunology*, *78*(2), 213–216. doi:10.1016/S1081-1206(10)63389-3 PMID:9048530

Anonymous. (n.d.). Retrieved 1 July 2014 from: http://thepaleodiet.com/vegetable-oil-fatty-acid-composition/

Antony, U., Sripriya, G., & Chandra, T. S. (1996). Effect of fermentation on the primary nutrients in finger millet (*Eleusine coracana*). *Journal of Agricultural and Food Chemistry*, *44*(9), 2616–2618. doi:10.1021/jf950787q

Apel, K., & Hirt, H. (2004). Reactive oxygen species: Metabolism, oxidative stress, and signal transduction. *Annual Review of Plant Biology*, *55*(1), 373–399. doi:10.1146/annurev.arplant.55.031903.141701 PMID:15377225

Arrigoni, E., Caprez, A., Amado, R., & Neukom, H. (1986). Chemical composition and physical properties of modified dietary fibre sources. *Food Hydrocolloids*, *1*(1), 57–64. doi:10.1016/S0268-005X(86)80007-8

Aruoma, O. I. (1998). Free radicals, oxidative stress, and antioxidants in human health and disease. *Journal of the American Oil Chemists' Society*, *75*(2), 199–212. doi:10.1007/s11746-998-0032-9

Arvidsson, K. (2009). *Factors affecting fatty acid composition in forage and milk*. (Doctoral Thesis). Swedish University of Agricultural Sciences.

Ascenso, A., Ribeiro, H., Marques, H. C., Oliveira, H., Santos, C., & Simões, S. (2014). Chemoprevention of photocarcinogenesis by lycopene. *Experimental Dermatology*, *23*(12), 874–878. doi:10.1111/exd.12491 PMID:25040310

Ashakiran & Deepthi, R. (2012). Fast Foods and their Impact on Health. *Journal of Krishna Institute of Medical Sciences University.*, *2*, 7–15.

Asp, N. G., Bjorck, I., & Nyman, M. (1986). Effects of processing on dietary fibre. In R. Amado & T. F. Schweizer (Eds.), *Nahrungsfasem dietary fibres* (pp. 177–189). London: Academic Press.

Association of Official Analytical Chemists. (1980). *Official methods of analysis* (11th ed.). Washington, DC: AOAC.

Atwater, W. O. (1900). *Discussion of the terms digestibility, availability and fuel value*. Twelfth Annual Report of the Storrs Agricultural Experimental Station.

Aurela, B., Ohra-Aho, & Söderhjelm, L. (n.d.). Migration of alkylbenzenes from packaging into food and Tenax®. *Packaging Technology and Science, 14*(2), 71–77.

Aureli, P., Costantini, A., & Zolea, S. (1992). Antimicrobial activity of some plant essential oils against *Listeria monocytogenes. Journal of Food Protection*, *55*, 344–348.

Awad, M. (1993). *Fisiologia Pós-colheita de frutos*. São Paulo, SP, Brasil: Nobel.

Azzura, A., & Paola, P. (2009). *Consumers' behaviours and attitudes toward healthy food products: The case of Organic and Functional foods*. Paper presented at 113th EAAE Seminar "A resilient European food industry and food chain in a challenging world", Chania, Crete, Greece.

Badei, A. Z., Hemeda, H. H., Hafez, S. A., & Hassanen, N. H. (2000). Effect of baking and storage on the essential oil components of anise and cumin biscuits. *Egyptian Journal of Agricultural Research.*, *78*, 321–334.

Bae, E. A., Han, M. J., & Kim, D. H. (1999). *In vitro* anti-Helicobacter pylori activity of some flavonoids and their metabolites. *Planta Medica*, *65*(05), 442–443. doi:10.1055/s-2006-960805 PMID:10454900

Bae, E. A., Han, M. J., & Kim, D. H. (2000). *In vitro* inhibitory effect of some flavonoids on rotavirus infectivity. *Biological & Pharmaceutical Bulletin*, *23*(9), 1122–1124. doi:10.1248/bpb.23.1122 PMID:10993220

Bagdia, A. B. G., Schmidtb, J., Szatmária, M., Schoenlechnerb, R., Berghoferb, E., & Tömösközia, S. (2011). Protein Characterization and Nutrient Composition of Hungarian Proso Millet Varieties and the Effect of Decortication. *Acta Alimentaria*, *40*(1), 128–141. doi:10.1556/AAlim.40.2011.1.15

Bajaj, S., Urooj, A., & Prabhasankar, P. (2006). Effect of incorporation of mint on texture, colour and sensory parameters of biscuits. *International Journal of Food Properties.*, *9*(4), 691–700. doi:10.1080/10942910600547632

Baker, G. C., Smith, J. J., & Cowan, D. A. (2003). Review and re-analysis of domain specific 16s primers. *Journal of Microbiological Methods*, *55*(3), 541–555. doi:10.1016/j.mimet.2003.08.009 PMID:14607398

Bala Ravi, S., Swain, S., Sengotuvel, D., & Parida, N. R. (2010). *Promoting nutritious millets for enhancing income and improved nutrition (p- 37). A case study from Tamil Nadu and Orissa*. Chennai, India: Minor Millets in South Asia.Published by Bioversity International, Rome, Italy and MSSRF.

Balakrishnan, R., Alagukannan, G., Kumar, N. A., Nambi, V. A., Balakrishnan, V., Balasubramanian, K., & Girigan, G. et al. (2002). *Rural and Tribal Women in Agrobiodiversity Conservation; An Indian Case Study, RAP Publication 2002/08*. Chennai, India: MS Swaminathan Research Foundation.

Balchin, M. L. (2006). Aromatherapy Science. In *A Guide for Healthcare Professionals* (1st ed.). USA: Pharmaceutical Press.

Ballabeni, V., Tognolinia, M., Bertonia, S., Brunib, R., Guerrinibm, A., Ruedac, G. M., & Barocellia, E. (2007). Antiplatelet and antithrombotic activities of essential oil from wild Ocotea quixos (Lam.) Kosterm. (Lauraceae) calices from Amazonian Ecuador. *Pharmacological Research*, *55*(1), 23–30. doi:10.1016/j.phrs.2006.09.009 PMID:17079160

Ballabeni, V., Tognolini, M., Chiavarini, M., Impicciatore, M., Bruni, R., Bianchi, A., & Barocelli, E. (2004). Novel antiplatelet and antithrombotic activities of essential oil from Lavandula hybrida Reverchon "grosso". *Phytomedicine*, *11*(7-8), 596–601. doi:10.1016/j.phymed.2004.01.002 PMID:15636172

Ballard, C., O'Brien, J., Reichelt, K., & Perry, E. (2002). Aromatherapy as a safe and effective treatment for the management of agitation in severe dementia: The results of a double blind, placebo controlled trial. *The Journal of Clinical Psychiatry*, *63*(7), 553–558. doi:10.4088/JCP.v63n0703 PMID:12143909

Ballmer-Weber, B. K., Vieths, S., Luttkopf, D., Heuschmann, P., & Wüthrich, B. (2000). Celery allergy confirmed by double-blind, placebo-controlled food challenge: A clinical study in 32 subjects with a history of adverse reactions to celery root. *The Journal of Allergy and Clinical Immunology*, *106*(2), 373–378. doi:10.1067/mai.2000.107196 PMID:10932083

Barbosa, L. N., Rall, V. L. M., Fernandes, A. A. F., Ushimaru, P. I., Probst, I. S., & Fernandes, A. (2009). Essential oils against foodborne pathogens and spoilage bacteria in minced meat. *Foodborne Pathogens and Disease*, *6*(6), 725–728. doi:10.1089/fpd.2009.0282 PMID:19580445

Barik, B. P., Yegneswaran, P. P., Tayung, K., & Sahu, H. K. (2011). Molecular Identification and in-vitro Antifungal Susceptibility of Fusarium sp. isolated from Corneal Scrape. *Journal of Life Science*, *3*(2), 127–130.

Baron, R. A. (1990). Environmentally-induced positive affect: Its impact on self efficacy, task performance, negotiation and conflict. *Journal of Applied Social Psychology*, *20*(5), 368–384. doi:10.1111/j.1559-1816.1990.tb00417.x

Baron, R. A., & Thomley, J. (1994). A whiff of reality. *Environment and Behavior*, *26*(6), 766–784. doi:10.1177/0013916594266003

Barreca, D., Laganà, G., Bruno, G., Magazù, S., & Bellocco, E. (2013). Diosmin binding to human serum albumin and its preventive action against degradation due to oxidative injuries. *Biochimie*, *95*(11), 2042–2049. doi:10.1016/j.biochi.2013.07.014 PMID:23886889

Bartke, A., Sun, L. Y., & Longo, V. (2013). Somatotropic signaling: Trade-offs between growth, reproductive development, and longevity. *Physiological Reviews*, *93*(2), 571–598. doi:10.1152/physrev.00006.2012 PMID:23589828

Bartlet, J. C., & Chapman, D. G. (1961). Butter adulteration, detection of hydrogenated fats in butter fat by measurement of cis-trans conjugated unsaturation. *Journal of Agricultural and Food Chemistry*, *9*(1), 50–53. doi:10.1021/jf60113a015

Bartolotta, S., Garcia, C. C., Candurra, N. A., & Damonte, E. B. (2001). Effect of fatty acids on adenavirus replication: Inhibition of virus production by lauric acid. *Archives of Virology*, *146*(4), 777–790. doi:10.1007/s007050170146 PMID:11402863

Bartram, T. (1995). *Encyclopaedia of herbal medicines*. Dorset, UK: Grace publishers.

Bassole, I. H., & Juliani, H. R. (2012). Essential oils in combination and their antimicrobial properties. *Molecules (Basel, Switzerland)*, *17*(4), 3989–4006. doi:10.3390/molecules17043989 PMID:22469594

Bauman, D. E., Everett, R. W., Weiland, W. H., & Collier, R. J. (1999). Production responses to bovine somatotropin in northeast dairy herds. *Journal of Dairy Science*, *82*(12), 2564–2573. doi:10.3168/jds.S0022-0302(99)75511-6 PMID:10629802

Becker, E. M., Nissen, L. R., & Skibsted, L. H. (2004). Antioxidant Evaluation Protocols: Food Quality or Health Effects. *European Food Research and Technology*, *219*(6), 561–571. doi:10.1007/s00217-004-1012-4

Bell, A.E., Sellers, L.A., Allen, A., Cunliffe, W.J., Morris, E.R., & Ross-Murphy, S.B. (1985). Properties of Gastric and Duodenal Mucus: Effect of Proteolysis, Disulfide Reduction, Bile, Acid, Ethanol, and Hypertonicity on Mucus Gel structure. *Gastroenterology, 88*(1), 269–280.

Bellanti, J. A., Sabra, A., & Zeligs, B. J. (2004). Gastrointestinal immunopathology and food allergy. *Annals of Allergy, Asthma & Immunology, 93*(5Suppl 3), S26–S32. doi:10.1016/S1081-1206(10)61729-2 PMID:15562871

Belletti, N., Kamdem, S.S., Patrignani, F., Lanciotti, R.., Covelli, A., & Gardini, F. (2007). *Antimicrobial activity of aroma compounds against* Saccharomyces cerevisiae *and improvement ofmicrobiological stability of soft drinks as assessed by logistic regression*. Academic Press.

Benjamin, S., Flotho, S., Börchers, T., & Spener, F. (2013). Conjugated linoleic acid isomers and their precursor fatty acids regulate peroxisome proliferator-activated receptor subtypes and major peroxisome proliferator responsive element-bearing target genes in HepG2 cell model. *Journal of Zhejiang University. Science. B., 14*(2), 115–123. doi:10.1631/jzus.B1200175 PMID:23365010

Benjamin, S., Hanhoff, T., Börchers, T., & Spener, F. (2005). An improved molecular test system for the screening of human PPAR transactivation by conjugated linoleic acid isomers and their precursor fatty acids. *European Journal of Lipid Science and Technology, 107*(10), 706–715. doi:10.1002/ejlt.200401041

Benjamin, S., Prakasan, P., Sreedharan, S., Wright, A. D. G., & Spener, F. (2015). Pros and cons of CLA consumption: An insight from clinical evidences. *Nutrition & Metabolosm, 12*(1), 4. doi:10.1186/1743-7075-12-4 PMID:25972911

Benjamin, S., & Spener, F. (2009). Conjugated linoleic acids as functional food: An insight into their health benefits. *Nutrition Metabolism, 6*(1), 36. doi:10.1186/1743-7075-6-36 PMID:19761624

Berjia, F. L., Poulsen, M., & Nauta, M. (2014). Burden of diseases estimates associated to different red meat cooking practices. *Food and Chemical Toxicology, 66*, 237–244. doi:10.1016/j.fct.2014.01.045 PMID:24491261

Bernard, E., Britz-McKibbin, P., & Gernigon, N. (2007). Resveratrol photoisomerization: An integrative-guide survey experiment. *Journal of Chemical Education, 84*(7), 1159. doi:10.1021/ed084p1159

Bernas, A., Kumar, N., Mäki-Arvela, P., Kul'kova, N. V., Holmbom, B., Salmi, T., & Murzin, D. Y. (2003). Isomerization of linoleic acid over supported metal catalysts. *Applied Catalysis A, General, 245*(2), 257–275. doi:10.1016/S0926-860X(02)00646-4

Bernd, Z., Ana, T., Lucija, H., & Hrvoje, F. (2010). Subcellular distribution of glutathione and cysteine in cyanobacteria. *Protoplasma, 246*(1-4), 65–72. doi:10.1007/s00709-010-0126-8 PMID:20349253

Bernhisel-Broadbent, J., Dintzis, H. M., Dintzis, R. Z., & Sampson, H. A. (1994). Allergenicity and antigenicity of chicken egg ovomucoid (Gal dIII) compared with ovalbumin (Gal d I) in children with egg allergy and in mice. *The Journal of Allergy and Clinical Immunology*, *93*(6), 1047–1059. doi:10.1016/S0091-6749(94)70054-0 PMID:8006309

Bertin, C., Rouau, X., & Thibault, I. F. (1988). Structure and properties of sugar beet fibres. *Science of Food and Agriculture*, (44), 15-29.

Beyer, K., Morrow, E., Li, X. M., Bardina, L., Bannon, G. A., Burks, A. W., & Sampson, H. A. (2001). Effects of cooking methods on peanut allergenicity. *The Journal of Allergy and Clinical Immunology*, *107*(6), 1077–1081. doi:10.1067/mai.2001.115480 PMID:11398088

Beyer, W., Imlay, J., & Fridovich, I. (1991). Superoxide dismutases. *Progress in Nucleic Acid Research*, *40*, 221–253. doi:10.1016/S0079-6603(08)60843-0 PMID:1851570

Biesalski, H. K. (2007). Polyphenols and inflammation: Basic interactions. *Current Opinion in Clinical Nutrition and Metabolic Care*, *10*(6), 724–728. doi:10.1097/MCO.0b013e3282f0cef2 PMID:18089954

Bigoniya, P., & Singh, K. (2014). Ulcer protective potential of standardized hesperidin, a citrus flavonoid isolated from *Citrus sinensis*. *Revista Brasileira de Farmacognosia*, *24*(3), 330–340. doi:10.1016/j.bjp.2014.07.011

Bishayee, K., & Khuda-Bukhsh, A. R. (2013). 5-Lipoxygenase Antagonist therapy: A new approach towards targeted cancer chemotherapy. *Acta Biochimica et Biophysica Sinica*, *45*(9), 709–719. doi:10.1093/abbs/gmt064 PMID:23752617

Bjelakovic, G., Nikolova, D., Gluud, L. L., Simonetti, R. G., & Gluud, C. (2007). Mortality in randomized trials of antioxidant supplements for primary and secondary revention: Systematic review and meta-analysis. *Journal of the American Medical Association*, *297*, 842–857. doi:10.1001/jama.297.8.842 PMID:17327526

Bjorck, I., Nyman, M., & Asp, N. G. (1984). Extrusion-cooking and dietary fiber. I. Effects on dietary fiber content and on degradation in the rat intestinal tract. *Cereal Chemistry*, *61*, 74–179.

Bloch, A. S. (2003). Nutrition for health promotion: Phytochemicals, functional foods, and alternative approaches to combat obesity. *Dental Clinics of North America*, *47*(2), 411–423. doi:10.1016/S0011-8532(02)00109-X PMID:12699239

Blokhina, O., & Fagerstedt, K. V. (2010). Oxygen deprivation, metabolic adaptations and oxidative stress. In S. Mancuso & S. Shabala (Eds.), *Waterlogging Signaling and Tolerance in Plants* (pp. 119–147). Berlin: Springer-Verlag. doi:10.1007/978-3-642-10305-6_7

Bock, S. A. (1987). Prospective appraisal of complaints of adverse reactions to foods in children during the first 3 years of life. *Pediatrics*, *79*, 683–688. PMID:3575022

Bock, S. A., & Atkins, F. M. (1989). The natural history of peanut allergy. *The Journal of Allergy and Clinical Immunology*, *83*(5), 900–904. doi:10.1016/0091-6749(89)90103-6 PMID:2715549

Bogsan, C. S., Florence, A. C. R., Perina, N., Hirota, C., Soares, F. A. S. M., Silva, R. C., & Oliveira, M. N. (2013). Survival of Bi fi dobacterium lactis HN019 and release of biogenic compounds in unfermented and fermented milk is affected by chilled storage at 4 C. *Journal of Probiotics and Health*, *4*(1).

Boire, N. A., Riedel, S., & Parrish, N. M. (2013). Essential Oils and Future Antibiotics: New Weapons against Emerging' Superbugs'? *Journal of Ancient Diseases & Preventive Remedies.*, *1*(2), 1–5. doi:10.4172/2329-8731.1000105

Bond, A., & Lader, M. (1974). The use of analogue scales in rating subjective feelings. *The British Journal of Medical Psychology*, *47*(3), 211–218. doi:10.1111/j.2044-8341.1974.tb02285.x

Bouhdid, S., Abrini, J., Amensour, M., Zhiri, A., Espuny, M. J., & Manresa, A. (2010). Functional and ultrastructural changes in *Pseudomonas aeruginosa* and *Staphylococcus aureus* cells induced by *Cinnamomum verum* essential oil. *Journal of Applied Microbiology*, *109*(4), 1139–1149. doi:10.1111/j.1365-2672.2010.04740.x PMID:20456525

Brackman, G., Defoirdt, T., Miyamoto, C., Bossier, P., Calenbergh, S. V., Nelis, H., & Coenye, T. (2008). Cinnamaldehyde and cinnamaldehyde derivatives reduce virulence in *Vibrio* spp. by decreasing the DNA-binding activity of the quorum sensing response regulator LuxR. *BMC Microbiology*, *8*(1), 149. doi:10.1186/1471-2180-8-149 PMID:18793453

Bradley, D. E., & Min, D. B. (1992). Singlet oxygen oxidation of foods. *Critical Reviews in Food Science and Nutrition*, *31*(3), 211–236. doi:10.1080/10408399209527570 PMID:1571085

Brafau, G., Canela, A. M., & Rafecas, M. (2008). Phytosterols: Physiologic and metabolic aspects related to cholesterol-lowering properties. *Nutrition Research (New York, N.Y.)*, *28*(4), 217–225. doi:10.1016/j.nutres.2008.02.003 PMID:19083411

Bravo, L. (1998). Polyphenols: Chemistry, dietary sources, metabolism and nutritional significance. *Nutrition Reviews*, *56*(11), 317–333. doi:10.1111/j.1753-4887.1998.tb01670.x PMID:9838798

Brewer, M. S. (2006). Natural Antioxidants: Sources, Compounds, Mechanisms of Action, and Potential Applications. *Comprehensive Reviews in Food Science and Food Safety*, *10*(4), 221–247. doi:10.1111/j.1541-4337.2011.00156.x

British Nutrition Foundation. (1990). *Complex carbohydrates in foods*. London: Chapman and Hall.

Britt, B., Freeman, A., & Amgen, C. (2013). Incorporated, thousand oaks, Dietary Composition and Obesity. *Digestive Diseases and Sciences*, *4*(3), 16–24.

Britton, G., Liaaen-Jensen, S., & Pfander, H. (2004). *Carotenoids Handbook*. Birkhäuser Basel. doi:10.1007/978-3-0348-7836-4

Brown, B. E., Ambarsari, I., Warner, M. E., Fitt, W. K., Dunne, R. P., Gibb, S. W., & Cummings, D. G. (1999). Diurnal changes in photochemical efficiency and xanthophyll concentrations in shallow water reef corals: Evidence for photoinhibition and photoprotection. *Coral Reefs*, *18*(2), 99–105. doi:10.1007/s003380050163

Bruni, R., Medici, A., Andreotti, E., Fantin, C., Muzzoli, M., Dehesa, M., & Sacchetti, G. et al. (2003). Chemical composition and biological activities of *Isphingo* essential oil, a traditional *Ecuadorian* spice from *Ocotea quixus* (Lam.) Kosterm. (Lauraceae) flower calices. *Food Chemistry, 85*(3), 415–421. doi:10.1016/j.foodchem.2003.07.019

Brush, S. B. (Ed.). (2000). Genes in the Field: On-Farm Conservation of Crop Diversity. RC/IPGRI/Lewis Publishers.

Bruulsema, T. W. (2000). Functional Food Components: A Role for Mineral Nutrients? *Better Crops., 84*(2), 4–5.

Buccioni, A., Minieri, S., Rapaccini, S., Antongiovanni, M., & Mele, M. (2011). Effect of chestnut and quebracho tannins on fatty acid profile in rumen liquid-and solid-associated bacteria: An in vitro study. *Animal, 5*(10), 1521–1530. doi:10.1017/S1751731111000759 PMID:22440342

Buck, L. B. (2000). The molecular architecture of odor and pheromone sensing in mammals. *Cell, 100*(6), 611–618. doi:10.1016/S0092-8674(00)80698-4 PMID:10761927

Bu, D. P., Wang, J. Q., Dhiman, T. R., & Liu, S. J. (2007). Effectiveness of oils rich in linoleic and linolenic acids to enhance conjugated linoleic acid in milk from dairy cows. *Journal of Dairy Science, 90*(2), 998–1007. doi:10.3168/jds.S0022-0302(07)71585-0 PMID:17235178

Budavari, S. (1996). *The Merck Index.* Merck and Co.

Buitrago-Lopez, A., Sanderson, J., Johnson, L., Warnakula, S., Wood, A., Di-Angelantonio, E., & Franco, O. H. (2011). Chocolate consumption and cardiometabolic disorders: Systematic review and meta-analysis. *British Medical Journal, 343*(1), d4488. doi:10.1136/bmj.d4488 PMID:21875885

Burkert, N.T., & Muckenhuber, J., Großscha, Ra´sky & Freidl, W. (2014). Nutrition and Health – The Association between Eating Behavior and Various Health Parameters: A Matched Sample Study. *PLoS ONE, 9*(2), e88278. PMID:24516625

Burr, G. O., & Burr, M. M. (1930). On the nature and role of the fatty acids essential in nutrition. *The Journal of Biological Chemistry, 86*(2), 587–621.

Burton, G. W., & Ingold, K. U. (1984). ß-carotene: An unusual type of lipid antioxidant. *Science, 224*(4649), 569–573. doi:10.1126/science.6710156 PMID:6710156

Butzke, C. E., & Bisson, L. F. (1997). *Ethyl Carbamate Preventative Action Manual.* Retrieved from http://www.cfsan.fda.gov/~frf/ecaction.html

Büyüktuncel, E., Porgal, E., & Çolak, C. (2014). Comparison of Total Phenolic Content and Total Antioxidant Activity in Local Red Wines Determined by Spectrophotometric Methods. *Food and Nutrition Sciences, 5*(17), 1660–1667. doi:10.4236/fns.2014.517179

Caillet, S., & Lacroix, M. (2006). Effect of gamma radiation and oregano essential oil on murein and ATP concentration of *Listeria monocytogenes. Journal of Food Protection, 69*, 2961–2969. PMID:17186665

Cai, Y., Zhao, L., Qin, Y., & He, Y. (2015). High dose of epigallocatechin-3-gallate inhibits proliferation and induces apoptosis of H9C2 cardiomyocytes through down-regulation of SIRT1. *Die Pharmazie*, *70*(1), 12–16. PMID:25975092

Calomme, M., Pieters, L., Vlietnick, A., & Berghe, D. V. (1996). Inibition of bacterial mutagenesis by Citurs flavonoids. *Planta Medica*, *62*(03), 222–226. doi:10.1055/s-2006-957864 PMID:8693033

Cameron, J. C., & Pakrasi, H. B. (2010). Essential Role of glutathione in acclimation to environmental and redox perturbations in the cyanobacterium *Synechocystis* sp. PCC 6803. *Plant Physiology*, *154*(4), 1672–1685. doi:10.1104/pp.110.162990 PMID:20935175

Caprez, A., Arrigoni, E., Amado, R., & Neukom, H. (1986). Influence of different type of thermal treatment on the chemical composition and physical properties of wheat bran. *Journal of Cereal Science*, *4*(4), 233–239. doi:10.1016/S0733-5210(86)80025-X

Carange, J., Longpré, F., Daoust, B., & Martinoli, M. G. (2011). 24-Epibrassinolide, a Phytosterol from the Brassinosteroid Family, Protects Dopaminergic Cells against MPP+-Induced Oxidative Stress and Apoptosis. *Journal of Toxicology*, *2011*, 13. doi:10.1155/2011/392859 PMID:21776258

Cardoso, F. S. P., Moro, A. V., & Correia, C. R. D. (2008, September). *Reação de Heck de estirenos com sais de diazônio: Síntese do Resveratrol e seus análogos*. Paper presented at XVI Congress Internal Scientific Initiation of Unicamp, Campinas, SP.

Cardó, X., Bergadà, O., Cesteros, Y., & Salagre, P. (2012). Effect of catalyst acidity and porosity on the catalytic isomerization of linoleic acid to obtain conjugated linoleic acids (CLAs). *Chemical Engineering Journal*, *183*, 459–465. doi:10.1016/j.cej.2011.12.088

Carpagnano, G. E., Kharitonov, S. A., Resta, O., Foschino-Barbaro, M. P., Gramiccioni, E., & Barnes, P. J. (2003). 8-Isoprostane, a marker of oxidative stress, is increased in exhaled breath condensate of patients with obstructive sleep apnea after night and is reduced by continuous positive airway pressure therapy. *Chest*, *124*(4), 1386–1392. doi:10.1378/chest.124.4.1386 PMID:14555570

Carvalho, W., Fonseca, M. E. N., Silva, H. R., Boiteux, L. S., & Giordano, L. B. (2005). Estimativa indireta de teores de licopeno em frutos genótipos de tomateiro via análise colorimétrica. *Horticultura Brasileira*, *23*(3), 819–825. doi:10.1590/S0102-05362005000300026

Castro, I. A., Barroso, L. P., & Sinnecker, P. (2005). Functional foods for coronary heart disease risk reduction: A meta-analysis using a multivariate approach. *The American Journal of Clinical Nutrition*, *82*(1), 32–40. PMID:16002797

Cavuoto, P., & Fenech, M. F. (2012). A review of methionine dependency and the role of methionine restriction in cancer growth control and life-span extension. *Cancer Treatment Reviews*, *38*(6), 726–736. doi:10.1016/j.ctrv.2012.01.004 PMID:22342103

Centers for Disease Control and Prevention (CDC). (2007). Fixed obstructive lung disease among workers in the flavor-manufacturing industry--California, 2004-2007. *MMWR Morb Mortal Wkly Rep.*, *56*(16), 389-93.

Chandrasekara, A., & Shahidi, F. (2010). Content of insoluble bound phenolics in millets and their contribution to antioxidant capacity. *Journal of Agricultural and Food Chemistry*, *58*(11), 6706–6714. doi:10.1021/jf100868b PMID:20465288

Chandrasekara, A., & Shahidi, F. (2011). Determination of antioxidant activity in free and hydrolyzed fractions of millet grains and characterization of their phenolic profiles by HPLC-DAD-ESI-MSn. *Journal of Functional Foods*, *3*(3), 144–158. doi:10.1016/j.jff.2011.03.007

Chandrasekara, A., & Shahidi, F. (2012). Bioaccessibility and antioxidant potential of millet grain phenolics as affected by simulated in vitro digestion and microbial fermentation. *J Funct Foods*, *4*(1), 226–237. doi:10.1016/j.jff.2011.11.001

Chang, H. C., Chen, T. G., Tai, Y. T., Chen, T. L., Chiu, W. T., & Chen, R. M. (2010). Resveratrol attenuates oxidized LDL-evoked Lox-1 signaling and consequently protects against apoptotic insults to cerebrovascular endothelial cells. *Journal of Cerebral Blood Flow and Metabolism*, *31*(3), 842–854. doi:10.1038/jcbfm.2010.180 PMID:20940732

Chang, M. C., & Morris, W. C. (2007). The Effect of Heat Treatments on Dietary Fiber as Assessed by Scanning Electron Microscopy. *Journal of Food Processing and Preservation*, *14*(5), 335–343. doi:10.1111/j.1745-4549.1990.tb00138.x

Chatterjee, S., Goswami, N., & Kothari, N. (2013). Evaluation of antioxidant activity of essential oil from Ajwain (Trachyspermum ammi) seeds. *International Journal of Green Pharmacy.*, *7*(2), 140–144. doi:10.4103/0973-8258.116396

Chen, F., Qian, L.-H., Deng, B., Liu, Z.-M., Zhao, Y., & Le, Y.-Y. (2013). Resveratrol Protects Vascular Endothelial Cells from High Glucose–Induced Apoptosis through Inhibition of NADPH Oxidase Activation–Driven Oxidative Stress. *CNS Neuroscience & Therapeutics*, *19*(9), 675–681. doi:10.1111/cns.12131 PMID:23731528

Cheng, C.-W., Adams, G. B., Perin, L., Wei, M., Zhou, X., Lam, B. S., & Longo, V. D. et al. (2014). Prolonged fasting reduces IGF-1/PKA to promote hematopoietic-stem-cell-based regeneration and reverse immunosuppression. *Cell Stem Cell*, *14*(6), 810–823. doi:10.1016/j.stem.2014.04.014 PMID:24905167

Chen, W. P., Chi, T. C., Chuang, L. M., & Su, M. J. (2007). Resveratrol enhances insulin secretion by blocking K(ATP) and K(V) channels of beta cells. *European Journal of Pharmacology*, *568*(1-3), 269–277. doi:10.1016/j.ejphar.2007.04.062 PMID:17573071

Chen, Y. X., Zhou, T., & Xie, K. P. (2013). Antibacterial Mechanism of Baicalein on Methicillin-resistant *Staphyloccocus aureus. Acta Veterinaria et Zootechnica Sinica*, *44*(12), 2000–2006.

Chhunchha, B., Fatma, N., Bhargavan, B., Kubo, E., Kumar, A., & Singh, D. P. (2011). Specificity protein, Sp1-mediated increased expression of Prdx6 as a curcumin-induced antioxidant defense in lens epithelial cells against oxidative stress. *Cell Death & Disease*, *2*(11), e234. doi:10.1038/cddis.2011.121 PMID:22113199

Chi, T., Ji, X., Xia, M., Rong, Y., Qiu, F., & Zou, L. (2009). Effect of six extractions from Wuhu decoction on isolated tracheal smoothe muscle in Guinea pig. *Zhongguo Shiyan Fangjixue Zazhi, 15*, 52–55.

Choi, J., Kang, O., Lee, Y., Oh, Y.-C., Chae, H.-S., Jang, H.-J., & Kwon, D.-Y. et al. (2009). Antibacterial activity of methylgallate isolated from Galla Rhois or carvacrol combined with nalidixic acid against nalidixic acid resistant bacteria. *Molecules (Basel, Switzerland), 14*(5), 1773–1780. doi:10.3390/molecules14051773 PMID:19471197

Choi, K., Jung, M. G., Lee, Y., Yoon, J. C., Kwon, S. H., Kang, H., & Yoon, H. et al. (2009). Epigallocatechin-3-Gallate, a Histone Acetyltransferase Inhibitor, Inhibits EBV-Induced B Lymphocyte Transformation via Suppression of RelA Acetylation. *Cancer Research, 69*(2), 583–592. doi:10.1158/0008-5472.CAN-08-2442 PMID:19147572

Choi, N. J., Imm, J. Y., Oh, S., Kim, B. C., Hwang, H. J., & Kim, Y. J. (2005). Effect of pH and oxygen on conjugated linoleic acid (CLA) production by mixed rumen bacteria from cows fed high concentrate and high forage diets. *Animal Feed Science and Technology, 123*, 643–653. doi:10.1016/j.anifeedsci.2005.04.054

Chopra, R. N., Nayar, S. L., & Chopra, I. C. (1965). Glossary of Indian Medicinal Plants with active principles Part-I (a-k). National Institute of Science Communication.

Christie, W. W. (2003). Analysis of conjugated linoleic acid: An overview. *Advances in Conjugated Linoleic Acid Research, 2*, 1–12.

Chun-Fai, Yu., Yu, P. H., Chan, P., Yan, Q., & Wong, P.-K. (2004). Two novel species of tetrodotoxin-producing bacteria isolated from toxic marine puffer fishes. *Toxicon, 44*(6), 641–647. doi:10.1016/j.toxicon.2004.07.021 PMID:15501290

Chun, Y. J., Kim, M. Y., & Guengerich, F. P. (1999). Resveratrol Is a Selective Human Cytochrome P450 1A1 Inhibitor. *Biochemical and Biophysical Research Communications, 262*(1), 20–24. doi:10.1006/bbrc.1999.1152 PMID:10448061

Cilla, A., Attanzio, A., Barberá, R., Tesoriere, L., & Livrea, M. A. (2015). Anti-proliferative effect of main dietary phytosterols and ß-cryptoxanthin alone or combined in human colon cancer Caco-2 cells through cytosolic Ca+2 and oxidative stress-induced apoptosis. *Journal of Functional Foods, 12*, 282–293. doi:10.1016/j.jff.2014.12.001

Cimanga, K., Kambu, K., Tona, L., Apers, S., DeBruyne, T., Hermans, N., & Tott, Ã. (2002). Correlation between chemical composition and antibacterial activity of essential oils of some aromatic medicinal plants growing in the Democratic Republic of Congo. *Journal of Ethnopharmacology, 79*(2), 213–220. doi:10.1016/S0378-8741(01)00384-1 PMID:11801384

Clydesdale, F. (2004). Functional foods: Opportunities and challenges. IFT Expert Panel Report. *Food Technology, 58*, 35–40.

Coakley, M., Ross, R. P., Nordgren, M., Fitzgerald, G., Devery, R., & Stanton, C. (2003). Conjugated linoleic acid biosynthesis by human-derived *Bifidobacterium* species. *Journal of Applied Microbiology*, *94*(1), 138–145. doi:10.1046/j.1365-2672.2003.01814.x PMID:12492934

Collins, M. D., & Jones, D. (1981). Distribution of isoprenoid quinone structural types in bacteria and their taxonomic implications. *Microbiological Reviews*, *45*, 316–354. PMID:7022156

Cooley, J. D., Wong, W. C., Jumper, C. A., & Straus, D. C. (1998). Correlation between the prevalence of certain fungi and sick building syndrome. *Occupational and Environmental Medicine*, *55*(9), 579–584. doi:10.1136/oem.55.9.579 PMID:9861178

Cordle, C. T. (2004). Soy protein allergy: Incidence and relative severity. *The Journal of Nutrition*, *134*(5), 1213S–1219S. PMID:15113974

Coulibaly, A., Kouakou, B., & Chen, J. (2011). Phytic acid in cereal grains: Structure, healthy or harmful ways to reduce phytic acid in cereal grains and their effects on nutritional quality. *Am. J. Plant Nutr. Fert. Technol*, *1*(1), 1–22. doi:10.3923/ajpnft.2011.1.22

Cousin, F. J., Mater, D. D., Foligne, B., & Jan, G. (2011). Dairy propionibacteria as human probiotics: A review of recent evidence. *Dairy Science & Technology*, *91*(1), 1–26.

Cowan, M. M. (1999). Plant products as antimicrobial agents. *Clinical Microbiology Reviews*, *12*, 564–582. PMID:10515903

Crespo, J. F., Pascual, C., Burks, A. W., Helm, R. M., & Martín Esteban, M. (1995a). Frequency of food allergy in a pediatric population from Spain. *Pediatric Allergy and Immunology*, *6*(1), 39–43. doi:10.1111/j.1399-3038.1995.tb00256.x PMID:7550764

Crespo, J. F., Pascual, C., Domínguez, C., Ojeda, I., Martín Muñoz, F., & Martín Esteban, M. (1995b). Allergic reactions associated with airborne fish particles in IgE-mediated fish hypersensitive patients. *Allergy*, *50*(3), 257–261. doi:10.1111/j.1398-9995.1995.tb01143.x PMID:7677242

Crevel, R. W. R., Ballmer-Weber, B. K., Holzhauser, T., Hourihane, J., Knulst, A. C., Mackie, A. R., & Taylor, S. L. et al. (2008). Thresholds for allergens and their value to different stakeholders. *Allergy*, *63*(5), 597–609. doi:10.1111/j.1398-9995.2008.01636.x PMID:18394134

Daley, C. A., Abbott, A., Doyle, P. S., Nader, G. A., & Larson, S. (2010). A review of fatty acid profiles and antioxidant content in grass-fed and grain-fed beef. *Nutrition Journal*, *9*(1), 10. doi:10.1186/1475-2891-9-10 PMID:20219103

Dalle-Donne, I., Rossi, R., Colombo, R., Giustarini, D., & Milzani, A. (2006). Biomarkers of oxidative damage in human disease. *Clinical Chemistry*, *52*(4), 601–623. doi:10.1373/clinchem.2005.061408 PMID:16484333

Damon, M., Flandre, O., Michel, F., Perdrix, L., Labrid, C., & Crastes de Paulet, A. (1987). Effect of chronic treatment with a purified flavonoid fraction on inflammatory granuloma in the rat. Study of prostaglandin E2 and F2 alpha and thromboxane B2 release and histological changes. *Arzneimittel-Forschung*, *37*(10), 1149–1153. PMID:3481266

Daniel, D. G. (2006). *Dietary Fiber*. Washington, DC: ILSI Press.

D'Archivio, M., Filesi, C., Vari, R., Scazzocchio, B., & Masella, R. (2010). Bioavailability of the polyphenols: Status and controversies. *International Journal of Molecular Sciences*, *11*(4), 1321–1342. doi:10.3390/ijms11041321 PMID:20480022

Das, S., Taygi, A. K., & Kaur, H. (2000). Cancer modulation by glucosinolates: A review. *Current Science*, *79*(12), 1665–1671.

Das, T., & Das, A. K. (2014). Inventory of the traditional rice varieties in farming system of southern Assam: A case study. *Indian Journal of Traditional Knowledge.*, *13*(1), 157–163.

Davies, K. J. A. (1987). Protein damage and degradation by oxygen radicals. I. General aspects. *The Journal of Biological Chemistry*, *162*, 9895–9901. PMID:3036875

Dawson, R. M., & Kemp, P. (1969). The effect of defaunation on the phospholipids and on the hydrogenation of unsaturated fatty acids in the rumen. *The Biochemical Journal*, *115*(2), 351–352. doi:10.1042/bj1150351 PMID:5378385

de Assis, J. S., Lima, R. A., Marques-Lima, J. P., Azevedo-Rodrigues, L. K., & Santiago, S. L. (2015). Effect of epigallocatechin-3-gallate application for remaining carious dentin disinfection. *Journal of Conservative Dentistry*, *18*(1), 51–55. doi:10.4103/0972-0707.148896 PMID:25657528

De Carvalho, M. D. C., & De Mesquita, J. F. (2013). Structural Modeling and In Silico Analysis of Human Superoxide Dismutase 2. *PLoS ONE*, *8*(6), e65558. doi:10.1371/journal.pone.0065558 PMID:23785434

De Souza, E. L., Barros, J. C., Oliveira, C. E. V., & Conceição, M. L. (2010). Influence of *Origanum vulgare* L. essential oil on enterotoxin production, membrane permeabliltiy and surface characteristics of *Staphylococcus aureus*. *International Journal of Food Microbiology*, *137*(2-3), 308–311. doi:10.1016/j.ijfoodmicro.2009.11.025 PMID:20015563

De Wet, J. M. J., Prasada Rao, K. E., Brink, D. E., & Mengesha, M. H. (1984). Systematic and Evolution of *Eleusine coracana*. *American Journal of Botany*, *71*(4), 550. doi:10.2307/2443330

Dean, B. J. (1978). Genetic toxicology of benzene, toluene, xylenes and phenols. *Mutation Research: Reviews in Genetic Toxicology*, *47*(2), 75–97. doi:10.1016/0165-1110(78)90014-3 PMID:415231

Debeaufort, F., Quezada-Gallo, J., & Voilley, A. (1998). Edible films and coatings: Tomorrow's packaging: A review. *Critical Reviews in Food Science and Nutrition*, *38*(4), 299–313. doi:10.1080/10408699891274219 PMID:9626488

Deepa, G., Singh, V., & Naidu, K. A. (2008). Nutrient composition and physico-chemical properties of Indian medicinal rice – Njavara. *Food Chemistry*, *106*(1), 165–171. doi:10.1016/j.foodchem.2007.05.062

Del Nobile, M. A., Corbo, M. R., Speranza, B., Sinigaglia, M., Conte, A., & Caroprese, M. (2009). Combined effect of MAP and active compounds on fresh blue fish burgher. *International Journal of Food Microbiology*, *135*(3), 281–287. doi:10.1016/j.ijfoodmicro.2009.07.024 PMID:19755204

DeLange, R. L., & Glazer, A. N. (1989). Phycoerythrin fluorescence based assay for peroxy radicals: A screen for biologically relevant protective agents. *Analytical Biochemistry*, *177*(2), 300–306. doi:10.1016/0003-2697(89)90056-0 PMID:2567129

DeLeve, L., & Kaplowitz, N. (1991). Glutathione metabolism and its role in hepatotoxicity. *Pharmacology & Therapeutics*, *52*(3), 287–305. doi:10.1016/0163-7258(91)90029-L PMID:1820580

Dembinska-Kiec, A., Mykkanen, O., Kiec-Wilk, B., & Mykkanen, H. (2008). Antioxidant phytochemicals against type 2 diabetes. *British Journal of Nutrition, 99*, ES109-117.

Demmig-Adams, B., & Adams, W. W. (1992). Photoprotection and other responses of plants to high light stress. Ann. Rev. *Plant Physiology*, *43*, 599–626.

Derache, R. (1990). *Toxicología y seguridad de los alimentos*. Barcelona, Spain: Ed. Omega.

Deschamps, J. D., Kenyoh, V. A., & Holman, T. R. (2006). Baicalein is a potent in vitro inhibitor against both reticulocyte 15-human and platelet 12-human lipoxygenases. *Bioorganic & Medicinal Chemistry*, *14*(12), 4294–4301. doi:10.1016/j.bmc.2006.01.057 PMID:16500106

Desideri, G., Kwik-Uribe, C., Grassi, D., Necozione, S., Ghiadoni, L., Mastroiacovo, D., & Ferri, C. et al. (2012). Benefits in cognitive function, blood pressure, and insulin resistance through cocoa flavanol consumption in elderly subjects with mild cognitive impairment: The Cocoa, Cognition, and Aging (CoCoA) study. *Hypertension*, *60*(3), 794–801. doi:10.1161/HYPERTENSIONAHA.112.193060 PMID:22892813

deSouza, E. L., Lima, E. O., Freire, K. R. L., & Sousa, C. P. (2005). Inhibitory action of some essential oils and phytochemicals on the growth of moulds isolated from foods. *Brazilian Archives of Biology and Technology.*, *48*(2), 245–250. doi:10.1590/S1516-89132005000200011

Destaillats, F., Trottier, J. P., Galvez, J. G., & Angers, P. (2005). Analysis of α-linolenic acid biohydrogenation intermediates in milk fat with emphasis on conjugated linolenic acids. *Journal of Dairy Science*, *88*(9), 3231–3239. doi:10.3168/jds.S0022-0302(05)73006-X PMID:16107413

Devillard, E., McIntosh, F. M., Duncan, S. H., & Wallace, R. J. (2007). Metabolism of linoleic acid by human gut bacteria: Different routes for biosynthesis of conjugated linoleic acid. *Journal of Bacteriology*, *189*(6), 2566–2570. doi:10.1128/JB.01359-06 PMID:17209019

Devillard, E., McIntosh, F. M., Newbold, C. J., & Wallace, R. J. (2006). Rumen ciliate protozoa contain high concentrations of conjugated linoleic acids and vaccenic acid, yet do not hydrogenate linoleic acid or desaturate stearic acid. *The British Journal of Nutrition*, *96*(04), 697–704. PMID:17010229

Devi, P. B., Vijayabharathi, R., Sathyabama, S., Malleshi, N. G., & Priyadarisini, V. B. (2011). Health benefits of finger millet (*Eleusine coracana* L.) polyphenols and dietary fiber: A review. *J. Food Science and Technology (Campinas.)*. doi:10.1007/s13197-011-0584-9

Dewdney, J. M., Maes, L., Raynaud, J. P., Blanc, F., Scheid, J. P., Jackson, T., & Verschueren, C. et al. (1991). Risk Assessment of antibiotic residues of ß–lactams and macrolides in food products with regard to their immunoallergic potential. *Food and Chemical Toxicology*, *29*(7), 477–483. doi:10.1016/0278-6915(91)90095-O PMID:1894215

Dewick. (2007). Medicinal Natural Products – A biosynthetic Approach. Chippenham, UK: Jhon Wiley & Sons.

Deyoe, C. W., Davies, R. E., Krishnan, R., Khaund, R., & Couch, J. R. (1962). Studies on the taste performance of chick. *Poultry Science*, *47*(3), 781–784. doi:10.3382/ps.0410781

Dhiman, T. R., Satter, L. D., Pariza, M. W., Galli, M. P., Albright, K., & Tolosa, M. X. (2000). Conjugated linoleic acid (CLA) content of milk from cows offered diets rich in linoleic and linolenic acid. *Journal of Dairy Science*, *83*(5), 1016–1027. doi:10.3168/jds.S0022-0302(00)74966-6 PMID:10821577

Di Santo, A., Mezzetti, A., Napoleone, E., Di Tommaso, R., Donati, M. B., De Gaetano, G., & Lorenzet, R. (2003). Resveratrol and quercetin down-regulate tissue factor expression by human stimulated vascular cells. *Journal of Thrombosis and Haemostasis*, *1*(5), 1089–1095. doi:10.1046/j.1538-7836.2003.00217.x PMID:12871381

Diaaz-Maroto, M. C., & Hidalgo, I. J. D. (2005). Saa nchez-Palomo, E. & Peä rez-Coello, M.S. (2005).Volatile components and key odorants of fennel (*Foeniculum vulgare* Mill.) and thyme (*Thymus vulgaris* L.) Oil extracts obtained by simultaneous distillation–extraction and supercritical fluid extraction. *Journal of Agricultural and Food Chemistry*, *53*(13), 5385–5389. doi:10.1021/jf050340+ PMID:15969523

Dias-Souza, M. V., Andrade, S., Aguiar, A. P., & Monteiro, A. S. (2013). Evaluation of Antimicrobial and Anti-biofilm activities of Anacardium occidentale stem bark extract. *Journal of Natural Products*, *26*, 198–205.

Dias-Souza, M. V., Caldoncelli, J. L., & Monteiro, A. S. (2013). *Annacardium occidentale* Stem Bark Extract can Decrease the Efficacy of Antimicrobial Drugs. *Revista Ciências Médicas e Biológicas*, *12*, 161–165.

Dillard, C. J., & Bruce German, J. (2000). Phytochemicals: Nutraceuticals and human health. *Journal of the Science of Food and Agriculture*, *80*(12), 744–1756. doi:10.1002/1097-0010(20000915)80:12<1744::AID-JSFA725>3.0.CO;2-W

Dinkova-Kostova, A. T., & Kostov, R. V. (2012). Glucosinolates and isothiocyanates in health and disease. *Trends in Molecular Medicine*, *18*(6), 337–347. doi:10.1016/j.molmed.2012.04.003 PMID:22578879

Directive of the European Union 1169/2011. (2011). *Regulation (EU) No 1169/2011 of the European Parliament and of the Council of 25 October 2011 on the provision of food information to consumers.*

Directive of the European Union 2003/89. (2003). *Directive 2003/89/EC of the European Parliament and of the Council of 10 November 2003 amending Directive 2000/13/EC as regards indication of the ingredients present in foodstuffs.*

Djenane, D., Yangüela, J., Roncalés, P., & Aider, M. (2013). Use of essential oils as natural food preservatives: Effect on the growth of *Salmonella Enteritidis* in liquid whole eggs stored under abuse refrigerated conditions. *Journal of Food Research.*, *2*(3), 65–78. doi:10.5539/jfr.v2n3p65

Dobson, G. (2003). Gas chromatography-mass spectrometry of conjugated linoleic acids and metabolites. *Advances in Conjugated Linoleic Acid Research*, *2*, 13–36.

Dolan, L. C., Matulka, R. A., & Burdock, G. A. (2010). Naturally Occurring Food Toxins. *Toxins*, *2*(9), 2289–2332. doi:10.3390/toxins2092289 PMID:22069686

Domadia, P., Swarup, S., Bhunia, A., Sivaraman, J., & Dasgupta, D. (2013). Inhibition of bacterial cell division protein FtsZ by cinnamaldehyde. *Biochemical Pharmacology*, *74*(6), 831–840. doi:10.1016/j.bcp.2007.06.029 PMID:17662960

Domínguez, A.R., & Hernández-Arana, A., Mendoza- Hernández, G. & Rendón, J.L. (1997). Thermal denaturation of glutathione reductase from cyanobacterium *Spirulina maxima. Biochemistry and Molecular Biology International*, *42*, 631–639. PMID:9247721

Dorman, H., & Deans, S. G. (2000). Antimicrobial agents from plants: Antibacterial activity of plant volatile oils. *Journal of Applied Microbiology*, *88*(2), 308–316. doi:10.1046/j.1365-2672.2000.00969.x PMID:10736000

Dos Santos, R. M., Pimenta-Freire, G., Figueiredo, F. J. B., Dias-Souza, M.V. (2016). Interference of flavonoids and carotenoids on the antimicrobial activity of some drugs against clinical isolates of Pseudomonas aeruginosa. International Food Research Journal, 23, 1268-1273.

Dos Santos, R. M., Pimenta-Freire, G., & Dias-Souza, M. V. (2016). Interference of flavonoids and carotenoids on the antimicrobial activity of some drugs against clinical isolates of *Pseudomonas aeruginosa. International Food Research Journal.*

Doyle, M. E. (2007). *Microbial food spoilage — losses and control strategies: a brief review of the literature*. FRI Briefings. Retrieved from www.wisc.edu/fri/

Dubal, S.A., Tilkari, Y.P., Momin, S.A. & Indrakant, V.B. (2008). Biotechnological routes in flavour industries. *Advanced Biotechnology*. 20-31.

Dubey, V., Ghosh, A. R., & Mandal, B. K. (2012). Appraisal of conjugated linoleic acid production by probiotic potential of *Pediococcus* spp. GS4. *Applied Biochemistry and Biotechnology*, *168*(5), 1265–1276. doi:10.1007/s12010-012-9855-9 PMID:22971829

Dutta, M., Phogat, B. S., & Dhillon, B. S. (2007). Genetic improvement and utilization of major underutilized crops in India. In Breeding of Neglected and nderutilized Crops, Spices and Herbs (pp. 251-298). Science Publishers.

Duttaroy, A. K., & Jorgensen, A. (2004). Effects of kiwi fruit consumption on platelet aggregation and plasma lipids in healthy human volunteers. *Platelets*, *15*(5), 287–292. doi:10.1080/09537100410001710290 PMID:15370099

Du, W.-X., Olsen, C. W., Avena-Bustillo, R. J., McHugh, T. H., Levin, C. E., Mandrell, R., & Friedman, M. (2009). Antibacterial effects of allspice, garlic and oregano essential oil in tomato films determined by overlay and vapour phase methods. *Journal of Food Science*, *74*(7), M390–M397. doi:10.1111/j.1750-3841.2009.01289.x PMID:19895486

Dykes, L., & Rooney, L. W. (2006). Sorghum and millet phenols and antioxidants. *Journal of Cereal Science*, *44*(3), 236–251. doi:10.1016/j.jcs.2006.06.007

Eastridge, M. L. (2006). Major advances in applied dairy cattle nutrition. *Journal of Dairy Science*, *89*(4), 1311–1323. doi:10.3168/jds.S0022-0302(06)72199-3 PMID:16537963

Edris, A. (2007). Pharmaceutical and Therapeutic Potentials of Essential Oils and Their Individual Volatile Constituents. *Phytotherapy Research*, *21*(4), 308–323. doi:10.1002/ptr.2072 PMID:17199238

Efeyan, A., Zoncu, R., & Sabatini, D. M. (2012). Amino acids and mTORC1: From lysosomes to disease. *Trends in Molecular Medicine*, *18*(9), 524–533. doi:10.1016/j.molmed.2012.05.007 PMID:22749019

Ehling-Schulz, M., Bilger, W., & Scherer, S. (1997). UV-B induced synthesis of photoprotective pigments and extracellular polysaccharides in the terrestrial cyanobacterium *Nostoc commune*. *Journal of Bacteriology*, *179*, 1940–1945. PMID:9068639

Elmali, N., Esenkaya, I., Harma, A., Ertem, K., Turkoz, Y., & Mizrak, B. (2005). Effect of resveratrol in experimental osteoarthritis in rabbits. *Inflammation Research*, *54*(4), 158–162. doi:10.1007/s00011-004-1341-6 PMID:15883738

Elson, C. E., Underbakke, G. L., Hanson, P., Shrago, E., Wainberg, R. H., & Qureshi, A. A. (1989). Impact of lemongrass oil, an essential oil, on serum cholesterol. *Lipids*, *24*(8), 677–679. doi:10.1007/BF02535203 PMID:2586227

Emiroğlu, Z. K., Yemiş, G. P., Coşkun, B. K., & Andoğan, K. (2010). Antimicrobial activity of soy edible films incorporated with thyme and oregano essential oils on fresh ground beef patties. *Meat Science*, *86*(2), 283–288. doi:10.1016/j.meatsci.2010.04.016 PMID:20580990

EPA-Attachment. (1997). *I-Final Risk Assessment of* Aspergillus oryzae. EPA.

Erlund, I., Koli, R., Alfthan, G., Marniemi, J., Puukka, P., Mustonen, P., & Jula, A. et al. (2008). Favorable effects of berry consumption on platelet function, blood pressure, and HDL cholesterol. *The American Journal of Clinical Nutrition*, *87*(2), 323–331. PMID:18258621

Espitia, P. J. P., Avena-Bustillos, R. J., Du, W. X., Chiou, B. S., Williams, T. G., Wood, D., & Soares, N. F. F. et al. (2014). Physical and Antibacterial Properties of Açaí Edible Films Formulated with Thyme Essential Oil and Apple Skin Polyphenols. *Journal of Food Science*, *79*(5), M903–M910. doi:10.1111/1750-3841.12432 PMID:24749789

Ewan, P. W. (1996). Clinical study of peanut and nut allergy in 62 consecutive patients: New features and associations. *British Medical Journal, 312*(7038), 1074–1078. doi:10.1136/bmj.312.7038.1074 PMID:8616415

Fabre, R., & Truhaut, R. (1976). Toxicología. Ed. Paraninfo.

Falguera, V., Quintero, J. P., Jiménez, A., Muñoz, J. A., & Ibarz, A. (2011). Edible films and coatings: Structures, active functions and trends in their use. *Trends in Food Science & Technology, 22*(6), 292–303. doi:10.1016/j.tifs.2011.02.004

FAO. (1991). Food and Agriculture Organization.Amino Acid Scoring Pattern. In: Protein quality evaluation. FAO/WHO Food and Nutrition Paper, Italy.

FAO. (2001). *Post harvest operations.* Millet: Kajuna.

FAO. (2009). *FAOSTAT. Food and Agriculture Organisation of the United Nations.* Retrieved from http://faostat.fao.org/site/339/default.aspx

FAO-WHO. (1965). *Food and Agriculture Organization of the United Nations.* World Health Organization.

Fardet, A., Rock, E., & Remesy, C. (2008). Is the in vitro antioxidant potential of whole-grain cereals and cereal products well reflected in vivo*? International Journal of Food Science & Technology, 43*(7), 1245–1252.

Farhath, S., Vijaya, P. P., & Manivannan, V. (2013). Immunomodulatory activity of geranial, geranial acetate, gingerol, and eugenol essential oils: Evidence for humoral and cell-mediated responses. *Avicenna Journal of Phytomedicine., 3*(3), 1–5. PMID:25050278

Farr, S. B., & Kogoma, T. (1991). Oxidative stress responses in *Escherichia coli* and *Salmonella typhimurium. Microbiological Reviews, 55*, 561–585. PMID:1779927

Fauser, J. K., Matthews, G. M., Cummins, A. G., & Howarth, G. S. (2013). Induction of apoptosis by the medium-chain length fatty acid lauric acid in colon cancer cells due to induction of oxidative stress. *Chemotherapy, 59*(3), 214–224. doi:10.1159/000356067 PMID:24356281

Fernandez, M. (2012). *Prevalence of allergies around the world: the big eight (ten, thirteen?).* Symposium on sensitizing properties of proteins, Prague, Czech Republic.

Fernandez-Lopez, R., Machón, C., Longshaw, C. M., Martin, S., Molin, S., Zechner, E. L., & de la Cruz, F. et al. (2005). Unsaturated fatty acids are inhibitors of bacterial conjugation. *Microbiology, 151*(11), 3517–3526. doi:10.1099/mic.0.28216-0 PMID:16272375

Figueiredo, F. J. B., Dias-Souza, M. V., Nascimento, E., & Lima, L. R. P. (2015). Physicochemical Characterization and Flavonoid Contents of Artisanal Brazilian Green Propolis. *International Journal of Pharmacy and Pharmaceutical Sciences, 7*, 64–68.

Fiore, G., Poli, A., Cosmo, A. D., D'ischia, M., & Palumbo, A. (2004). Dopamine in the ink defence system of *Sepia officinalis*: Biosynthesis, vesicular compartmentation in mature ink gland cells, nitric oxide (NO)/cGMP-induced depletion and fate in secreted ink. *The Biochemical Journal, 378*(3), 785–791. doi:10.1042/bj20031864 PMID:14670074

Fisher, K., & Phillips, C. (2008). Potential antimicrobial uses of essential oils in food:is citrus the answer? *Trends in Food Science & Technology, 19*(3), 156–164. doi:10.1016/j.tifs.2007.11.006

Fitzgerald, D. J., Stratford, M., Gasson, M. J., & Narbad, A. (2005). Structure-function analysis o f the vanillin molecule and its antifungal properties. *Journal of Agricultural and Food Chemistry, 53*(5), 1769–1775. doi:10.1021/jf048575t PMID:15740072

Flint, A. J., Hu, F. B., Glynn, R. J., Jensen, M. K., Franz, M., Sampson, L., & Rimm, E. B. (2009). Whole grains and incident hypertension in man. *The American Journal of Clinical Nutrition, 90*(3), 493–498. doi:10.3945/ajcn.2009.27460 PMID:19571218

Flourie, B. (1992). The Influence of Dietary Fibre on Carbohydrate Digestion and Absorption. In T. F. Schweizer et al. (Eds.), *Dietary Fibre - A Component of Food* (pp. 40–54). Springer-Verlag London Limited. doi:10.1007/978-1-4471-1928-9_10

Ford, E. S., Giles, W. H., & Dietz, W. H. (2002). Prevalence of the metabolic syndrome among US adults: Findings from the third National Health and Nutrition Examination Survey. *Journal of the American Medical Association, 287*(3), 356–359. doi:10.1001/jama.287.3.356 PMID:11790215

Fotsis, T., Pepper, M. S., Montesano, R., Aktas, E., Breit, S., Schweigerer, L., & Adlercreutz, H. et al. (1998). 7Phytoestrogens and inhibition of angiogenesis. *Bailliere's Clinical Endocrinology and Metabolism, 12*(4), 649–666. doi:10.1016/S0950-351X(98)80009-8

Fox, M., Krueger, E., Putterman, L., & Schroeder, R. (2012). The Effect of Peppermint on Memory Performance. *Journal of Advanced Student Science., 01*, 1–7.

Foyer, C. H., & Halliwell, B. (1976). The presence of glutathione and glutathione reductase in chloroplasts: A proposed role in ascorbic acid metabolism. *Planta, 133*(1), 21–25. doi:10.1007/BF00386001 PMID:24425174

Foyer, C. H., & Noctor, G. (2003). Redox sensing and signaling associated with reactive oxygen in chloroplasts, peroxisomes and mitochondria. *Physiologia Plantarum, 119*(3), 355–364. doi:10.1034/j.1399-3054.2003.00223.x

Franck, P., Kanny, G., Dousset, B., Nabet, P., & Moneret-Vautrin, D. A. (2000). Lettuce allergy. *Allergy, 55*(2), 201–202. doi:10.1034/j.1398-9995.2000.00373.x PMID:10726743

Frankel, E. N. (1985). Chemistry of free radical and singlet oxidation of lipids. *Progress in Lipid Research, 23*(4), 197–221. doi:10.1016/0163-7827(84)90011-0 PMID:6100997

Fremont, L. (2014). Efeitos biológicos de resveratrol. *Ciências da Vida, 66*, 663–673.

Frewer, L., Scholderer, J., & Lambert, N. (2003). Consumer acceptance of functional foods: Issues for the future. *British Food Journal, 105*(10), 714–731. doi:10.1108/00070700310506263

Fryer, M. J. (1992). The antioxidant effects of thylakoid vitamin E (α-tocopherol). *Plant, Cell & Environment*, *15*(4), 381–392. doi:10.1111/j.1365-3040.1992.tb00988.x

Fu, Z., Wang, H., Hu, X., Sun, Z., & Han, C. (2013). The Pharmacological Properties of *Salvia* Essential Oils. *Journal of Applied Pharmaceutical Science*, *3*(07), 122–127.

Galhano, V., Peixoto, F., & Gomes-Laranjo, J. (2011). Exposure of the cyanobacterium *Nostoc muscorum* from Portuguese rice fields to Molinate: Effects on the antioxidant system and fatty acid profile. *Aquatic Toxicology (Amsterdam, Netherlands)*, *101*(2), 367–376. doi:10.1016/j.aquatox.2010.11.011 PMID:21216347

Galli, F. (2007). Interactions of polyphenolic compounds with drug disposition and metabolism. *Current Drug Metabolism*, *8*(8), 830–838. doi:10.2174/138920007782798180 PMID:18220564

Gammon, C. S., Kruger, R., Minihane, A. M., Conlon, C. A., von Hurst, P. R., & Stonehouse, W. (2013). Kiwifruit consumption favourably affects plasma lipids in a randomised controlled trial in hypercholesterolaemic men. *The British Journal of Nutrition*, *109*(12), 2208–2218. doi:10.1017/S0007114512004400 PMID:23151354

Gangidi, R. R., & Proctor, A. (2004). Photochemical production of conjugated linoleic acid from soybean oil. *Lipids*, *39*(6), 577–582. doi:10.1007/s11745-004-1266-7 PMID:15554158

Gangur, V., Kelly, C., & Navuluri, L. (2005). Sesame allergy: A growing food allergy of global proportions? *Annals of Allergy, Asthma & Immunology*, *95*(1), 4–11. doi:10.1016/S1081-1206(10)61181-7 PMID:16095135

Ganz, M. B., & Seftel, A. (2000). Glucose-induced changes in protein kinase C and nitric oxide are prevented by vitamin E. *American Journal of Physiology. Endocrinology and Metabolism*, *278*(1), E146–E152. PMID:10644549

Gao, Q., & Garcia-Pichel, F. (2011). Microbial ultraviolet sunscreens. *Nature Reviews. Microbiology*, *9*(11), 791–802. doi:10.1038/nrmicro2649 PMID:21963801

García Ara, M. C., Boyano, M. T., Díaz Pena, J. M., Martín Muñoz, F., Pascual, C., García, G., & Martín Esteban, M. (2003). Incidencia de alergia a proteínas de leche de vaca en el primer año de vida y su repercusión en el consumo de hidrolizados. *Anales de Pediatria (Barcelona, Spain)*, *58*(2), 100–105. doi:10.1016/S1695-4033(03)78012-6

Garcia-Robaina, J. C., Eraso, E., Martinez, J., Martinez, A., De la Torre Morin, F., Hernandez-Nieto, L., & Guisantes, J. et al. (1997). Sensitization to *Blomia kulagini* in a general population of a sub-tropical region of Spain (Canary Islands). *Allergy*, *52*(7), 727–731. doi:10.1111/j.1398-9995.1997.tb01229.x PMID:9265987

Gardini, F., Lanciotti, R., & Guerzoni, M. E. (2001). Effect of trans-2-hexenal on the growth of *Aspergillus flavus* in relation to its concentration, temperature and water activity. *Letters in Applied Microbiology*, *33*(1), 50–55. doi:10.1046/j.1472-765X.2001.00956.x PMID:11442815

Gardner, P. R., & Fridovich, I. (1991). Superoxide sensitivity of *Escherichia coli* 6-phosphogluconate dehydratose. *The Journal of Biological Chemistry*, *266*, 1478–1483. PMID:1846355

Garg, A., Garg, S., Zaneveld, L. J. D., & Singla, A. K. (2001). Chemistry and pharmacology of the citrus bioflavonoid hesperidin. *Phytotherapy Research*, *15*(8), 655–669. doi:10.1002/ptr.1074 PMID:11746857

Garg, P., Gopinathan, U., Choudhary, K., & Rao, G. N. (2000). Keratomycosis: Clinical and microbiologic experience with dematiaceous fungi. *Ophthalmology*, *107*(3), 574–580. doi:10.1016/S0161-6420(99)00079-2 PMID:10711898

Gaunt, L., Higgins, S., & Hughes, J. (2005). Decontamination of surface borne bacteria by ionized antimicrobial vapours. *Journal of Electrostatics*, *63*(6-10), 809–814. doi:10.1016/j.elstat.2005.03.076

Geerwani, P., & Eggum, B. O. (1989). Nutrient composition and protein quality of minor millets. *Plant Foods for Human Nutrition (Dordrecht, Netherlands)*, *39*(2), 201–208. doi:10.1007/BF01091900 PMID:2548175

Gélinas, P., McKinnon, C. M., Mena, M. C. & Méndez, E. (2008). *Gluten contamination of cereal*. Academic Press.

Giampieri, F., Forbes-Hernandez, T. Y., Gasparrini, M., Alvarez-Suarez, J. M., Afrin, S., Bompadre, S., & Battino, M. et al. (2015). Strawberry as a health promoter: An evidence based review. *Food & Function*, *6*(5), 1386–1398. doi:10.1039/C5FO00147A PMID:25803191

Gill, A. O., & Holley, R. A. (2006). Inhibition of membrane bound ATPases of *Escherichia coli* and *Listeria monocytogenes* by plant oil aromatics. *International Journal of Food Microbiology*, *111*(2), 170–174. doi:10.1016/j.ijfoodmicro.2006.04.046 PMID:16828188

Gladyshev, V. N. (2014). The free radical theory of aging is dead. Long live the damage theory. *Antioxidants & Redox Signalling*, *20*(4), 727–731. doi:10.1089/ars.2013.5228 PMID:24159899

Gonçalves, A. B., Russell, R., & Paterson, M. (2006). Survey and significance of filamentous fungi from tap water. *International Journal of Hygiene and Environmental Health*, *209*(3), 257–264. doi:10.1016/j.ijheh.2005.12.001 PMID:16459143

González de la Pena, M. A., Villalba, M., Garcia-Lopez, J. L., & Rodriguez, R. (1993). Cloning and expression of the major allergen from yellow mustard seeds Sen a1. *Biochemical and Biophysical Research Communications*, *190*(2), 648–653. doi:10.1006/bbrc.1993.1097 PMID:8093997

González, R., Varela, J., Carreira, J., & Polo, F. (1995). Soybean hydrophobic protein and soybean hull allergy. *Lancet*, *346*(8966), 48–49. doi:10.1016/S0140-6736(95)92676-3 PMID:7603155

Götz, T., Windhovel, U., Böger, P., & Sandmann, G. (1999). Protection of photosynthesis against UV-B radiation by carotenoids in transformants of the cyanobacterium *Synechococcus* PCC 7942. *Plant Physiology*, *120*(2), 599–604. doi:10.1104/pp.120.2.599 PMID:10364412

Gould, J. M., Jasberg, B. K., Dexter, L. B., Hsu, J. T., Lewis, S. M., Fahey, G. C. (1989). High fiber, non-caloric flour substitute for baked food properties of alkaline peroxide-treated lignocellulose. *Cereal Chemistry*, (66), 201-205.

Gould, S. W., Fielder, M. D., Kelly, A. F., & Naughton, D. P. (2009). Anti-microbial activities of pomegranate rind extracts: Enhancement by cupric sulphate against clinical isolates of *S. aureus*, MRSA and PVL positive CA-MSSA. *BMC Complementary and Alternative Medicine*, *9*(23). PMID:19635137

Green, B. J., Mitakakis, T. Z., & Tovey, E. R. (2002). Allergen detection from 11 fungal species before and after germination. *The Journal of Allergy and Clinical Immunology*, *111*(2), 285–289. doi:10.1067/mai.2003.57 PMID:12589346

Griinari, J. M., Corl, B. A., Lacy, S. H., Chouinard, P. Y., Nurmela, K. V. V., & Bauman, D. E. (2000). Conjugated linoleic acid is synthesized endogenously in lactating dairy cows by Δ9-desaturase. *The Journal of Nutrition*, *130*(9), 2285–2291. PMID:10958825

Grynbaum, M. D., Hentschel, P., Putzbach, K., Rehbein, J., Krucker, M., Nicholson, G., & Albert, K. (2005). Unambiguous detection of astaxanthin and astaxanthin fatty acid esters in krill (*Euphausia superba* Dana). *Journal of Separation Science*, *28*(14), 1685–1693. doi:10.1002/jssc.200500152 PMID:16224962

Gugler, K., Piscitelli, C., & Dennis, J. (2013). Hidden dangers in the kitchen: Common foods toxic to dogs and cats. *Compend Contin Educ Vet*, *35*(7), E2. PMID:23677840

Gulmez, M., Oral, N., Guven, A., Vatansever, L., & Baz, E. (2006). Antibacterial activity of oregano tea and a commercial oregano water against *Escherichia coli* O157/:H7, *Listeria monocytogenes* 4b, *Staphylococcus aureus* and *Yersinia enterocolitica* O3. *Internet Journal of Food Safety*, *8*, 7–13.

Gunstone, F. D., & Padley, F. B. (1997). *Lipid technology and applications*. New York, NY: Marcel Dekker Inc.

Guo, J., Huo, H., Zhao, B., Liu, H., Li, L., Ma, Y., & Jiang, T. et al. (2005). Cinnamaldehyde reduces IL-1β-induced cyclooxygenase-2 activity in rat cerebral microvascular endothelial cells. *European Journal of Pharmacology*, *537*(1-3), 174–180. doi:10.1016/j.ejphar.2006.03.002 PMID:16624280

Gu, X., Creasy, L., Kester, A., & Zeece, M. (1999). Capillary Electrophoretic Determination of Resveratrol in Wines. *Journal of Agricultural and Food Chemistry*, *47*(8), 3223–3227. doi:10.1021/jf981211e PMID:10552635

Gu, X., & Manautou, J. E. (2012). Molecular mechanisms underlying chemical liver injury. *Expert Reviews in Molecular Medicine*, *14*, e4. doi:10.1017/S1462399411002110 PMID:22306029

Hadimani, N. A., & Malleshi, N. G. (1993). Studies on milling, physico-chemical properties, nutrient composition and dietary fiber content of millets. *Journal of Food Science and Technology*, *30*, 17–20.

Hagerman, A. E., Riedl, K. M., Jones, G. A., Sovik, K. N., Ritchard, N. T., Hartzfeld, P. W., & Riechel, T. L. (2015). High Molecular Weight Plant Polyphenolics (Tannins) as Biological Antioxidants. *Journal of Agricultural and Food Chemistry*, *46*(5), 1887–1892. doi:10.1021/jf970975b

Halliwell, B., & Gutteridge, J. M. C. (1999). Free radicals in biology and medicine. In Free radicals in biology and medicine (3rd ed.). Clarendon Press.

Halliwell, B., & Gutteridge, J. M. C. (1989). *Free Radicals in Biology and Medicine*. Oxford, UK: Clarendon Press.

Hammersley, R., & Reid, M. (2009). Theorising transient mood after ingestion. *Neuroscience and Biobehavioral Reviews*, *33*(3), 213–222. doi:10.1016/j.neubiorev.2008.07.010 PMID:18775746

Hancock, J. T., Desikan, R., & Neill, S. J. (2001). Role of Reactive Oxygen Species in Cell Signaling Pathways. *Biochemical and Biomedical Aspects of Oxidative Modification*, *29*(2), 345–350. PMID:11356180

Hanhineva, K., Torronen, R., Bondia-Pons, I., Pekkinen, J., Kolehmainen, M., Mykkanen, H., & Poutanen, K. (2010). Impact of dietary polyphenols on carbohydrate metabolism. *International Journal of Molecular Sciences*, *11*(4), 1365–1402. doi:10.3390/ijms11041365 PMID:20480025

Hanieh, H., Narabara, K., Piao, M., Gerile, C., Abe, A., & Kondo, Y. (2010). Modulatory effects of two levels of dietary Alliums on immune response and certain immunological variables, following immunization, in White Leghorn chickens. *Animal Science Journal*, *81*(6), 673–680. doi:10.1111/j.1740-0929.2010.00798.x PMID:21108687

Hansen, M., Flatt, T., & Aguilaniu, H. (2013). Reproduction, fat metabolism, and life span: What is the connection? *Cell Metabolism*, *17*(1), 10–19. doi:10.1016/j.cmet.2012.12.003 PMID:23312280

Hark, L., & Deen, D. (2005). *Saúde e Nutrição. S.l.* DK Civilização.

Harman, D. (1956). Aging: A theory based on free radical and radiation chemistry. *Journal of Gerontology*, *11*(3), 298–300. doi:10.1093/geronj/11.3.298 PMID:13332224

Harpole, J. L., Tucci, M., & Benghuzzi, H. (2015). Pathophysiological Effects of Thymoquinone and Epigallocatechin-3-Gallate on SK-OV-3 Ovarian Cancer Like Cell Line. *Biomedical Sciences Instrumentation*, *51*, 31–39. PMID:25996696

Harrison, D. E., Strong, R., Sharp, Z. D., Nelson, J. F., Astle, C. M., Flurkey, K., & Miller, R. A. et al. (2009). Rapamycin fed late in life extends lifespan in genetically heterogeneous mice. *Nature*, *460*, 392–395. PMID:19587680

Hasler, C. M. (2002). Functional Foods: Benefits, Concerns and Challenges—A Position Paper from the American Council on Science and Health. *The Journal of Nutrition*, *132*(12), 3772–3781. PMID:12468622

Havsteen, B. (1983). Flavonoids, class of natural of high pharmacological potency. *Biochemical Pharmacology*, *32*(7), 1141–1148. doi:10.1016/0006-2952(83)90262-9 PMID:6342623

Health Benefits of Orange Essential Oil. (n.d.). Retrieved from: https://www.organicfacts.net/health-benefits/essential-oils/orange-essential-oil.html

Hegde, P. S., Chandrakasan, G., & Chandraa, T. S. (2002). Inhibition of collagen glycation and crosslinking in vitro by methanolic extracts of Finger millet (*Eleusine coracana)* and Kodo millet (*Paspalum scrobiculatum*). *The Journal of Nutritional Biochemistry*, *13*(9), 517–521. doi:10.1016/S0955-2863(02)00171-7 PMID:12231421

Hegde, P. S., & Chandra, T. S. (2005). ESR spectroscopic study reveals higher free radical quenching potential in kodo millet (*Paspalum scrobiculatum*) compared to other millets. *Food Chemistry*, *92*, 177–182. doi:10.1016/j.foodchem.2004.08.002

Helander, I. M., Alakomi, H. L., Latva-Kala, K., Mattila-Sandholm, T., Pol, I., Smid, E. J., & von Wright, A. et al. (1998). Characterization of the action of selected essential oil components on Gram-negative bacteria. *Journal of Agricultural and Food Chemistry*, *46*(9), 3590–3595. doi:10.1021/jf980154m

Heller, S. N., Rivers, J. M., & Hackler, L. R. (1977). Dietary fiber: The effect of particle size and pH on its measurement. *Journal of Food Science*, *42*(2), 436–439. doi:10.1111/j.1365-2621.1977.tb01517.x

Hennessy, A. A., Barrett, E., Ross, R. P., Fitzgerald, G. F., Devery, R., & Stanton, C. (2012). The production of conjugated α-linolenic, γ-linolenic and stearidonic acids by strains of *bifidobacteria* and *propionibacteria*. *Lipids*, *47*(3), 313–327. doi:10.1007/s11745-011-3636-z PMID:22160449

Henry, G. E., Momin, R. A., Nair, M. G., & Dewitt, D. L. (2002). Antioxidant and cyclooxygenase activities of fatty acids found in food. *Journal of Agricultural and Food Chemistry*, *50*(8), 2231–2234. doi:10.1021/jf0114381 PMID:11929276

Hess, J. L. (1993). Vitamin E, α-tocopherol. In R. G. Alscher & J. L. Hess (Eds.), *Antioxidants in Higher Plants* (pp. 111–134). Boca Raton, FL: CRC Press.

Hinneberg, I., Dorman, D. H. J., & Hiltunen, R. (2006). Antioxidant activities of extracts from selected culinary herbs and spices. *Food Chemistry*, *97*(1), 122–129. doi:10.1016/j.foodchem.2005.03.028

Hirata, T., Tanaka, M., Ooike, M., Tsunomura, T., & Sakaguchi, M. (2000). Antioxidant activities of phycocyanobilin prepared from Spirulina platensis. *Journal of Applied Phycology*, *12*(3/5), 435–439. doi:10.1023/A:1008175217194

Hitoshi, A. (2012). Beneficial Effects of Fragrances. In *Beverages on Human Health, Nutrition, Well-Being and Health*. Retrieved from http://www.intechopen.com/books/nutrition-well-being-and-health/beneficial-effects-of-fragrances-in-beverages-on-human-health

Horváth, G., Kemény, Á., Barthó, L., Molnár, P., Deli, J., Szente, L., & Helyes, Z. et al. (2015). Effects of some natural carotenoids on TRPA1- and TRPV1-induced neurogenic inflammatory processes *in vivo* in the mouse skin. *Journal of Molecular Neuroscience*, *56*(1), 113–121. doi:10.1007/s12031-014-0472-7 PMID:25645682

Hosseini, M. S., Nasari, M., Zarai, A., Lotfollahian, H., Riyazi, S. R., & Meimandipour, A. (2013). Effects of lemon essential oil on gastrointestinal tract, blood parameter and immune responses in broilers. *Annals of Biological Research*, *4*(10), 47–51. Retrieved from http://patents.justia.com/patent/20140010768

Houba, R., Doekes, G., & Heederik, D. (1998). Occupational respiratory allergy in bakery workers: A review of the literature. *American Journal of Industrial Medicine*, *34*(6), 529–546. doi:10.1002/(SICI)1097-0274(199812)34:6<529::AID-AJIM1>3.0.CO;2-I PMID:9816411

Hou, N. S., & Taubert, S. (2012). Function and regulation of lipid biology in caenorhabditis elegans aging. *Frontiers in Physics*, *3*, 143. PMID:22629250

Hristov, A. N., Kennington, L. R., McGuire, M. A., & Hunt, C. W. (2005). Effect of diets containing linoleic acid-or oleic acid-rich oils on ruminal fermentation and nutrient digestibility, and performance and fatty acid composition of adipose and muscle tissues of finishing cattle. *Journal of Animal Science*, *83*(6), 1312–1321. PMID:15890808

Hui, K. M., Wang, X. H., & Xue, H. (2000). Interaction of Flavones from the Roots of *Scutellaria baicalensis* with the Benzodiazepine Site. *Planta Medica*, *66*(1), 91–93. doi:10.1055/s-0029-1243121 PMID:10705749

Hulse, J. H., Liang, E. M., & Pearson, O. E. (1980in press). *Sorghum and the millets: Their composition and nutritive value*. London: Academic Press.

Hurst, W. J., Glinski, J. A., Miller, K. B., Apgar, J., Davey, M. H., & Stuart, D. A. (2008). Survey of the trans-Resveratrol and trans-Piceid Content of Cocoa-Containing and Chocolate Products. *Journal of Agricultural and Food Chemistry*, *56*(18), 8374–8378. doi:10.1021/jf801297w PMID:18759443

Hwang, D., & Lim, Y. H. (2015, May5). Resveratrol antibacterial activity against Escherichia coli is mediated by Z-ring formation inhibition via suppression of FtsZ expression. *Scientific Reports*, *5*, 10029. doi:10.1038/srep10029 PMID:25942564

Hyldgard, M., Mygind, T., & Meyer, R. L. (2012). Essential oils in food preservation: Mode of action, synergies, and interactions with food matrix components. *Frontiers in Microbiology*, *2*(12), 1–24.

ICAR. (2013). *Handbook of Agriculture*. New Delhi: Indian Council of Agricultural Research.

Ichihashi, M., Ueda, M., Budiyanto, A., Bito, T., Oka, M., Fukunaga, M., & Horikawa, T. et al. (2003). UV-induced skin damage. *Toxicology*, *189*(1-2), 21–39. doi:10.1016/S0300-483X(03)00150-1 PMID:12821280

ICRISAT & FAO. (1996). *The world sorghum and millets economies: Facts, trends and outlook, joint study report by ICRISAT and FAO*. ICRISAT.

Imlay, J. A., & Linn, S. (1986). DNA damage and oxygen radical toxicity. *Science*, *240*(4857), 1302–1309. doi:10.1126/science.3287616 PMID:3287616

Indian Standard Institution (ISI). (1985). Method for Estimation Of total Dietary Fibre in Foodstuffs. Author.

International Programme on Chemical Safety (IPCS). (1988). *Environmental health criteria 80 - pyrrolizidine alkaloids*. Geneva, Switzerland: World Health Organization.

Islam, S. N., Begum, P., Ahsan, T., Huque, S., & Ahsan, M. (2004). Immunosuppressive and cytotoxic properties of *Nigella sativa. Phytotherapy Research*, *18*(5), 395–398. doi:10.1002/ptr.1449 PMID:15174000

Izadi, Z., Nasirpour, A., Izadi, M., & Izadi, T. (2012). Reducing blood cholesterol by a healthy diet. *Int. Food Res. J*, *19*(1), 29–37.

Jain, V. P., Proctor, A., & Lall, R. (2008). Pilot-scale production of conjugated linoleic acid-rich soy oil by photoirradiation. *Journal of Food Science*, *73*(4), 183–192. doi:10.1111/j.1750-3841.2008.00718.x PMID:18460128

Jamroz, D., Wertelecki, T., Houszka, M., & Kamel, C. (2006). Influence of diet type on the inclusion of plant origin active substances on morphological and histochemical characteristics of the stomach and jejunum walls in chicken. *Journal of Animal Physiology and Animal Nutrition*, *90*(5-6), 255–268. doi:10.1111/j.1439-0396.2005.00603.x PMID:16684147

Jang, I. S., Ko, Y. H., Kang, S. Y., & Lee, C. Y. (2007). Effect of a commercial essential oil on growth performance, digestive enzyme activity and intestinal microflora population in broiler chickens. *Animal Feed Science and Technology*, *134*(3-4), 304–315. doi:10.1016/j.anifeedsci.2006.06.009

Jansen, J. J. N., Kardinaal, A. F. M., Huijbers, G., Viieg-Boerstra, B. J., Martens, B. P. M., & Ockhuizen, T. (1994). Prevalence of food allergy and intolerance in the adult Dutch population. *The Journal of Allergy and Clinical Immunology*, *93*(2), 446–456. doi:10.1016/0091-6749(94)90353-0 PMID:8120272

Jarvis, D. I., Padoch, C., & Cooper, H. D. (Eds.). (2007). *Managing Biodiversity in Agricultural ecosystems*. Bioversity International, Rome, Italy.

Jayaprakasam, B., Vareed, S. K., Olson, L. K., & Nair, M. G. (2005). Insulin secretion by bioactive anthocyanins and anthocyanidins present in fruits. *Journal of Agricultural and Food Chemistry*, *53*(1), 28–31. doi:10.1021/jf049018+ PMID:15631504

Jenkins, T. C., AbuGhazaleh, A. A., Freeman, S., & Thies, E. J. (2006). The production of 10-hydroxystearic and 10-ketostearic acids is an alternative route of oleic acid transformation by the ruminal microbiota in cattle. *The Journal of Nutrition*, *136*(4), 926–931. PMID:16549452

Jiang, F., Hellman, U., Sroga, G. E., Bergman, B., & Mannervik, B. (1995). Cloning, sequencing, and regulation of the glutathione reductase gene from the cyanobacterium *Anabaena* PCC 7120. *The Journal of Biological Chemistry*, *270*(39), 22882–22889. doi:10.1074/jbc.270.39.22882 PMID:7559423

Jiang, J., Björck, L., & Fonden, R. (1998). Production of conjugated linoleic acid by dairy starter cultures. *Journal of Applied Microbiology*, *85*(1), 95–102. doi:10.1046/j.1365-2672.1998.00481.x PMID:9721660

Jiang, J., Wolk, A., & Vessby, B. (1999). Relation between the intake of milk fat and the occurrence of conjugated linoleic acid in human adipose tissue. *The American Journal of Clinical Nutrition*, *70*(1), 21–27. PMID:10393134

Jingju, N. L. Z. C., Huiyuan, Y., & Ying, X. (2007). "Optimization of stress medium enhance hydroxyl radical inhibition by water-soluble protein from germinated millet." LWT – *Fd Sci. Technol*, *40*, 1630–1636.

Johnson, S. C., Rabinovitch, P. S., & Kaeberlein, M. (2013). mTOR is a key modulator of ageing and age-related disease. *Nature*, *493*(7432), 338–345. doi:10.1038/nature11861 PMID:23325216

Johnston, K., Sharp, P., Clifford, M., & Morgan, L. (2005). Dietary polyphenols decrease glucose uptake by human intestinal Caco-2 cells. *FEBS Letters*, *579*(7), 1653–1657. doi:10.1016/j.febslet.2004.12.099 PMID:15757656

Joint FAO/WHO Expert Committee on Food Additives. Meeting. (2009). *Safety evaluation of certain food additives*. Author.

Jung, E. H., Kim, S. R., Hwang, I. K., & Ha, T. Y. (2007). Hypoglycemic effects of a phenolic acid fraction of rice bran and ferulic acid in C57BL/KsJ-db/db mice. *Journal of Agricultural and Food Chemistry*, *55*(24), 9800–9804. doi:10.1021/jf0714463 PMID:17973443

Kadwe, S. K., Bhamre, M. A., Naukudkar, V. J., & Barhate, M. D. (2015). Effect of antioxidants on free radicals. *International Journal of Pharmaceutical Research & Development*, *6*(12), 57–60.

Kaefer, C. M., & Milner, J. A. (2008). The Role of Herbs and Spices in Cancer Prevention. *The Journal of Nutritional Biochemistry*, *19*(6), 347–361. doi:10.1016/j.jnutbio.2007.11.003 PMID:18499033

Kamal-Eldin, A., & Appelqvist, L. (1996). The chemistry and antioxidant properties of tocopherols and tocotrienols. *Lipids*, *31*(7), 671–701. doi:10.1007/BF02522884 PMID:8827691

Kamaljeet, D. N., Thakur, N., Tomar, S., Lalit, S., & Thakur, R. (2012). *Trachyspermum ammi* (Ajwain): A comprehensive Review. *International Research Journal of Pharmacy.*, *3*(5), 133–138.

Kamatou, G. P. P., & Viljoen, A. M. (2010). A review of the application and pharmacological properties of α-bisabolol and α-bisabolol-rich oils. *Journal of the American Oil Chemists' Society*, *87*(1), 1–7. doi:10.1007/s11746-009-1483-3

Kanny, G., Moneret-Vautrin, D. A., Flabbee, J., Beaudouin, E., Morisset, M., & Thevenin, F. (2001). Population study of food allergy in France. *The Journal of Allergy and Clinical Immunology*, *108*(1), 133–140. doi:10.1067/mai.2001.116427 PMID:11447395

Kan, Y., Ucan, U. S., Kartal, M., Altun, M. L., Aslan, S., Sayar, E., & Ceyhan, T. (2006). GC-MS analysis and antibacterial activity of cultivated *Satureja cuneifolia* Ten. essential oil. Turkish. *Journal of Chemistry*, *30*, 253–259.

Karlson-Stiber C., Perssons H. (2003). Cytotoxic fungi--an overview. *Toxicon.*, *42*(4), 339-49.

Karni, L., Moss, S. J., & Tel-Or, E. (1984). Glutathione reductase activity in heterocysts and vegetative cells of *Nostoc muscorum*. *Archives of Microbiology*, *140*(2-3), 215–217. doi:10.1007/BF00454930

Kaur, S., Modi, N. H., Panda, D., & Roy, N. (2010). Probing the binding site of curcumin in *Escherichia coli* and *Bacillus subtilis* FtsZ--a structural insight to unveil antibacterial activity of curcumin. *European Journal of Medicinal Chemistry*, *45*(9), 4209–4214. doi:10.1016/j.ejmech.2010.06.015 PMID:20615583

Kearney, J. (2010). Food consumption trends and drivers. *Philosophical Transitions of the Royal Society*, *365*(1554), 2793–2807. doi:10.1098/rstb.2010.0149 PMID:20713385

Kemp, P., & Lander, D. J. (1983). The hydrogenatrion of Gamma-linoleic acids by pure culture of two rumen bacteria. *The Biochemical Journal*, *216*(2), 519–522. doi:10.1042/bj2160519 PMID:6318740

Kemp, P., Lander, D. J., & Gunstone, F. D. (1984). The hydrogenation of some cis-and trans-octadecenoic acids to stearic acid by a rumen *Fusocillus* sp. *The British Journal of Nutrition*, *52*(01), 165–170. doi:10.1079/BJN19840083 PMID:6743636

Kemp, P., Lander, D. J., & Holman, R. T. (1984). The hydrogenation of the series of methylene-interrupted cis, cis-octadecadienoic acids by pure cultures of six rumen bacteria. *The British Journal of Nutrition*, *52*(01), 171–177. doi:10.1079/BJN19840084 PMID:6743637

Kennedy, D. O., Dodd, F. L., Robertson, B. C., Okello, E. J., Reay, J. L., Scholey, A. B., & Haskell, C. F. (2011). Monoterpenoid extract of sage (*Salvia lavandulaefolioa*) with cholinesterase injhibiting properties improves cognitive performance and mood in healthy adults. *Journal de Pharmacologie*, *25*(8), 1088–1100. PMID:20937617

Kepler, C. R., Hirons, K. P., McNeill, J. J., & Tove, S. B. (1966). Intermediates and products of the biohydrogenation of linoleic acid by *Butyrivibrio fibrisolvens*. *The Journal of Biological Chemistry*, *241*(6), 1350–1354. PMID:5936712

Kepler, C. R., & Tove, S. B. (1967). Biohydrogenation of unsaturated fatty acids III. Purification and properties of a linoleate Δ12-cis, Δ11-trans-isomerase from Butyrivibrio fibrisolvens. *The Journal of Biological Chemistry*, *242*(24), 5686–5692. PMID:5633396

Kesheri, M., Richa, & Sinha, R.P. (2011). Antioxidants as natural arsenal against multiple stresses in cyanobacteria. *International Journal Pharma and Bioscience*, *2*(2), B-168-B-187.

Kesheri, M., Kanchan, S., Chowdhury, S., & Sinha, R. P. (2015). Secondary and Tertiary Structure Prediction of Proteins: A Bioinformatic Approach. In Q. Zhu & A. T. Azar (Eds.), *Studies in Fuzziness and Soft Computing* (pp. 541–569). Springer Verlag. doi:10.1007/978-3-319-12883-2_19

Kesheri, M., Kanchan, S., Richa, , & Sinha, R. P. (2014). Isolation and in silico analysis of Fe-superoxide dismutase in the cyanobacterium Nostoc commune. *Gene*, *553*(2), 117–125. doi:10.1016/j.gene.2014.10.010 PMID:25303871

Khan, M. S. A., Zahin, M., Hasan, S., Husain, F. M., & Ahmad, I. (2009). Inhibition of quorum sensing regulated bacterial functions by plant essential oils with special reference to clove oil. *Letters in Applied Microbiology*, *49*(3), 354–360. doi:10.1111/j.1472-765X.2009.02666.x PMID:19627477

Khiaosa-Ard, R., Bryner, S. F., Scheeder, M. R. L., Wettstein, H. R., Leiber, F., Kreuzer, M., & Soliva, C. R. (2009). Evidence for the inhibition of the terminal step of ruminal α-linolenic acid biohydrogenation by condensed tannins. *Journal of Dairy Science*, *92*(1), 177–188. doi:10.3168/jds.2008-1117 PMID:19109277

Kima, C. (2015). *The Psychology of Overeating. Food and the Culture of Consumerism. Bloomsbury Academic*. New York: Bloomsbury Publishing.

Kim, E. Y., Ham, S. K., Shigenaga, M. K., & Han, O. (2008). Bioactive dietary polyphenolic compounds reduce nonheme iron transport across human intestinal cell monolayers. *The Journal of Nutrition*, *138*(9), 1647–1651. PMID:18716164

Kim, J., Maurice, R. M., & Wei, C. (1995). Antibacterial Activity of some essential oil components against five food borne pathogens. *Journal of Agricultural and Food Chemistry*, *43*(11), 2839–2845. doi:10.1021/jf00059a013

Kim, Y. J., Liu, R. H., Rychlik, J. L., & Russell, J. B. (2002). The enrichment of a ruminal bacterium (Megasphaera elsdenii YJ-4) that produces the trans-10, cis-12 isomer of conjugated linoleic acid. *Journal of Applied Microbiology*, *92*(5), 976–982. doi:10.1046/j.1365-2672.2002.01610.x PMID:11972704

Kirkwood, T. B., & Kowald, A. (2012). The free-radical theory of ageing—older, wiser and still alive. *BioEssays*, *34*(8), 692–700. doi:10.1002/bies.201200014 PMID:22641614

Kirsh, S., Fourdrilis, S., Dobson, R., Scippo, M.-L., Rogister, G. M., & De Pauw, E. (2009). Quantitative methods for food allergens, a review. *Analytical and Bioanalytical Chemistry*, *395*(1), 57–67. doi:10.1007/s00216-009-2869-7 PMID:19543718

Kishino, S., Ogawa, J., Omura, Y., Matsumura, K., & Shimizu, S. (2002). Conjugated linoleic acid production from linoleic acid by lactic acid bacteria. *Journal of the American Oil Chemists' Society*, *79*(2), 159–163. doi:10.1007/s11746-002-0451-4

Kishino, S., Ogawa, J., Yokozeki, K., & Shimizu, S. (2009). Microbial production of conjugated fatty acids. *Lipid Technology*, *21*(8-9), 177–181. doi:10.1002/lite.200900044

Kita, T., Ima, S., Sawada, H., Kumagai, H., & Seto, H. (2008). The Biosynthetic Pathway of Curcuminoid in Turmeric (Curcuma longa) as Revealed by 13C-Labeled Precursors. *Bioscience, Biotechnology, and Biochemistry*, *72*(7), 1789–1798. doi:10.1271/bbb.80075 PMID:18603793

Klaassen, C. D., Casarett, L. J., & Amdur, M. O. (1986). *Toxicology: the basic science of poisons*. Ed Macmillan.

Kordsardouei, H., Barzegar, M., & Sahari, M. A. (2013). Application of *Zataria multiflora* Boiss. and *Cinnamon zeylanicum* essential oils as two natural preservatives in cake. *Avicenna Journal of Phytomedicine.*, *3*(3), 238–247. PMID:25050280

Kotsonis, F. N., Tschanz, C., Butchko, H. H., & Stargel, W. W. (1996). The Clinical Evaluation of a Food Additive: Assessment of Aspartame. CRC Press.

Krewson, C. F., & Naghski, J. (2006). Some physical properties of rutin. *Journal of the American Pharmaceutical Association*, *41*(11), 582–587. doi:10.1002/jps.3030411106 PMID:12999623

Krishan, G., & Narang, A. (2014). Use of essential oils in poultry nutrition: A new approach. *Journal of Advanced Veterinary and AnimalResearch.*, *1*(4), 156–162.

Krishnan, R., Dharmaraj, U., & Malleshi, N. G. (2011). Quality characteristics of biscuits prepared from finger millet seed coat based composite flour. *Food Chemistry*, *129*(2), 499–506. doi:10.1016/j.foodchem.2011.04.107

Książek, K. (2010). Let's stop overlooking bacterial aging. *Biogerontology*, *11*(6), 717–723. doi:10.1007/s10522-010-9278-3 PMID:20440559

Kuhnt, K., Flotho, S., Benjamin, S., Boerchers, T., Schubert, R., Jahreis, G., & Spener, F. (2009). Gene expression after dietary intervention with trans fatty acids (trans-11/trans-12 18: 1) in humans. *European Journal of Lipid Science and Technology*, *111*(5), 442–450. doi:10.1002/ejlt.200800217

Kumar, K. K., & Parmeswaran, K. P. (1999). Characterization of storage protein from selected varieties of foxtail millet (*Setaria italica* L. Beauv). *Journal of the Science of Food and Agriculture*, *77*(4), 535–542. doi:10.1002/(SICI)1097-0010(199808)77:4<535::AID-JSFA77>3.0.CO;2-G

Kumar, S., & Pandey, A. K. (2013). Chemistry and Biological Activities of Flavonoids: An Overview. *TheScientificWorldJournal*, *29*, 162750. PMID:24470791

Kuzuyama, T., Noel, J. P., & Richard, S. B. (2005). Structural basis for the promiscuous biosynthetic prenylation of aromatic natural products. *Nature*, *435*(7044), 983–987. doi:10.1038/nature03668 PMID:15959519

Kwon, J. A., Yu, C. B., & Park, H. D. (2003). Bacteriocidal effects and inhibition of cell separation of cinnamicaldehyde on *Bacillus cereus*. *Letters in Applied Microbiology*, *37*(1), 61–65. doi:10.1046/j.1472-765X.2003.01350.x PMID:12803558

Laczkowski, M. S., & Laczkowski, I. M. (2013, October). *Microencapsulaçcão de curcumina com maltodextrin, avaliação daestabilidade e aplicação em alimentos*. Paper presented at VIII Meeting of Scientific Production and Technology, Paraná, Brasil.

Lagouge, M., Argmann, C., Gerhart-Hines, Z., Mezaine, H., Lerin, C., Daussin, F., & Auwerx, J. et al. (2006). Resveratrol Improves Mitochondrial Function and Protects against Metabolic Disease by Activating SIRT1 and PGC-1a. *Cell, 127*(6), 1109–1122. doi:10.1016/j.cell.2006.11.013 PMID:17112576

Lai, L. S., Chou, S. T., & Chao, W. W. (2001). Studies on the antioxidative activities of hsian-tsao (Mesona procumbens Hemsl) leaf gum. *Journal of Agricultural and Food Chemistry, 49*(2), 963–968. doi:10.1021/jf001146k PMID:11262057

Lakshmi, B. S., & Naidu, K. C. (2010). Antimicrobial efficacy of essential oil *Syzygium aromaticum* against common infectants of storage cereals and fruits. *Journal of Pharmacy Research, 3*(10), 2544.

Lakshmi, S. V., Padmaja, G., Kuppusamy, P., & Kutala, V. K. (2009). Oxidative stress in cardiovascular disease. *Indian Journal of Biochemistry & Biophysics, 46*(6), 421–440. PMID:20361706

Lapidot, T., Walker, M. D., & Kanner, J. (2002). Antioxidant and prooxidant effects of phenolics on pancreatic β-cells in vitro. *Journal of Agricultural and Food Chemistry, 50*(25), 7220–7225. doi:10.1021/jf020615a PMID:12452635

Larry Branen, A., Davidson, P. M., Salminen, S., & Thorngate, J. H. III, (Eds.). (2002). *Food Additives*. New York: Marcel Dekker, Inc.

Latha, M., Abdul Nizar, M., Abraham, Z., Joseph John, K., Asokan Nair, R., Mani, S., & Dutta, M. (2013). Rice landraces of Kerala State of India: A documentation. *International Journal of Biodiversity and Conservation., 5*(4), 250–263.

Ledl, F., & Schleicher, E. (2003). New Aspects of the Maillard Reaction in Foods and in the Human Body. *Angewandte Chemie International Edition in English, 29*(6), 565–594. doi:10.1002/anie.199005653

Lee, C., Raffaghello, L., Brandhorst, S., Safdie, F. M., Bianchi, G., Martin-Montalvo, A., & Longo, V. D. et al. (2012). Fasting cycles retard growth of tumors and sensitize a range of cancer cell types to chemotherapy. *Science Translational Medicine, 4*(124), 124–127. doi:10.1126/scitranslmed.3003293 PMID:22323820

Lee, K. W., Everts, H., & Beynen, A. C. (2004). Essential oils in broiler nutrition. *International Journal of Poultry Science, 3*(12), 738–752. doi:10.3923/ijps.2004.738.752

Lee, W. J., Shim, J., & Zhu, B. T. (2005). Mechanisms for the Inhibition of DNA Methyltransferases by Tea Catechins and Bioflavonoids. *Molecular Pharmacology, 68*(4), 1019–1030. doi:10.1124/mol.104.008367 PMID:16037419

Lejonklev, J., Storm, A. C., Larsen, M. K., Mortensen, G., & Weisbjerg, M. R. (2013). Differences in rate of ruminal hydrogenation of C18 fatty acids in clover and ryegrass. *Animal, 7*(10), 1607–1613. doi:10.1017/S1751731113001286 PMID:23842207

Lemay, M. J., Choquette, J., Delaquis, P. J., Gariépy, C., Rodrigue, N., & Saucier, L. (2002). Antimicrobial effect of natural preservatives in a cooked and acidified chicken meat model. *International Journal of Food Microbiology*, *78*(3), 217–226. doi:10.1016/S0168-1605(02)00014-4 PMID:12227640

Leung, P. S., Chow, W. K., Duffey, S., Kwan, H. S., Gershwin, M. E., & Chu, K. H. (1996). IgE reactivity against a crossreactive allergen in crustacea and mollusca: Evidence for tropomyosin as the common allergen. *The Journal of Allergy and Clinical Immunology*, *98*(5), 954–961. doi:10.1016/S0091-6749(96)80012-1 PMID:8939159

Levine, A. S., & Labuza, T. P. (1990). Food systems: The relationship between health and food science/technology. *Environmental Health Perspectives*, *86*, 233–238. doi:10.1289/ehp.9086233 PMID:2401259

Leyva, E., Navarro-Tovar, G., Loredo-Carrillo, S.E., & Santos Díaz, M.D.S. (2011). Biosíntesis y actividad biológica de fitoestrógenos y fitoesteroides. *Bol. Soc. Quím. Méx.*, *5*(2-3), 35-43.

Li, L., Liu, W. Y., Feng, F., Wu, C. Y., & Xie, N. (2013). Synthesis and *in vitro* cytotoxicity evaluation of baicalein amino acid derivatives. *Chinese Journal of Natural Medicine*, *11*(3), 284–288. doi:10.1016/S1875-5364(13)60030-8 PMID:23725843

Ling, Z., Wang, J., Bao, Y., Fuy, Y., Liu, B., & An, L. (2007). Selection of Enterobacter aerogenes mutant with High Productivity of Diacetyl and Analysis of Fermentation Kinetics. Biotechnology.

Lin, S. J., & Austriaco, N. (2014). Aging and cell death in the other yeasts, Schizosaccharomyces pombe and Candida albicans. *FEMS Yeast Research*, *14*(1), 119–135. doi:10.1111/1567-1364.12113 PMID:24205865

Lin, T. Y. (2000). Conjugated linoleic acid concentration as affected by lactic cultures and additives. *Food Chemistry*, *69*(1), 27–31. doi:10.1016/S0308-8146(99)00218-6

Lin, T. Y. (2006). Conjugated linoleic acid production by cells and enzyme extract of *Lactobacillus delbrueckii* ssp. *bulgaricus* with additions of different fatty acids. *Food Chemistry*, *94*(3), 437–441. doi:10.1016/j.foodchem.2004.11.032

Lin, T. Y., Hung, T. H., & Cheng, T. S. (2005). Conjugated linoleic acid production by immobilized cells of *Lactobacillus delbrueckii* ssp. *bulgaricus* and *Lactobacillus acidophilus*. *Food Chemistry*, *92*, 23–28. doi:10.1016/j.foodchem.2004.07.003

Lipinski, C. A., Lombardo, F., Dominy, B. W., & Feeney, P. J. (1997). Experimental and computational approaches to estimate solubility and permeability in drug discovery and development settings. *Advanced Drug Delivery Reviews*, *23*(1-3), 3–25. doi:10.1016/S0169-409X(96)00423-1 PMID:11259830

Lipson, S. M., Ozen, F. S., Louis, S., & Karthikeyan, L. (2015). Comparison of a-glucosyl hesperidin of citrus fruits and epigallocatechin gallate of green tea on the Loss of Rotavirus Infectivity in Cell Culture. *Frontiers in Microbiology*, *6*, e359. doi:10.3389/fmicb.2015.00359

Liu, A., Wang, W., Fang, H., Yang, Y., Jiang, X., Liu, S., & Dirsch, O. et al. (2015). Baicalein protects against polymicrobial sepsis-induced liver injury via inhibition of inflammation and apoptosis in mice. *European Journal of Pharmacology*, *748*, 45–53. doi:10.1016/j.ejphar.2014.12.014 PMID:25533331

Liu, D., Sheng, J., Qi, H., & Zhang, W. (2015). Anti-aging activities of polysaccharides from *Athyrium multidentatum* (Doll.) Ching. *Journal of Chemical and Pharmaceutical Research*, *7*(1), 386–389.

Liu, P., Shen, S. R., Ruan, H., Zhou, Q., Ma, L. L., & He, G. Q. (2011). Production of conjugated linoleic acids by *Lactobacillus plantarum* strains isolated from naturally fermented Chinese pickles. *Journal of Zhejiang University. Science. B.*, *12*(11), 923–930. doi:10.1631/jzus.B1100072 PMID:22042657

Lockie & Carpenter. (2011). *Agriculture, Biodiversity and Markets. Livelihoods and agroecology in comparative perspective*. London: Earthscan publishers.

Lonneborg, A., Lind, L. K., Kalla, S. R., Gustafsson, P., & Öquist, G. (1985). Acclimatation process in the light harvesting system of cyanobacterium *Anacystis nidulans* following a light shift from white light to red light. *Plant Physiology*, *78*(1), 110–114. doi:10.1104/pp.78.1.110 PMID:16664182

Lopez-Torrejon, G., Salcedo, G., Martin-Esteban, M., Diaz-Perales, A., Pascual, C. Y., & Sanchez-Monge, R. (2003). Lenc 1, a major allergen and vicilin from lentil seeds: Protein isolation and cDNA cloning. *The Journal of Allergy and Clinical Immunology*, *112*, 1208–1215. doi:10.1016/j.jaci.2003.08.035 PMID:14657885

Luckey, T. D., & Venugopal, B. (1977). Metal Toxicity in Mammals. *Human Ecology*, *7*(1), 99–101.

Luo, R., Wang, J., Zhao, L., Lu, N., You, Q., Guo, Q., & Li, Z. (2014). Synthesis and biological evaluation of baicalein derivatives as potent antitumor agents. *Bioorganic & Medicinal Chemistry Letters*, *24*(5), 1334–1338. doi:10.1016/j.bmcl.2014.01.053 PMID:24507925

Lupton, J. R. (2010). Codex definition of dietary fibre and issues requiring resolution. In Dietary fibre: new frontiers for food and health. Texas A&M University.

Lu, T., Sheng, H., Wu, J., Cheng, Y., Zhu, J., & Chen, Y. (2012). Cinnamon extract improves fasting blood glucose and glycosylated hemoglobin level in Chinese patients with type 2 diabetes. *Nutrition Research (New York, N.Y.)*, *32*(6), 408–412. doi:10.1016/j.nutres.2012.05.003 PMID:22749176

Lv, F., Liang, H., Yuan, Q., & Li, C. (2011). antimicrobial effects and mechanism of action of selected plant essential oil combinations against four food-related microorganisms. *Food Research International*, *44*(9), 3057–3064. doi:10.1016/j.foodres.2011.07.030

MacDonald, T. T., & Di Sabatino, A. (2009). The Immunologic Basis for Gastrointestinal Food Allergy. *Current Opinion in Gastroenterology*, *25*(6), 521–526. doi:10.1097/MOG.0b013e3283306236 PMID:19654542

Maen, A., & Cock, I. E. (2015). Inhibitory activity of Australian culinary herb extracts against the bacterial triggers of selected autoimmune diseases. *Pharmacognosy Communications.*, *5*(2), 130–139. doi:10.5530/pc.2015.2.4

Maftoonazad, N., & Badii, F. (2009). Use of Edible Films and Coatings to Extend the Shelf Life of Food Products. *Recent Patents on Food. Nutrition & Agriculture.*, *1*(2), 162–170.

Mahmood, T., Bibi, Y., Ishaq, H., Mahmood, I., Wahab, A., & Sherwani, S. (2013). Complexation and Antimicrobial activities of ß sitosterol with trace metals.(Cu (II), Co (II), and Fe (III)). *European Academic Research*, *1*(5), 677–685.

Mahmood, T., Bibi, Y., Zafar, R., Wahab, A., Mahmood, I., Arshad, N., & Sherwani, S. K. (2015). Report: Complexation of ß-sitosterol with tris (dibenzylideneacetone) dipalladium and its antimicrobial activity. *Pakistan Journal of Pharmaceutical Sciences*, *28*(2), 631–634. PMID:25730794

Maia, M. R., Chaudhary, L. C., Figueres, L., & Wallace, R. J. (2007). Metabolism of polyunsaturated fatty acids and their toxicity to the microflora of the rumen. *Antonie van Leeuwenhoek*, *91*(4), 303–314. doi:10.1007/s10482-006-9118-2 PMID:17072533

Makkar, H. P. S. (2003). Effects and fate of tannins in ruminant animals, adaptation to tannins, and strategies to overcome detrimental effects of feeding tannin-rich feeds. *Small Ruminant Research*, *49*(3), 241–256. doi:10.1016/S0921-4488(03)00142-1

Mal, B., & Padulosi, S. (2013). Best Practices, Methods and Tools in Minor Millets Value Chains and Uptaking Processes. Bioversity International.

Mal, B. (2007). Neglected and underutilized crop genetic resources for sustainable agriculture. *J. Plant Genet. Resour*, *20*(1), 1–14.

Mal, B., Padulosi, S., & Ravi, S. B. (2010). Minor millets in South Asia: learnings from IFAD-NUS Project in India and Nepal. *Swaminathan Research Foundation*, *32*(2), 1–185.

Malik, T., & Singh, P. (2010). Antimicrobial effects of essential oils against uropathogens with varying sensitivity to antibiotics. *Asian Journal of Biological Sciences.*, *3*(2), 92–98. doi:10.3923/ajbs.2010.92.98

Malik, T., & Singh, P. (2015a). Antimicrobial activity of aromachemicals against uropathogens. 2015. *Journal of Environmental and Applied Research.*, *03*(02), 86–91.

Malik, T., Singh, P. S., Pant, S., Chauhan, N., & Lohani, H. (2011). Potentiation of antimicrobial activity of ciprofloxacin by *Pelargonium graveolens* essential oil against selected uropathogens. *Phytotherapy Research*, *25*(8), 1225–1228. doi:10.1002/ptr.3479 PMID:21618302

Malik, T., Singh, P., Pant, S., Chauhan, N., Kumar, V., & Swarup, S. (2015b). Inhibition of swarming behavior in P. mirabilis by Pelargonium graveolens L her Essential oil. *Bangladesh Journal of Medical Sciences*, *14*(4), 384. doi:10.3329/bjms.v14i4.20004

Malik, T., Singh, P., Pant, S., Kumar, N., Chauhan, N., & Lohani, H. (2008). Antimicrobial activity of essential oils on pathogens associated with food borne infections. *Journal of Medicinal and Aromatic Plant Sciences*, *30*, 314–319.

Malleshi, N. G. (2014). *Post-harvest processing of millets for value addition.* Retrieved from http://isites.harvard.edu /fs/docs/icb.topic868074

Malleshi, N. G., & Hadimani, N. A. (1993). Nutritional and technological characteristics of small millets and preparation of value added products from them. In Advances in Small Millets (pp. 271-287). Oxford IBH Publishing Co. Pvt. Ltd.

Manach, C., Mazur, A., & Scalbert, A. (2005). Polyphenols and prevention of cardiovascular diseases. *Current Opinion in Lipidology*, *16*(1), 77–84. doi:10.1097/00041433-200502000-00013 PMID:15650567

Manach, C., Scalbert, A., Morand, C., Remesy, C., & Jimenez, L. (2004). Polyphenols: Food sources and bioavailability. *The American Journal of Clinical Nutrition*, *79*(5), 727–747. PMID:15113710

Mandallaz, M. M., de Weck, A. L., & Dahinden, C. A. (1988). Bird-egg syndrome. Cross-reactivity between bird antigens and egg-yolk livetins in IgE-mediated hypersensitivity. *International Archives of Allergy and Immunology*, *87*(2), 143–150. doi:10.1159/000234664 PMID:3192303

Man, G., Mauro, T. M., Zhai, Y., Kim, P. L., Cheung, C., Hupe, M., & Man, M. Q. et al. (2015). Topical hesperidin enhances epidermal function in an aged murine model. *The Journal of Investigative Dermatology*, *135*(4), 1184–1187. doi:10.1038/jid.2014.486 PMID:25402552

Mangena, T., & Muyima, N. Y. O. (1999). Comparative evaluation of the antimicrobial activities of essential oils of *Artemisia afra, Pteronia incana* and *Rosamarinus officinalis* on selected bacteria and yeast strains. *Letters in Applied Microbiology*, *28*(4), 291–296. doi:10.1046/j.1365-2672.1999.00525.x PMID:10212442

Manolova, Y., Deneva, V., Antonov, L., Drakalsa, E., Momekova, D., & Lambov, N. (2014). The effect of the water on the curcumin tautomerism: A quantitative approach. *Spectrochimica Acta. Part A: Molecular and Biomolecular Spectroscopy*, *132*, 815–820. doi:10.1016/j.saa.2014.05.096 PMID:24973669

Manzan, A. C. C. M., Toniolo, F. S., Bredow, E., & Povh, N. P. (2003, November). Extration of essential oil and pigments from *Curcuma longa L.* by steam distillation and extraction with volatile solvents. *Journal of Agricultural and Food Chemistry*, *51*(23), 6802–6807. doi:10.1021/jf030161x PMID:14582978

Manzanilla, E. G., Perez, J. F., Martin, M., Kamel, C., Baucells, F., & Gasa, J. (2004). Effect of plant extracts and formic acid on the intestinal equilibrium of early-weaned pigs. *Journal of Animal Science*, *82*, 3210–3218. PMID:15542467

Marambuad, P., Zhao, H., & Davies, P. (2005). Resveratrol Promotes Clearance of Alzheimer's Disease Amyloid-β Peptides. *The Journal of Biological Chemistry*, *280*(45), 37377–37382. doi:10.1074/jbc.M508246200 PMID:16162502

Marçal, P. H. F., Dias-Souza, M. V., Villela, E. G., Luz, L. M., Pereira, M. K., Vale, C. H. B., & Rabelo, F. L. A. (2014). Qualidade Físico-Química, Microbiológica e Microscópica de Polpas de Frutas Congeladas Comercializadas no Município de Governador Valadares, MG. Nova. *Revista Científica, 2*, 1–10.

Marchal, J., Pifferi, F., & Aujard, F. (2013). Resveratrol in mammals: Effects on aging biomarkers, age-related diseases, and life span. *Annals of the New York Academy of Sciences, 1290*(1), 67–73. doi:10.1111/nyas.12214 PMID:23855467

Maritim, A. C., Sanders, R. A., & Watkins, J. B. III. (2003). Diabetes, oxidative stress, and antioxidants: A review. *Journal of Biochemical and Molecular Toxicology, 17*(1), 24–38. doi:10.1002/jbt.10058 PMID:12616644

Markham, K. R. (1982). *Techniques of flavonoid identification*. New York, NY: Academic Press.

Martín Esteban, M. (2006). Alergia a fórmulas de sustitución en alérgicos a proteínas de leche de vaca. *Pediátrika, 1*, 12–15.

Martinez-Oyanedel, J., Contreras-Martel, C., Bruna, C., & Bunster, M. (2004). Stuctural-functional analysis of the oligomeric protein R-phycoerythrin. *Biological Research, 37*(4), 733–745. doi:10.4067/S0716-97602004000500003 PMID:15586822

Martin, G. N. (1996). Olfactory remediation: Current evidence and possible applications. *Social Science & Medicine, 43*(1), 63–70. doi:10.1016/0277-9536(95)00334-7 PMID:8816011

Martin, S. A., & Jenkins, T. C. (2002). Factors affecting conjugated linoleic acid and trans-C18: 1 fatty acid production by mixed ruminal bacteria. *Journal of Animal Science, 80*, 3347–3352. PMID:12542176

Matan, N. (2012). Antimicrobial activity of edible film incorporated with essential oils to preserve dried fish (*Decapterus maruadsi*). *International Food Research Journal., 19*(4), 1733–1738.

Mathanghi, S.K. & Sudha, K. (2012). Functional and phytochemical properties of Finger Millet _*Eleusine coracana* L.) for health. *International Journal of Pharmaceutical, Chemical and Biological Sciences, 2*(4), 431-438.

Mathis, P., & Kleo, J. (1973). The triplet state of ß-carotene and of analog polyenes of different length. *Photochemistry and Photobiology, 18*(4), 343–346. doi:10.1111/j.1751-1097.1973.tb06431.x

Matsui, T., Ebuchi, S., Kobayashi, M., Fukui, K., Sugita, K., Terahara, N., & Matsumoto, K. (2002). Anti-hyperglycemic effect of diacylated anthocyanin derived from Ipomoea batatas cultivar Ayamurasaki can be achieved through the alpha-glucosidase inhibitory action. *Journal of Agricultural and Food Chemistry, 50*(25), 7244–7248. doi:10.1021/jf025913m PMID:12452639

Mbithi-Mwikya, S., Ooghe, W., Van Cam, J., Nagundi, D., & Huyghebaert, A. (2000). Amino acid profile after sprouting, autoclaving and lactic acid fermentation of finger millet (*Elusine coracana*) and kidney beans (*Phaseolus vulgaris* L.). *Journal of Agricultural and Food Chemistry, 48*(8), 3081–3085. doi:10.1021/jf0002140 PMID:10956072

McCarty, M. F., Barroso-Aranda, J., & Contreras, F. (2009). The low-methionine content of vegan diets may make methionine restriction feasible as a life extension strategy. *Medical Hypotheses*, *72*(2), 125–128. doi:10.1016/j.mehy.2008.07.044 PMID:18789600

McDonough, C. M., Rooney, L. W., & Serna-Saldivar, S. O. (2000). The Millets. In Handbook of Cereal Science and Technology (2nd ed.; pp. 177–210). CRC Press.

McKain, N., Shingfield, K. J., & Wallace, R. J. (2010). Metabolism of conjugated linoleic acids and 18: 1 fatty acids by ruminal bacteria: products and mechanisms. *Microbiology*, *156*(2), 579–588. doi:10.1099/mic.0.036442-0 PMID:19926650

Meamarbashi, A. (2014). Instant effects of peppermint essential oil on the physiological parameters and exercise performance. *Avicenna Journal of Phytomedicine.*, *4*(1), 72–78. PMID:25050303

Mechanick, J. I., Brett, E. M., Chausmer, A. B., Dickey, R. A., & Wallach, S. (2003). American Association of Clinical Endocrinologists medical guidelines for the clinical use of dietary supplements and nutraceuticals. *Endocrine Practice*, *9*(5), 417–470. doi:10.4158/EP.9.5.417 PMID:14583426

Meister, A. (1989). Metabolism and function of glutathione. In D. Dolphin, R. Poulson, & R. Auramovic (Eds.), *Glutathione: chemical, biochemical, and medical aspects* (pp. 367–474). New York: John Wiley and Sons.

Mejlholm, O., & Dalgaard, P. (2002). Antimicrobial effect of essential oils on the seafood spoilage micro-organism *Photobacterium phosphoreum* in liquid media and fish products. *Letters in Applied Microbiology*, *34*(1), 27–31. doi:10.1046/j.1472-765x.2002.01033.x PMID:11849488

Melby, E. C., & Altman, N. H. (Eds.). (1976). *Handbook of Laboratory Animal Science* (Vol. 2). Cleveland, Ohio, USA: IIICRC Press.

Melis, A., Mamdori, A., Glick, R. E., Ghirardi, M. L., McCauly, S. W., & Neal, P. J. (1985). The mechanism of photosynthetic membrane adaptation to environmental stress conditions; a hypothesis on the role of electron transport capacity and of ATP/NADPH pool in regulation of thylakoid membrane organization and function. *Physiologie Vegetale*, *23*, 757–765.

Menrad, K. (2003). Market and marketing of functional food in Europe. *Journal of Food Engineering*, *56*(2-3), 181–188. doi:10.1016/S0260-8774(02)00247-9

Metcalfe, D. (1984). Food hypersensitivity. *The Journal of Allergy and Clinical Immunology*, *73*(6), 749–762. doi:10.1016/0091-6749(84)90442-1 PMID:6609945

Midio, A. F. M. (2000). *Toxicologia de Alimentos*. São Paulo, SP: Livraria Varella.

Miele, M., Dondero, R., Ciarallo, G., & Mazzei, M. (2001). Methyleugenol in Ocimum basilicum L. Cv. Genovese Gigante. *Journal of Agricultural and Food Chemistry*, *49*(1), 517–521. doi:10.1021/jf000865w PMID:11170620

Miguel, M. G. (2010). Antioxidant and Anti-Inflammatory Activities of Essential Oils. *Molecules (Basel, Switzerland)*, *15*(12), 9252–9287. doi:10.3390/molecules15129252 PMID:21160452

Miksusanti, H., & Masril, K. I. (2013). Antibacterial and Antioxidant of Uwi (Dioscorea Alata L) Starch Edible Film Incorporated with Ginger Essential Oil. *International Journal of Bioscience. Biochemistry and Bioinformatics.*, *3*(4), 354–356.

Mirisola, M. G., Taormina, G., Fabrizio, P., Wei, M., Hu, J., & Longo, V. D. (2014). Serine- and threonine/valine-dependent activation of PDK and Tor orthologs converge on Sch9 to promote aging. *PLOS Genetics*, *10*(2), e1004113. doi:10.1371/journal.pgen.1004113 PMID:24516402

Miri, V. H., Tyagi, A. K., Ebrahimi, S. H., & Mohini, M. (2013). Effect of cumin (Cuminum cyminum) seed extract on milk fatty acid profile and methane emission in lactating goat. *Small Ruminant Research*, *113*(1), 66–72. doi:10.1016/j.smallrumres.2013.01.015

Mir, P. S., Bittman, S., Hunt, D., Entz, T., & Yip, B. (2006). Lipid content and fatty acid composition of grasses sampled on different dates through the early part of the growing season. *Canadian Journal of Animal Science*, *86*(2), 279–290. doi:10.4141/A05-050

Mishra, N., & Rizvi, S. I. (2012). Quercetin modulates Na(+)/K(+) ATPase and sodium hydrogen exchanger in type 2 diabetic erythrocytes. *Cellular and Molecular Biology (Noisy-Le-Grand)*, *58*(1), 148–152. PMID:23273205

Mishra, P., Kale, R. K., & Kar, A. (2008). Chemoprevention of mammary tumorigenesis and chemomodulation of the antioxidative enzymes and peroxidative damage in prepubertal Sprague Dawley rats by Biochanin A. *Molecular and Cellular Biochemistry*, *312*(1-2), 1–9. doi:10.1007/s11010-008-9714-8 PMID:18273562

Mithen, R. F., Dekker, M., Verkerk, R., Rabot, S., & Jhonson, T. (2000). The nutritional significance, biosynthesis and bioavailability of glucosinolates in human foods. *Journal of the Science of Food and Agriculture*, *80*(7), 967–984. doi:10.1002/(SICI)1097-0010(20000515)80:7<967::AID-JSFA597>3.0.CO;2-V

Mitropoulou, G., Fitsiou, E., Stavropoulou, E., Papavassilopoulou, E., Vamvakias, M., Pappa, A., Oreopoulou, A., & Kourkoutas, Y. (2015).Composition, antimicrobial, antioxidant, and antiproliferative activity of *Origanum dictamnus*(dittany) essential oil. *Microbial Ecology in Health & Disease, 26*, 26543-26552.

Moeller, R. E., Gilroy, S., Williamson, C. E., Grad, G., & Sommaruga, R. (2005). Dietary acquisition of photoprotective compounds (mycosporine-like amino acids, carotenoids) and acclimation to ultraviolet radiation in a freshwater copepod. *Limnology and Oceanography*, *50*(2), 427–439. doi:10.4319/lo.2005.50.2.0427

Mohamed, S. H. S., Zaky, W. M., Kassem, J. M., Abbas, H. M., Salem, M. M. E., & Said-Al Ahl, H. A. H. (2013). Impact of antimicrobial properties of some essential oils on cheese yoghurt quality. *World Applied Sciences Journal*, *27*(4), 497–507.

Mohiuddin, M., & Chowdhry, M.J., Alam, & Hossain, M.K. (2012). Chemical composition of essential oils of four flavouring plants used by the tribal people of Bandarban hill district in Bangladesh. *International Journal of Medicinal & Aromatic Plants.*, *2*(1), 106–113.

Moneret-Vautrin, D. A., & Kanny, G. (2004). Update on threshold doses of food allergens: Implications for patients and the food industry. *Current Opinion in Allergy and Clinical Immunology*, *4*(3), 215–219. doi:10.1097/00130832-200406000-00014 PMID:15126945

Monforte, M. T., Trovato, A., Kirjavainen, S., Forestieri, A. M., Galati, E. M., & Lo Curto, R. B. (1995). Biological effects of hesperidin, a citrus flavonoid. (note II): Hypolipidemic activity on experimental hypercholesterolemia in rat. *Pharmacology*, *50*(9), 595–599. PMID:7495469

Monnier, V. M. (1990). Nonenzymatic glycosylation, the Maillard reaction and the aging process. *Journal of Gerontology*, *45*(4), 105–111. doi:10.1093/geronj/45.4.B105 PMID:2195101

Monsalve, R. I., González de la Peña, M. A., Menéndez-Arias, L., López-Otín, C., Villalba, M., & Rodríguez, R. (1993). Characterization of a new oriental-mustard (Brassica juncea) allergen, Bra j IE: Detection of an allergenic epitope. *The Biochemical Journal*, *293*(3), 625–632. doi:10.1042/bj2930625 PMID:7688955

Monteiro, P. V., Sudharshana, L., & Ramchandra, G. (1987). Japanese barnyard millet (*Echinochloa frumentacea*): Protein content, quality and SDSPAGE of protein fractions. *Journal of the Science of Food and Agriculture*, *43*(1), 17–25. doi:10.1002/jsfa.2740430104

Monu, E., Blank, G., Holley, R., & Zawistowski, J. (2008). Phytosterol effects on milk and yogurt microflora. *Journal of Food Science*, *73*(3), 121–126. doi:10.1111/j.1750-3841.2008.00668.x PMID:18387114

Morisset, M., Moneret-Vautrin, D. A., Kanny, G., Guénard, L., Beaudouin, E., Flabbée, J., & Hatahet, R. (2003). Thresholds of clinical reactivity to milk, egg, peanut and sesame in immunoglobulin E-dependent allergies: Evaluation by double-blind or single blind placebo-controlled oral challenges. *Clinical and Experimental Allergy*, *33*(8), 1046–1051. doi:10.1046/j.1365-2222.2003.01734.x PMID:12911777

Morvan, B., & Joblin, K. N. (1999). Hydration of Oleic Acid by Enterococcus gallinarum, Pediococcus acidilactici andLactobacillus sp. Isolated from the Rumen. *Anaerobe*, *5*(6), 605–611. doi:10.1006/anae.1999.0306

Mosley, E. E., McGuire, M. K., Williams, J. E., & McGuire, M. A. (2006). Cis-9, trans-11 conjugated linoleic acid is synthesized from vaccenic acid in lactating women. *The Journal of Nutrition*, *136*(9), 2297–2301. PMID:16920844

Mosley, E. E., Powell, G. L., Riley, M. B., & Jenkins, T. C. (2002). Microbial biohydrogenation of oleic acid to trans isomers in vitro. *Journal of Lipid Research*, *43*(2), 290–296. PMID:11861671

Moss, M., Cook, J., Wesnes, K., & Duckett, P. (2003). Aromas of rosemary and lavender essential oils differentially affect cognition and mood in healthy adults. *The International Journal of Neuroscience*, *113*(1), 15–38. doi:10.1080/00207450390161903 PMID:12690999

Moss, M., Hewitt, S., Moss, L., & Wesnes, K. (2008). Modulation of cognitive performance and mood by aromas of peppermint and Ylang-Ylang. *The International Journal of Neuroscience*, *118*(1), 59–77. doi:10.1080/00207450601042094 PMID:18041606

Mottram, D. S., Bronislaw, L. W., & Dodson, A. T. (2002). Food chemistry: Acrylamide is formed in the Maillard reaction. *Nature*, *419*(6906), 448–449. doi:10.1038/419448a PMID:12368844

Munné-Bosch, S., & Alegre, L. (2002). The function of tocopherols and tocotrienols in plants. *Critical Reviews in Plant Sciences*, *21*(1), 31–57. doi:10.1080/0735-260291044179

Muraki, I., Imamura, F., Manson, J. E., Hu, F. B., Willett, W. C., Van Dam, R. M., & Sun, Q. (2013). Fruit consumption and risk of type 2 diabetes: Results from three prospective longitudinal cohort studies. *British Medical Journal*, *347*(1), f5001. doi:10.1136/bmj.f5001 PMID:23990623

Myrie, S., Jones, P., & Saarela, M. (2011). Functional foods and obesity. In *Functional foods: concept to product*, (pp. 234-260).

NABARD. (2007). *Millets in your meals (ppt – 21)*. NABARD.

Nadakarni, A. K. (1973). *Indian Meteria Medica*. Mumbai. *Popular Prakashan*, *1*(1), 72.

Nadesapanicker, A. K., Gopi, G., & Prajeesh, P. (2010). Genetic Erosion and Degradation of Ecosystem Services of Wetland Rice Fields: A Case Study From Western Ghats, India.

Nagengast, F. M. (1992). Dietary Fibre and Bile Acid Metabolism. Academic Press.

Nakamura, C. V., Ueda-Nakamura, T., Bando, E., & Negr, Ã. (1999). Antibacterial activity of *Ocimum gratissimum* L. essential oil. *Memorias do Instituto Oswaldo Cruz*, *94*(5), 675–678. doi:10.1590/S0074-02761999000500022 PMID:10464416

Nakatsuji, T., Kao, M. C., Fang, J.-Y., Zouboulis, C. C., Zhang, L., Gallo, R. L., & Huang, C.-M. (2009). Antimicrobial Property of Lauric Acid Against *Propionibacterium acnes*: Its Therapeutic Potential for Inflammatory Acne Vulgaris. *The Journal of Investigative Dermatology*, *129*(10), 2480–2488. doi:10.1038/jid.2009.93 PMID:19387482

Nam, I. S., & Garnsworthy, P. C. (2007). Factors influencing biohydrogenation and conjugated linoleic acid production by mixed rumen fungi. *Journal of Microbiology (Seoul, Korea)*, *45*(3), 199. PMID:17618224

Nam, S. Y., Chang, M. H., Don, Z. J. S., Seo, H. J., & Oh, H. K. (2008). Essential oil of niaoulipreferentially potentiates antigen-specific cellular immunity and cytokine production by macrophages. *Immunopharmacology and Immunotoxicology*, *30*(3), 459–474. doi:10.1080/08923970802135187 PMID:18668393

Nehir, E. I. S., & Simsek, S. (2012). Food technological applications for optimal nutrition: An Overview of opportunities for the Food Industry. *Comprehensive Reviews in Food Science and Food Safety*, *11*(1), 1–11. doi:10.1111/j.1541-4337.2011.00167.x

Nguefack, J., Tamgue, O., Dongmo, J. B. L., Dakole, C. D., Leth, V., Vis-mer, H. F., & Nkeng-fack, A. E. et al. (2012). Synergistic action between fractions of essential oils from *Cymbopogon citratus, Ocimum gratissimum* and *Thymus vulgaris* against *Penicillium expansum*. *Food Control*, *23*(2), 377–383. doi:10.1016/j.foodcont.2011.08.002

Niu, S., Afre, S., & Gilbert, E. S. (2006). Sub inhibitory concentrations of cinnamaldehyde interfere with quorum sensing. *Letters in Applied Microbiology*, *43*(5), 489–494. doi:10.1111/j.1472-765X.2006.02001.x PMID:17032221

Noel, P., Briand, E., & Dumont, J. P. (1990). Role of nitrite in flavour development in uncooked cured meat products: Sensory assessment. *Meat Science*, *28*(1), 1–8. doi:10.1016/0309-1740(90)90015-X PMID:22055434

Norberto, S., Silva, S., Meireles, M., Faria, A., Pintado, M., & Calhau, C. (2013). Blueberry anthocyanins in health promotion: A metabolic overview. *Journal of Functional Foods*, *5*(4), 1518–1528. doi:10.1016/j.jff.2013.08.015

Nordlee, J. A., Taylor, S. L., Townsend, J. A., Thomas, L. A., & Bush, R. K. (1996). Identification of a Brazil-nut allergen in transgenic soybeans. *The New England Journal of Medicine*, *334*(11), 688–692. doi:10.1056/NEJM199603143341103 PMID:8594427

Nowak-Wegrzyn, A., Assa'ad, A. H., Bahna, S. L., Bock, S. A., Sicherer, S. H., & Teuber, S. S. (2009). Work Group report: Oral food challenge testing. *The Journal of Allergy and Clinical Immunology*, *123*(6), S365–S383. doi:10.1016/j.jaci.2009.03.042 PMID:19500710

Nugent, A. P. (2005). Health properties of resistant starch. *Nutrition Bulletin*, *30*(1), 27–54. doi:10.1111/j.1467-3010.2005.00481.x

Obilana, A. B., & Manyasa, E. (2002). Millets. In P. S. Belton & J. R. N. Taylor (Eds.), Pseudo cereals and less common cereals: Grain properties and utilization potential (pp. 177–217). Springer-Verlag.

O'Bryan, C. A., Crandall, P. G., Chalova, V. I., & Ricke, S. C. (2008). Orange essential oils antimicrobial activities against Salmonella spp. *Journal of Food Science*, *73*(6), M264–M267. doi:10.1111/j.1750-3841.2008.00790.x PMID:19241555

Ogawa, J., Matsumura, K., Kishino, S., Omura, Y., & Shimizu, S. (2001). Conjugated linoleic acid accumulation via 10-hydroxy-12-octadecaenoic acid during microaerobic transformation of linoleic acid by *Lactobacillus acidophilus*. *Applied and Environmental Microbiology*, *67*(3), 1246–1252. doi:10.1128/AEM.67.3.1246-1252.2001 PMID:11229917

Ohkawa, H., Ohishi, N., & Yagi, K. (1979). Assay for lipid peroxidase in animal tissues by thiobarbituric acid reaction. *Analytical Biochemistry*, *95*(2), 351–358. doi:10.1016/0003-2697(79)90738-3 PMID:36810

Okonkwo, C., & Assumpta, O. (2014). Nutritional Evaluation of Some Selected Spices Commonly Used in the South-Eastern Part of Nigeria. *Journal of Biology. Agriculture and Healthcare*, *15*(4), 97–103.

Okumura, N., Masamoto, N., & Wada, H. (1997). The *gshB* gene in the cyanobacterium *Synechococcus* sp. PCC 7942 encodes a functional glutathione synthetase. *Microbiology*, *143*(9), 2883–2890. doi:10.1099/00221287-143-9-2883 PMID:9308172

Oleinick, N. L., Chiu, S., Ramakrishnan, N., & Xue, L. (1986). The formation, identification, and significance of DNA-protein cross-links in mammalian cells. *British Journal of Cancer*, *55*, 135–140. PMID:3477283

ONU/UNEP/POPS. (2014). *Tenth meeting of the Persistent Organic Pollutants Review Committee (POPRC.10)*. FAO Headquarters. Retrieved from http://chm.pops.int/TheConvention/POPsReviewCommittee/Meetings/POPRC10/Overview/tabid/3779/mctl/ViewDetails/EventModID/871/EventID/514/xmid/11873/Default.aspx

Opara, E. I., Diaaz-Maroto, M. C., & Hidalgo, I. J. D. (2014). Culinary Herbs and Spices: Their Bioactive Properties, the Contribution of Polyphenols and the Challenges in Deducing Their True Health Benefits. *International Journal of Molecular Sciences*, *15*(10), 19183–19202. doi:10.3390/ijms151019183 PMID:25340982

Orhan, D. D., Ozçelik, B., Ozgen, S., & Ergun, F. (2010). Antibacterial, antifungal, and antiviral activities of some flavonoids. *Microbiological Research*, *165*(6), 496–504. doi:10.1016/j.micres.2009.09.002 PMID:19840899

Or-Rashid, M. M., AlZahal, O., & McBride, B. W. (2008). Studies on the production of conjugated linoleic acid from linoleic and vaccenic acids by mixed rumen protozoa. *Applied Microbiology and Biotechnology*, *81*(3), 533–541. doi:10.1007/s00253-008-1690-0 PMID:18797866

Or-Rashid, M. M., AlZahal, O., & McBride, B. W. (2011). Comparative studies on the metabolism of linoleic acid by rumen bacteria, protozoa, and their mixture in vitro. *Applied Microbiology and Biotechnology*, *89*(2), 387–395. doi:10.1007/s00253-010-2865-z PMID:20865258

Ortolani, C., Ballmer-Weber, B. K., Hansen, K. S., Ispano, M., Wüthrich, B., Bindslev-Jensen, C., & Pastorello, E. A. et al. (2000). Hazelnut allergy: A double-blind, placebo-controlled food challenge multicenter study. *The Journal of Allergy and Clinical Immunology*, *105*(3), 577–581. doi:10.1067/mai.2000.103052 PMID:10719310

O'Shea, E. F., Cotter, P. D., Stanton, C., Ross, R. P., & Hill, C. (2012). Production of bioactive substances by intestinal bacteria as a basis for explaining probiotic mechanisms: Bacteriocins and conjugated linoleic acid. *International Journal of Food Microbiology*, *152*(3), 189–205. doi:10.1016/j.ijfoodmicro.2011.05.025 PMID:21742394

Otoni, C. G., Silvania, F. O. P., Medeiros, E.A.A., & Soares, N. de F. F. (2014). Edible Films from Methylcellulose and Nanoemulsions of Clove Bud art *Syzygium aromaticum* and Oregano (*Origanum vulgare*) Essential Oils as Shelf Life Extenders for Sliced Bread. *J. Agric. Food Chemistry, 62*(22), 5214–5219.

Oyaizu, M. (1986). Studies on products of browning reactions: Antioxidative activities of products of browning reaction prepared from glucosamine. *Japanese Journal of Nutrition*, *44*(6), 307–315. doi:10.5264/eiyogakuzashi.44.307

Padulosi, S., Mal, B., King, O., & Gotor, E. (2015). Minor Millets as a Central Element for Sustainably Enhanced Incomes, Empowerment, and Nutrition in Rural India. *Sustainability*, *7*(7), 8904–8933. doi:10.3390/su7078904

Pakdeechanuan, P. S., Salaemae, A., & Odpiban, S. (2010). Effect of reducing propylene glycol content on conjugated linoleic acid production from sunflower oil. *KKU Science Journal, 38*, 532–543.

Palanisamy Bruntha Devi, R. V., Sathyabama, Malleshi, & Priyadarisini. (2011). Health benefits of finger millet (*Eleusine coracana* L.) polyphenols and dietary fiber: a review. *J Food Sci Technol.*

Pallett, K. E., & Young, A. J. (1993). Caratenoids. In R. G. Alscher & J. L. Hess (Eds.), *Antioxidants in Higher Plants* (pp. 91–110). Boca Raton, FL: CRC Press.

Palosuo, K. (2003). Update on wheat hypersensitivity. *Current Opinion in Allergy and Clinical Immunology, 3*(3), 205–209. doi:10.1097/00130832-200306000-00009 PMID:12840704

Pandey, K. B., & Rizvi, S. I. (2009). Plant polyphenols as dietary antioxidants in human health and disease. *Oxidative Medicine and Cellular Longevity, 2*(5), 270–278. doi:10.4161/oxim.2.5.9498 PMID:20716914

Parameswaran, K., & Sadasivam, S. (1994). Changes in the carbohydrates and nitrogenous components during germination of proso millet (*Panicum miliaceum*). *Plant Foods for Human Nutrition (Dordrecht, Netherlands), 45*(2), 97–102. doi:10.1007/BF01088466 PMID:8153070

Parejo, I., Iadomat, V., Bastida, J., Rosas-romero, A., Flerlage, N., Burillo, J., & Codina, C. (2002). Comparison between the Radical Scavenging Activity and Antioxidant Activity of Six Distilled and Nondistilled Mediterranean Herbs and Aromatic Plants. *Journal of Agricultural and Food Chemistry, 50*(23), 6882–6890. doi:10.1021/jf020540a PMID:12405792

Parisi, G. C., Zilli, M., Miani, M. P., Carrara, M., Bottona, E., Verdianelli, G., & Leandro, G. et al. (2002). High-fiber diet supplementation in patients with irritable bowel syndrome (IBS): A multicenter, randomized, open trial comparison between wheat bran diet and partially hydrolyzed guar gum (PHGG). *Digestive Diseases and Sciences, 47*(8), 1697–1704. doi:10.1023/A:1016419906546 PMID:12184518

Park, B. J., Morikawa, T., Ogata, T., Washida, K., Iwamoto, M., Nakamura, H., & Miyazaki, Y. (2009). Physiological effects of ingesting eucalyptus EO with milk casein peptide. *Silva Fennica, 43*(1), 173–179. doi:10.14214/sf.223

Park, E. K., Ryu, M. H., Kim, Y. H., Lee, Y. A., Lee, S. H., Woo, D. H., & Kim, K. S. et al. (2006). Anti-inflammatory effect of an ethanolic extract from Clematis mandshurica Rupr. *Journal of Ethnopharmacology, 108*(1), 142–147. doi:10.1016/j.jep.2006.04.025 PMID:16787723

Park, H. G., Cho, S. D., Kim, J. H., Lee, H., Chung, S. H., Kim, S. B., & Kim, Y. J. et al. (2009). Characterization of conjugated linoleic acid production by *Bifidobacterium breve* LMC 520. *Journal of Agricultural and Food Chemistry, 57*(16), 7571–7575. doi:10.1021/jf9014813 PMID:20349924

Park, S. J., Ahmad, F., Philp, A., Baar, K., Williams, T., Luo, H., & Chung, J. H. et al. (2012). Resveratrol ameliorates aging-related metabolic phenotypes by inhibiting cAMP phosphodiesterases. *Cell, 148*(3), 421–433. doi:10.1016/j.cell.2012.01.017 PMID:22304913

Pascual, C., Martín Esteban, M., & Fernández Crespo, J. (1992). Fish allergy: Evaluation of the importance of cross-reactivity. *The Journal of Pediatrics*, *121*(5), S29–S34. doi:10.1016/S0022-3476(05)81403-9 PMID:1447631

Pasqua, R. D., Feo, V. D., Francesco, V., & Mauriello, G. (2005). *In vitro* antimicrobial activity of essential oils from Mediterranean Apiaceae, Verbenaceae and Lamiaceae food borne pathogens and spoilage bacteria. *Annals of Microbiology*, *55*(2), 139–143.

Pastorello, E. A., Farioli, L., Pravettoni, V., Ispano, M., Scibola, E., Trambaioli, C., & Ortolani, C. et al. (2000). The maize major allergen, which is responsible for food-induced allergic reactions, is a lipid transfer protein. *The Journal of Allergy and Clinical Immunology*, *106*(4), 744–751. doi:10.1067/mai.2000.108712 PMID:11031346

Pastorello, E. A., Vieths, S., Pravettoni, V., Farioli, L., Trambaioli, C., Fortunato, D., & Conti, A. et al. (2002). Identification of hazel-nut major allergens in sensitive patients with positive double-blind, placebo- controlled food challenge results. *The Journal of Allergy and Clinical Immunology*, *109*(3), 563–570. doi:10.1067/mai.2002.121946 PMID:11898007

Paul, S., Dubey, R. C., Maheswari, D. K., & Kang, S. C. (2011). *Trachyspermum ammi* (L.) fruit essential oil influencing on membrane permeability and surface characteristics in inhibiting food–borne pathogens. *Food Control*, *22*(5), 725–731. doi:10.1016/j.foodcont.2010.11.003

Peña-Llopis, S., Peña, J. B., Sancho, E., Fernández-Vega, C., & Ferrando, M. D. (2001). Glutathione-dependent resistance of the European eel *Anguilla anguilla* to the herbicide molinate. *Chemosphere*, *45*(4-5), 671–681. doi:10.1016/S0045-6535(00)00500-2 PMID:11680763

Pennington, J. A. T. (1998). Dietary exposure models for nitrates and nitrites. *Food Control*, *9*(6), 385–395. doi:10.1016/S0956-7135(98)00019-X

Percival, M. (1998). Antioxidants. *Clinical Nutrition Insight*, *31*, 1–4.

Perdones, Á., Vargas, M., Atarés, L., & Chiralt, A. (2011). Physical, Antioxidant and Antimicrobial Properties of Chitosan-Cinnamon Leaf oil Films as Affected by Oleic Acid. *Food Hydrocolloids*, *36*, 256–264. doi:10.1016/j.foodhyd.2013.10.003

Pereira, M. J., Belver, M. T., Pascual, C. Y., & Martin Esteban, M. (2002). The allergenic significance of legumes. *Allergologia et Immunopathologia*, *30*, 346–353. doi:10.1016/S0301-0546(02)79152-0 PMID:12464170

Perez-Gago, M. B., Serra, M., & del R'ıo, M. A. (2006). Color change of fresh-cut apples coated with whey protein concentrate-based edible coatings. *Postharvest Biology and Technology*, *39*(1), 84–92. doi:10.1016/j.postharvbio.2005.08.002

Perricone, M., Arace, E., Corbo, M. R., Sinigaglia, M., & Bevilacqua, A. (2015). Bioactivity of essential oils:a review on their interaction with food components. *Frontiers in Micribiology.*, *6*(76), 1–7. PMID:25709605

Pittman, C. I., Pendleton, S., Bisha, B., O'Bryan, C. A., Belk, K. E., Goodridge, L., & Ricke, S. C. et al. (2011). Activity of citrus essential oils against *Escherichia coli* O157:H7 and *Salmonella* spp. and effects on beef subprimal cuts under refrigeration. *Journal of Food Science, 76*(6), M433–M438. doi:10.1111/j.1750-3841.2011.02253.x PMID:22417514

Platel, K., & Srinivasan, K. (2001). Studies on the influence of dietary spices on food transit time in experimental rats. *Nutrition Research (New York, N.Y.), 21*(9), 1309–1314. doi:10.1016/S0271-5317(01)00331-1

Polivka, T., & Sundström, V. (2004). Ultrafast dynamics of carotenoid excited states- from solution to natural and artificial systems. *Chemical Reviews, 104*(4), 2021–2071. doi:10.1021/cr020674n PMID:15080720

Ponce, A. G., Roura, S. I., Del valle, C. E., & Moreira, M.R. (2008). Antimicrobial and Antioxidant Activities of Edible Coatings Enriched with Natural Plant Extracts: In Vitro and In Vivo Studies. Postharvest Biology and Technolog., 49(2), 294-300.

Prabhakaran, T. R., Das, Balaravi, & King. (2012). *Assessing farmers willingness to participate in the on-farm conservation of minor millet using direct compensation payment.* Working Paper 73/2012.

Prabuseenivasan, S., Jayakumar, M., & Ignacimuthu, S. (2006). *In vitro* antibacterial activity of some plant essential oil. *BMC Complementary and Alternative Medicine, 6*(1), 1–8. doi:10.1186/1472-6882-6-39 PMID:16412227

Prasanna, R., Sood, A., Jaiswal, P., Nayak, S., Gupta, V., Chaudhary, V., & Natarajan, C. et al. (2010). Rediscovering cyanobacteria as valuable sources of bioactive compounds. *Prikladnaia Biokhimiia i Mikrobiologiia, 46*(2), 133–147. PMID:20391755

Priya, B., Sivaprasanth, R. K., Jensil, V. D., Uma, L., Subramanian, G., & Prabaharan, D. (2010). Characterization of manganese superoxide dismutase from a marine cyanobacterium *Leptolyngbya valderiana* BDU20041. *Saline Systems, 6*(1), 1–10. doi:10.1186/1746-1448-6-6 PMID:20525290

Priya, P., Kesheri, M., Sinha, R. P., & Kanchan, S. (2016). Molecular dynamics simulations for Biological Systems. In W. B. A. Karâa & N. Dey (Eds.), *Biomedical Image Analysis and Mining Techniques for Improved Health Outcomes, Advances in Bioinformatics and Biomedical Engineering (ABBE) Series* (pp. 286–313). IGI Global. doi:10.4018/978-1-4666-8811-7.ch014

Pryce, J. E., Wales, W. J., De Haas, Y., Veerkamp, R. F., & Hayes, B. J. (2014). Genomic selection for feed efficiency in dairy cattle. *Animal, 8*(01), 1–10. doi:10.1017/S1751731113001687 PMID:24128704

Quintin, J., & Lewin, G. (2004). Semisynthesis of linarin, acacetin and 6-iodoapiagenin derivatives from diosmin. *Journal of Natural Products, 67*(9), 1624–1627. doi:10.1021/np040079b PMID:15387678

Racette, S. B., Lin, X., Ma, L., & Ostlund, R. E. (2015). Natural Dietary Phytosterols. *Journal of AOAC International, 98*(3), 679–684. PMID:26086252

Ragaee, S., Abdel-Aal, E. M., & Noaman, M. (2006). Antioxidant activity and nutrient composition of selected cereals for food use. *Food Chemistry*, *98*(1), 32–38. doi:10.1016/j.foodchem.2005.04.039

Rahimi, S., Zadeh, T., Karimi, M. A., Omidbaigi, R., & Rokni, H. (2011). Effect of the three herbal extracts on growth performance, immune system, blood factors and intestinal selected bacterial population in broiler chickens. *Journal of Agriculture Science and Technology.*, *13*, 527–539.

Rainio, A., Vahvaselkä, M., Suomalainen, T., & Laakso, S. (2001). Reduction of linoleic acid inhibition in production of conjugated linoleic acid by *Propionibacterium freudenreichii* ssp. *shermanii. Canadian Journal of Microbiology*, *47*(8), 735–740. doi:10.1139/cjm-47-8-735 PMID:11575500

Rajukkannu, K., Sathya, A., & Quintal, O. (2009). The diversity of traditional rice varieties in India-A focus on Tamil Nadu. PANAP. Rice sheets, Penang, Malaysia. 1-11.

Ralet, M. C., Thibault, J. F., & Della, V. G. (1991). Solubilisation of sugar beet cell wall polysaccharides by extrusion-cooking. *Lebensmittel-Wissenschaft + [i.e. Und] Technologie. Food Science + Technology. Science + Technologie Alimentaire*, *24*, 107–112.

Ramprasath, V. R., & Awad, A. B. (2015). Role of Phytosterols in Cancer Prevention and Treatment. *Journal of AOAC International*, *98*(3), 735–738. PMID:26086253

Ranganna, S. (1995). *Handbook of Analysis and Quality control for fruit and vegetable project*. New Delhi: McGraw-Hill.

Rao, A., Zhang, Y., Muend, S., & Rao, R. (2010). Mechanism of anti- fungal activity of terpenoid phenols resembles calcium stress and inhibition of the TOR pathway. *Antimicrobial Agents and Chemotherapy*, *54*(12), 5062–5069. doi:10.1128/AAC.01050-10 PMID:20921304

Rašković, A., Milanović, I., Pavlović, N., Ćebović, T., Vukmirović, S., & Mikov, M. (2014). Antioxidant activity of rosemary (*Rosmarinus officinalis* L.) essential oil and its hepatoprotective potential. *BMC Complementary and Alternative Medicine*, *14*(1), 225–234. doi:10.1186/1472-6882-14-225 PMID:25002023

Rasooli, I. (2007). Food Preservation – A Biopreservative Approach. *Food*, *1*(2), 111–136.

Rather, M. A., Dar, B. A., Sofi, S. N., Bhat, B. A., & Qurishi, M. A. (2012). Volatile components and key odorants of fennel (Foeniculum vulgare Mill.) and thyme (Thymus vulgaris L.) Oil extracts obtained by simultaneous distillation–extraction and supercritical fluid extraction. *Journal of Agricultural and Food Chemistry*, *53*, 5385–5389. PMID:15969523

Ratnam, D. V., Ankola, D. D., Bhardwaj, V., Sahana, D. K., & Kumar, M. N. V. R. (2006). Role of Antioxidants in Prophylaxis and Therapy: A Pharmaceutical Perspective. *Journal of Controlled Release*, *113*(3), 189–207. doi:10.1016/j.jconrel.2006.04.015 PMID:16790290

Rattan, S. I., Kryzch, V., Schnebert, S., Perrier, E., & Nizard, C. (2013). Hormesis-based anti-aging products: A case study of a novel cosmetic. *Dose-Response*, *11*(1), 99–108. doi:10.2203/dose-response.11-054.Rattan PMID:23548988

Ravikumar, Y. S., Mahadevan, K. M., Manjunatha, H., & Satyanarayana, N. D. (2010). Antiproliferative, apoptotic and antimutagenic activity of isolated compounds from Polyalthia cerasoides seeds. *Phytomedicine*, *17*(7), 513–518. doi:10.1016/j.phymed.2009.09.005 PMID:19879119

Raybaudi-Massilia, R. M., Mosqueda-Melgar, J., & Martin-Belloso, O. (2006). Antimicrobial activity of essential oils on *Salmonella enteritidis, Escherichiacoli*, and *Listeriainnocua* in fruit-juices. *Journal of Food Protection*, *69*, 1579–1586. PMID:16865889

Raybaudi-Massilia, R. M., Mosqueda-Melgar, J., Sobrino-Lopez, A., Soliva-Fortuny, R., & Martín-Belloso, O. (2009). Use of malic acid and other quality stabilizing compounds to assure the safety of freshcut"fuji" apples by inactivation of *Listeria monocytogenes, Salmonella Enteridis*, and *Escherichia coli* O157:H7. *Journal of Food Safety*, *29*(2), 236–252. doi:10.1111/j.1745-4565.2009.00153.x

Read, N. W., & Eastwood, M. A. (1992). Gastro-intestinal physiology and function. In T. F. Schweizer et al. (Eds.), *Dietary Fibre - A Component of Food* (pp. 40–54). Springer-Verlag London Limited. doi:10.1007/978-1-4471-1928-9_5

Reche, M., Pascual, C. Y., Vicente, J., Caballero, T., Martín Muñoz, F., Sánchez, S., & Martín Esteban, M. (2001). Tomato allergy in children and young adults: Cross-reactivity with latex and potato. *Allergy*, *56*(12), 1197–1201. doi:10.1034/j.1398-9995.2001.00279.x PMID:11736750

Reis-Sobreiro, M., Gajate, C., & Mollinedo, F. (2009). Involvement of mitochondria and recruitment of Fas/CD95 signaling in lipid rafts in resveratrol-mediated antimyeloma and antileukemia actions. *Oncogene*, *28*(36), 3221–3234. doi:10.1038/onc.2009.183 PMID:19561642

Repetto, M. (1981). *Toxicología Avanzada* (D. de Santos, Ed.). Madrid, Spain.

Richa, Rastogi, R.P., Kumari, S., Singh, K.L., Kannaujiya, V.K., Singh, G., …Sinha, R.P. (2011). Biotechnological potential of mycosporine-like amino acids and phycobiliproteins of cyanobacterial origin. *Biotechnolgy Bioinformatics and Bioengineering*, *1*(2), 159–171.

Robbers, E. J. (1997). *Farmacognosia e Farmacobiotecnologia*. São Paulo, SP, Brasil: Premier.

Rocks, N., Bekaert, S., Coia, I., Paulissen, G., Gueders, M., Evrard, B., & Cataldo, D. et al. (2012). Curcumin-cyclodextrin complexes potentiate gemcitabine effects in an orthotopic mouse model of lung cancer. *British Journal of Cancer*, *107*(7), 1083–1092. doi:10.1038/bjc.2012.379 PMID:22929882

Rodriguez, E. B., Flavier, M. E., Rodriguez-Amaya, D. B., & Amaya-Farfán, J. (2006). Phytochemicals and functional foods. Current situation and prospect for developing countries. *Segurança Alimentar e Nutricional, Campinas*, *13*(1), 1–22.

Rojas-Grau¨, M. A., & Roberto, J. (2006). Mechanical, Barrier, and Antimicrobial Properties of Apple Puree Edible Films Containing Plant. *Journal of Agricultural and Food Chemistry*, *54*(24), 9262–9267. doi:10.1021/jf061717u PMID:17117819

Rojas-Hijazo, B., Garces, M. M., Caballero, M. L., Alloza, P., & Moneo, I. (2006). Unsuspected lupin allergens hidden in food. *International Archives of Allergy and Immunology*, *141*(1), 47–50. doi:10.1159/000094181 PMID:16804325

Rosberg-Cody, E., Ross, R. P., Hussey, S., Ryan, C. A., Murphy, B. P., Fitzgerald, G. F., & Stanton, C. (2004). Mining the microbiota of the neonatal gastrointestinal tract for conjugated linoleic acid-producing bifidobacteria. *Applied and Environmental Microbiology*, *70*(8), 4635–4641. doi:10.1128/AEM.70.8.4635-4641.2004 PMID:15294796

Rosen, G. M., Pou, S., Ramos, C. L., Cohen, M. S., & Britigan, B. E. (1995). Free radicals and phagocytic cells. *The FASEB Journal*, *9*, 200–209. PMID:7540156

Rossander, L., Sandbergv, A. S., & Sandstrom, B. (1992). The influence of dietary fibre on mineral absorption and utilization. In T. F. Schweizer et al. (Eds.), *Dietary Fibre - A Component of Food* (pp. 40–54). Springer-Verlag London Limited. doi:10.1007/978-1-4471-1928-9_11

Rouse, M. S., Rotger, M., Piper, K. E., Steckelberg, J. M., Scholz, M., Andrews, J., & Patel, R. (2005). *In Vitro* and *In Vivo* Evaluations of the Activities of Lauric Acid Monoester Formulations against *Staphylococcus aureus*. *Antimicrobial Agents and Chemotherapy*, *49*(8), 3187–3191. doi:10.1128/AAC.49.8.3187-3191.2005 PMID:16048923

Rudrappa, T., & Bais, H. P. (2008). Curcumin, a known phenolic from *Curcuma longa*, attenuates the virulence of *Pseudomonas aeruginosa* PAO1 in whole plant and animal pathogenicity models. *Journal of Agricultural and Food Chemistry*, *56*(6), 1955–1962. doi:10.1021/jf072591j PMID:18284200

Saavedra, M. J., Borges, A., Dias, C., Aires, A., Bennett, R. N., Rosa, E. S., & Simões, M. (2010). Antimicrobial activity of phenolics and glucosinolate hydrolysis products and their synergy with streptomycin against pathogenic bacteria. *Medicinal Chemistry (Shariqah, United Arab Emirates)*, *6*(3), 174–183. doi:10.2174/157340641100603 0174 PMID:20632977

Sahib, N. J., Anwar, F., Gilani, A. H., Hamid, A. A., Saari, A., & Khalid, M. (2012). Coriander (Coriandrum sativum L.): A PotentialSource of High-Value Components for Functional Foods and Nutraceuticals- A Review. *Phytotherapy Research*, *27*(10), 1439–1456. PMID:23281145

Sakuradani, E., Ogawa, J., Kishino, S., Ando, A., Yokozeki, K., & Shimizu, S. (2010). Oils, microbial production. Encyclopedia of Industrial Biotechnology.

Saleh, A. S. M., Zhang, Q., Chen, J., & Shen, Q. (2013). Millet Grains: Nutritional Quality, Processing, and Potential Health Benefits. *Comprehensive Reviews in Food Science and Food Safety*, *12*(3), 281–295. doi:10.1111/1541-4337.12012

Saleh, M. O., Clark, S., Woodward, B., & Deolo-Sobogun, S. A. (2010). Antioxidant and free radical scavenging of essential oils. *Ethnicity & Disease*, *20*, 78–82. PMID:20521390

Salem, M. L. (2005). Immunomodulatory and therapeutic properties of the *Nigella sativa* L. seed. *International Immunopharmacology*, *5*(13-14), 1749–1770. doi:10.1016/j.intimp.2005.06.008 PMID:16275613

Salem, M. L., & Hossain, M. S. (2000). Protective effect of black seed oil from *Nigella sativa* against murine cytomegalovirus infection. *International Journal of Immunopharmacology*, *22*(9), 729–740. doi:10.1016/S0192-0561(00)00036-9 PMID:10884593

Sampson, H. A. (2004). Update on Food allergy. *Current Reviews of Allergy and Clinical Immunology*, *113*(5), 805–819. doi:10.1016/j.jaci.2004.03.014 PMID:15131561

Sánchez-González, L., Pastor, C., Vargas, M., Chiralt, A., González-Martínez, C., & Cháfer, M. (2011). Effect of Hydroxypropylmethylcellulose and Chitosan Coatings with and Without Bergamot Essential Oil on Quality and Safety of Cold-Stored Grapes. *Postharvest Biology and Technology*, *60*(1), 57–63. doi:10.1016/j.postharvbio.2010.11.004

Santhakumar, A. B., Bulmer, A. C., & Singh, I. (2014). A review of the mechanisms and effectiveness of dietary polyphenols in reducing oxidative stress and thrombotic risk. *Journal of Human Nutrition and Dietetics*, *27*(1), 1–21. doi:10.1111/jhn.12177 PMID:24205990

Santhakumar, A. B., Kundur, A. R., Fanning, K., Netzel, M., Stanley, R., & Singh, I. (2015). Consumption of anthocyanin-rich Queen Garnet plum juice reduces platelet activation related thrombogenesis in healthy volunteers. *Journal of Functional Foods*, *12*(0), 11–22. doi:10.1016/j.jff.2014.10.026

Sanz Ortega, J., Martorell Aragonés, A., & Michavila Gómez, A. (2001). Estudio de la incidencia de alergia mediada por IgE frente a la proteína de la leche de vaca en el primer año de vida. *Anales Espanoles de Pediatria*, *545*, 36–39.

Sarada, R., Pillai, M. G., & Ravishankar, G. A. (1999). Phycocyanin from *Spirullina* sp.: Influence of processing of biomass on phycocyanin yield, analysis of efficiency of extraction methods and stability studies on phycoyanin. *Process Biochemistry*, *34*(8), 795–801. doi:10.1016/S0032-9592(98)00153-8

Sato, M., Tanaka, H., Tani, N., Nagayama, M., & Yamaguchi, R. (2006). Different antibacterial actions of isoflavones isolated from *Erythrina poeppigiana* against methicillin-resistant *Staphylococcus aureus*. *Letters in Applied Microbiology*, *43*(3), 243–248. doi:10.1111/j.1472-765X.2006.01963.x PMID:16910926

Scalbert, A. (1991). Antimicrobial properties of tannins. *Phytochemistry*, *30*(12), 3875–3883. doi:10.1016/0031-9422(91)83426-L

Scalbert, A., Manach, C., Morand, C., Remesy, C., & Jimenez, L. (2005). Dietary polyphenols and the prevention of diseases. *Critical Reviews in Food Science and Nutrition*, *45*(4), 287–306. doi:10.1080/1040869059096 PMID:16047496

Scherzberg, M. C., Kiehl, A., Zivkovic, A., Stark, H., Stein, J., Fürst, R., & Ulrich-Rückert, S. et al. (2015). Structural modification of resveratrol leads to increased anti-tumor activity, but causes profound changes in the mode of action. *Toxicology and Applied Pharmacology*, *287*(1), 67–76. PMID:26044878

Schmid, B., Einsle, O., Chiu, H. J., Willing, A., Yoshida, M., Howard, J. B., & Rees, D. C. (2002). Biochemical and structural characterization of the cross-linked complex of nitrogenase: Comparison to the ADP-AlF4--stabilized structure. *Biochemistry*, *41*(52), 15557–15565. doi:10.1021/bi026642b PMID:12501184

Season & crop report. (2012). Chennai: Department of Economics and Statistics, Government of India.

Sehgal, A., & Kwatra, A. (2003). Processing and utilization of pearl millet for Nutrition Security. In *Proceeding of national seminar on Recent Trend in Millet Processing and Utilization.*

Selman, C. J., McLaren, S., Collins, A. R., Duthie, G. G., & Speakman, J. R. (2013). Deleterious consequences of antioxidant supplementation on lifespan in a wild-derived mammal. *Biology Letters*, *9*(4), 20130432. doi:10.1098/rsbl.2013.0432 PMID:23825087

Serrano, A., Rivas, J., & Losada, M. (1984). Purification and properties of glutathione reductase from the cyanobacterium *Anabaena* sp. strain 7119. *Journal of Bacteriology*, *158*, 317–324. PMID:6425264

Seruga, M., Novak, I., & Jakobek, L. (2011). Determination of Polyphenols Content and Antioxidant Activity of Some Red Wines by Differential Pulse Voltammetry, HPLC and Spectrophotometric Methods. *Food Chemistry*, *124*(3), 1208–1216. doi:10.1016/j.foodchem.2010.07.047

Shareck, J., Nantel, A., & Belhumeur, P. (2011). Conjugated linoleic acid inhibits hyphal growth in *Candida albicans* by modulating Ras1p cellular levels and downregulating TEC1 expression. *Eukaryotic Cell*, *10*(4), 565–577. doi:10.1128/EC.00305-10 PMID:21357478

Shelton, B. G., Kirkland, K. H., Flanders, W. D., & Morris, G. K. (2002). Profiles of Airborne Fungi in Buildings and Outdoor Environments in the United States. *Applied and Environmental Microbiology*, *68*(4), 1743–1753. doi:10.1128/AEM.68.4.1743-1753.2002 PMID:11916692

Shen, J., Niijima, A., Tanida, M., Horii, Y., Maeda, K., & Kastuya, N. (2005a). Olfactory stimulation with scent of grapefruitoil affects autonomic nerves, lipolysis and appetite in rats. *Neuroscience Letters*, *380*(3), 289–294. doi:10.1016/j.neulet.2005.01.058 PMID:15862904

Shen, J., Niijima, A., Tanida, M., Horii, Y., Maeda, K., & Nagai, K. (2005b). Olfactory stimulation with scent of lavender oil affects autonomic nerves, lipolysis and appetite in rats. *Neuroscience Letters*, *383*(1-2), 188–193. doi:10.1016/j.neulet.2005.04.010 PMID:15878236

Shipradeep, K. S., Khare, R.S., Ojha, S., Kundu, K., & Kundu, S. (2012). Development of Probiotic Candidate in Combination with Essential Oils from Medicinal Plant and Their Effect on Enteric Pathogens: A Review. Gastroenterology Research and Practice.

Shobana, S., & Malleshi, N. G. (2007). Preparation and functional properties of decorticated finger millet (*Eleusine coracana*). *Journal of Food Engineering*, *79*(2), 529–538. doi:10.1016/j.jfoodeng.2006.01.076

Si, D., Wang, Y., Zhou, Y., Guo, Y., Wang, J., Zhou, H., & Fawcett, J. P. et al. (2009). Mechanism of CYP2C9 inhibition by flavones and flavonols. *Drug Metabolism and Fawcett*, *37*(3), 629–634. doi:10.1124/dmd.108.023416 PMID:19074529

Sikkema, J., DeBont, J. A. M., & Poolman, B. (1995). Mechanisms of membrane toxicity of hydrocarbons. *Microbiological Reviews*, *59*, 201–222. PMID:7603409

Silveira e Sá, R. C., Andrade, L. N., Oliveira, R. R. B., & Sousa, D. P. (2014). A Review on Anti-Inflammatory Activity of Phenylpropanoids Found in Essential Oils. *Molecules (Basel, Switzerland)*, *19*(2), 1459–1480. doi:10.3390/molecules19021459 PMID:24473208

Simeray, J., Mandin, D., & Chaumont, J.-P.Impact on the Study of Allergies. (1995). Variations in the Distribution of Fungal Spores in the Atmosfere of Bakehouses. Impact on the Study of Allergies. *Grana*, *34*(4), 269–274. doi:10.1080/00173139509429056

Sindhu, E. R., Preethi, K. C., & Kuttan, R. (2010). Antioxidant activity ofcarotenoid luteinin vitroandin vivo. *Indian Journal of Experimental Biology*, *48*, 843–848. PMID:21341544

Singh, A., Singh, R. K., Bhunia, A. K., & Singh, N. (2004). Efficacy of plant essential oils as antimicrobial agents against *Listeria monocytogenes* in hot-dogs. *LWT-Food Science & Technology*, *36*(8), 787–794. doi:10.1016/S0023-6438(03)00112-9

Singh, G., & Maurya, S. (2005). Antimicrobial, antifungal and insecticidal investigations on essential oils – an overview. *Natural Product Radiance*, *4*(3), 179–192.

Singh, I., Turner, A. H., Sinclair, A. J., Li, D., & Hawley, J. A. (2007). Effects of gamma-tocopherol supplementation on thrombotic risk factors. *Asia Pacific Journal of Clinical Nutrition*, *16*(3), 422–428. PMID:17704022

Singh, K. P., Mishram, H. N., & Saham, S. (2012). Changes during accelerated storage in millet–wheat composite flours for bread. *Food and Bioprocess Technology Journal*, *5*(5), 2003–2011. doi:10.1007/s11947-011-0769-2

Singh, M. P., & Bhatia, A. (2011). Role of functional foods in periodontal health and disease. *Indian Journal of Dental Advancements*, *3*(3), 587–592. doi:10.5866/3.3.587

Singh, M., Govindarajan, R., Rawat, A. K. S., & Khare, P. B. (2008). Antimicrobial Flavonoid Rutin from *Pteris vittata L.* Against Pathogenic Gastrointestinal Microflora. *American Fern Journal*, *98*(2), 98–103. doi:10.1640/0002-8444(2008)98[98:AFRFPV]2.0.CO;2

Singh, P., & Malik, T. (2008). Essence of plants: essential oils as antimicrobials. In P. Parihar & L. Parihar (Eds.), *Advances in Applied Microbiology* (pp. 137–148). Bikaner, India: Agrobios Publishers.

Singh, P., & Raghuvanshi, R. S. (2012). Finger millet for food and nutritional security. *African Journal of Food Science*, *6*(4), 77–84.

Sinha, R. P., Klisch, M., Gröniger, A., & Häder, D.-P. (1998). Ultraviolet absorbing/screening substances in cyanobacteria, phytoplankton and macroalgae. *Journal of Photochemistry and Photobiology. B, Biology*, *47*(2-3), 83–94. doi:10.1016/S1011-1344(98)00198-5

Sinha, S., Jothiramajayam, M., Ghosh, M., & Mukherjee, A. (2014). Evaluation of toxicity of essential oils palmarosa, citronella, lemongrass and vetiver in human lymphocytes. *Food and Chemical Toxicology*, *68*, 71–77. doi:10.1016/j.fct.2014.02.036 PMID:24650756

Škrinjar, M. M., & Neme, N. T. (2009). Antimicrobial effects of spices and herbs essential oils. *Acta Periodica Technologica.*, *40*(40), 195–209. doi:10.2298/APT0940195S

Skrivanová, E., Marounek, M., Dlouhá, G., & Kanka, J. (2005). Susceptibility of *Clostridium perfringens* to C-C fatty acids. *Letters in Applied Microbiology*, *41*(1), 77–81. doi:10.1111/j.1472-765X.2005.01709.x PMID:15960756

Slavin, J. (2013). Health aspects of dietary fiber. In J. Slavin (Ed.), *Fibre- rich and wholegrain foods* (pp. 234–239). New York: Woodhead Publishing Limited. doi:10.1533/9780857095787.1.61

Smadja, J. (2009). Essential oils: chemical composition and localization. In Essential oils and green extractions and applications (pp. 194-213). Har Krishan Bhalla and Sons.

Smith-Palmer, A., Stewart, J., & Fyfe, L. (2001). The potential application of plant essential oils as natural food preservatives in soft cheese. *Food Microbiology*, *18*(4), 463–470. doi:10.1006/fmic.2001.0415

Smith, R. C., Prézelin, B. B., Baker, K. S., Bidigare, R. R., Boucher, N. P., Coley, T., & et, et al.. (1992). Ozone depletion: Ultraviolet radiation and phytoplankton biology in Antarctic waters. *Science*, *255*(5047), 952–959. doi:10.1126/science.1546292 PMID:1546292

Smith, R.L., Cohen, S.M., Doull, J., Feron, V.J., Goodman, J.I., & Marnett, L.J, Porto Ghese, P.S., & Adams, T.B. (2005). A procedure for the safety evaluation of natural flavor complexes used as ingredients in food: Essential oils. *Food and Chemical Toxicology*, *43*(3), 345–363. PMID:15680674

Solon-Biet, S. M., McMahon, A. C., Ballard, J. W. O., Ruohonen, K., Wu, L. E., Cogger, V. C., & Simpson, S. J. et al. (2014). The ratio of macronutrients, not caloric intake, dictates cardiometabolic health, aging, and longevity inad libitum-fed mice. *Cell Metabolism*, *19*(3), 418–430. doi:10.1016/j.cmet.2014.02.009 PMID:24606899

Speranza, B., & Corbo, M. R. (2010). Essential oils for preserving perishable foods: possibilities and limitations. In Application of Alternative Food Preservation Technologies to Enhance Food Safety and Stability, (pp. 35-57). Sharjah, UAE: Bentham Publisher.

Srinivasan, S., & Pari, L. (2012). Ameliorative effect of diosmin, a citrus flavonoid against streptozotocin-nicotinamide generated oxidative stress induced diabetic rats. *Chemico-Biological Interactions*, *195*(1), 43–51. doi:10.1016/j.cbi.2011.10.003 PMID:22056647

Stanly, Raj, & Shanmugam. (2013). A study on millets based cultivation and consumption in India. *International Journal of Marketing, Financial Services & Management Research*, *2*(4), 49-58.

Steffen, L. M., Jacobs, D. R., Stevens, J., Shahar, E., Carithers, T., & Folsom, A. R. (2003). Associations of WholeGrain, Refined-Grain, and Fruit and Vegetable Consumption with Risks of All-Cause Mortality and Incident Coronary Artery Disease and İschemic Stroke: The Atherosclerosis Risk in Communities (ARIC) Study. *The American Journal of Clinical Nutrition*, *78*, 383–390. PMID:12936919

Steinberg, D., Feldman, M., Ofek, I., & Weiss, E. I. (2005). Cranberry high molecular weight constituents promote *Streptococcus sobrinus* desorption from artificial biofilm. *International Journal of Antimicrobial Agents*, *25*(3), 247–251. doi:10.1016/j.ijantimicag.2004.10.014 PMID:15737520

Stobiecki, M. (2000). Application of mass spectrometry for identification and structural studies of flavonoid glycosides. *Phytochemistry*, *54*(3), 237–256. doi:10.1016/S0031-9422(00)00091-1 PMID:10870178

Stockholm Convention on POPs. (2001). Available in: http://chm.pops.int/TheConvention/POPsReviewCommittee/ReportsandDecisions/tabid/3309/Default.aspx

Stout, M. B., Tchkonia, T., Pirtskhalava, T., Palmer, A. K., List, E. O., Berryman, D. E., & Kirkland, J. L. et al. (2014). Growth hormone action predicts ge-related white adipose tissue dysfunction and senescent cell burden in mice. *Aging*, *6*(7), 575–586. doi:10.18632/aging.100681 PMID:25063774

Subramanian, S., & Viswanathan, R. (2003). Thermal properties of minor millet grains and flours. *Biosystems Engineering*, *84*(3), 289–296. doi:10.1016/S1537-5110(02)00222-2

Sudharshana, L., Monteiro, P. V., & Ramchandra, G. (1987). Studies on proteins of kodo millet (*Paspalum scroculatum*). *Journal of the Science of Food and Agriculture*, *42*(4), 315–323. doi:10.1002/jsfa.2740420405

Sumalan, R. M., Alexa, E., & Poiana, M. A. (2013). Assessment of inhibitory potential of essential oils on natural mycoflora and *Fusarium* mycotoxins production in wheat. *Chemistry Central Journal*, *7*(32), 1–12. PMID:23409841

Sun, L. M., Zhang, C. L., & Li, P. (2011). Characterization, antimicrobial activity, and mechanism of a high-performance (-)-epigallocatechin-3-gallate (EGCG)-CuII/polyvinyl alcohol (PVA) nanofibrous membrane. *Journal of Agricultural and Food Chemistry*, *59*(9), 5087–5092. doi:10.1021/jf200580t PMID:21417240

Sun, L., Wang, S., Chen, L., & Gong, X. (2003). Promising fluorescent probes from phycobiliproteins. *IEEE Journal of Select Topics in Quantam Electronics*, *9*(2), 177–188. doi:10.1109/JSTQE.2003.812499

Suomalainen, H., & Ronkainen, P. (1968). The production of aroma compounds by yeast. *J. Insl. Brew*, *85*, 149-156.

Svoboda, K. P., Ingli, A., Hampson, J., Galambosi, B., & Asakawa, Y. (1998). Biomass production, essential oil yield and composition of *Myrica gale* L. harvested from wild populations in Scotland and Finland. *Flavour and Fragrance Journal*, *13*(6), 367–372. doi:10.1002/(SICI)1099-1026(199811/12)13:6<367::AID-FFJ724>3.0.CO;2-M

Szabo, M. A., Vagra, G. J., Hohmann, J., Schelz, Z., Szegedi, E. E., Amaral, L., & Molnar, J. (2012). Inhibition of quorum sensing signals by essential oils. *Phytotherapy Research*, *24*(5), 782–786. doi:10.1002/ptr.3010 PMID:19827025

Szocs, K. (2004). Endothelial dysfunction and reactive oxygen species production on ischemia/reperfusion and nitrate tolerance. *General Physiology and Biophysics*, *23*, 265–295. PMID:15638116

Szöllőskei, G., Wagner, L., Németh, S., & Husvéth, F. (2005). In sacco studies of conjugated linoleic acid production from various oils in the rumen of sheep. *Acta Veterinaria Hungarica*, *53*(4), 411–423. doi:10.1556/AVet.53.2005.4.2 PMID:16363143

Tahir, M., Rehman, M. U., Lateef, A., Khan, A. Q., Khan, R., Qamar, W., & Sultana, S. et al. (2013). Diosmin abrogates chemically induced hepatocarcinogenesis via alleviation of oxidative stress, hyperproliferative and inflammatory markers in murine model. *Toxicology Letters*, *220*(3), 205–218. doi:10.1016/j.toxlet.2013.04.004 PMID:23665045

Taiz, L., & Zeiger, E. (2002). *Plant physiology* (3rd ed.). Sinauer Associates Inc Publishers.

Tajuddin, A. S., & Latif, A. (2005). An experimental study of sexual function improving effect of *Myristica fragrans* Houtt. *BMC Complementary and Alternative Medicine*, *5*(1), 16. doi:10.1186/1472-6882-5-16 PMID:16033651

Tajuddin, S., Ahmed, S., & Latif, A. (2003). Aphrodisiac activity of 50% ethanolic extracts of *Myristica fragrans* houtt and *Syzygium aromatican* (L) Merr. And Perry (clove) in male mice. A comparative study. *BMC Complementary and Alternative Medicine*, *3*(1), 6. doi:10.1186/1472-6882-3-6 PMID:14567759

Takaoka, M. (1939). Resveratrol, a new phenolic compound, from *Veratrum grandiflorum. Journal of the Chemical Society of Japan*, *60*(1), 1090–1100.

Tanabe, H., Yoshida, M., & Tomita, N. (2002). Comparison of the antioxidant activities of 22 commonly used culinary herbs and spices on the lipid oxidation of pork meat. *Animal Science Journal*, *73*(5), 389–393. doi:10.1046/j.1344-3941.2002.00054.x

Tandeau de Marsac, N., & Houmard, J. (1988). Complementary chromatic adaptation: Physiological conditions and action spectra. *Methods in Enzymology*, *167*, 318–328. doi:10.1016/0076-6879(88)67037-6

Tanikawa, K., & Torimura, T. (2006). Studies on oxidative stress in liver diseases: Important future trends in liver research. *Medical Molecular Morphology*, *39*(1), 22–27. doi:10.1007/s00795-006-0313-z PMID:16575511

Tapsell, L.C., Hemphill, I., Cobiac, L., Sullivan, D.R., Fenech, M., & Patch, C.S., Roodenrys, ... Inge, K.E. (2006). Health benefits of herbs and spices: The past, the present, the future. *The Medical Journal of Australia*, *185*, S1–S24. PMID:17022438

Tareke, E., Rydberg, P., Karlsson, P., Eriksson, S., & Törnqvist, M. (2000). Acrylamide: A Cooking Carcinogen? *Chemical Research in Toxicology*, *13*(6), 517–522. doi:10.1021/tx9901938 PMID:10858325

Tassou, C., Drosinos, E. H., & Nychas, G. J. E. (1996). Inhibition of resident microbial flora and pathogen inocula on cold fresh fish fillets in olive oil, oregano, and lemon juice under modified atmosphere or air. *Journal of Food Protection*, *59*, 31–34.

Taylor, S. L., Hefle, S. L., Bindslev-Jensen, C., Atkins, F. M., Andre, C., Bruijnzeel-Koomen, C., . . . Abbott, P. (2004). *A consensus protocol for the determination of the threshold doses for allergenic foods: how much is too much?* Faculty Publications in Food Science and Technology. Retrieved from http://digitalcommons.unl.edu/foodsciefacpub/36

Taylor, S. L., Straton, J. E., & Nordlee, J. A. (1989). Histamine poisoning (scombroid fish poisoning): An allergy-like intoxication. *Journal of Toxicology. Clinical Toxicology*, *27*(4-5), 225–240. doi:10.3109/15563658908994420 PMID:2689658

Tchkonia, T., Morbeck, D. E., Von Zglinicki, T., Van Deursen, J., Lustgarten, J., Scrable, H., & Kirkland, J. L. et al. (2010). Fat tissue, aging, and cellular senescence. *Aging Cell*, *9*(5), 667–684. doi:10.1111/j.1474-9726.2010.00608.x PMID:20701600

Thibault, J. F., Lahaye, M., & Guillon, F. (1992). Physico-chemical properties of food plant cell walls. In T. F. Schweizer et al. (Eds.), *Dietary Fibre - A Component of Food* (pp. 40–54). Springer-Verlag London Limited. doi:10.1007/978-1-4471-1928-9_2

Thomas, S. C., Beveridge, T. H. J., & Drover, J. C. G. (2006). Phytosterol content of sea buckthorn (*Hippophae rhamnoides L.*) seed oil: Extraction and identification. *Food Chemistry*, *101*(4), 1633–1639.

Thompson, A., Meah, D., Ahmed, N., Conniff-Jenkins, R., Chileshe, E., Phillips, C. O., & Row, P. E. et al. (2013). Comparison of the antibacterial activity of essential oils and extracts of medicinal and culinary herbs to investigate potential new treatments for irritable bowel syndrome. *BMC Complementary and Alternative Medicine*, *13*(1), 338–350. doi:10.1186/1472-6882-13-338 PMID:24283351

Threlfall, D. R., & Whistance, G. R. (1971). Biosynthesis of isoprenoid quinones and chromanols. In T. W. Goodwin (Ed.), *Aspects of Terpenoid Chemistry and Biochemistry* (pp. 357–404). London: Academic Press.

Timmers, S., Auwerx, J., & Schrauwen, P. (2012). The journey of resveratrol from yeast to human. *Aging*, *4*(3), 146–158. doi:10.18632/aging.100445 PMID:22436213

Tongnuanchan, P., Benjakul, S., & Prodpran, T. (2014). Physico Chemical Properties, Morphology and Antioxidant Activity of Film from Fish Skin Gelatin Incorporated with Root Essential Oils. *Journal of Food Engineering*, *117*(3), 350–360. doi:10.1016/j.jfoodeng.2013.03.005

Towne, G., Nagaraja, T. G., Brandt, R. T., & Kemp, K. E. (1990). Ruminal ciliated protozoa in cattle fed finishing diets with or without supplemental fat. *Journal of Animal Science*, *68*(7), 2150–2155. PMID:2117004

Trebst, A., Depka, B., Jager, J., & Oettmeier, W. (2004). Reversal of the inhibition of photosynthesis by herbicides affecting hydroxyphenylpyruvate dioxygenase by plastoquinone and tocopheryl derivatives in *Chlamydomonas reinhardtii*. *Pest Management Science*, *60*(7), 669–674. doi:10.1002/ps.847 PMID:15260297

Tripathi, K. D. (1994). Essentials of Medical Pharmacology. Jaypee Brothers Medical Publishers.

Trombetta, D., Castelli, F., Sarpietro, M. G., Venuti, V., Cristani, M., Daniele, C., & Bisignano, G. et al. (2005). Mechanisms of antibacterial action of three monoterpenes. *Antimicrobial Agents and Chemotherapy*, *49*(6), 2474–2478. doi:10.1128/AAC.49.6.2474-2478.2005 PMID:15917549

Tsao, R. (2010). Chemistry and biochemistry of dietary polyphenols. *Nutrients*, *2*(12), 1231–1246. doi:10.3390/nu2121231 PMID:22254006

Turpeinen, A. M., Mutanen, M., Aro, A., Salminen, I., Basu, S., Palmquist, D. L., & Griinari, J. M. (2002). Bioconversion of vaccenic acid to conjugated linoleic acid in humans. *The American Journal of Clinical Nutrition*, *76*(3), 504–510. PMID:12197992

Tyagi, A. K., Bukvicki, D., Gottardi, D., Tabanelli, G., Montanari, C., Malik, A., & Guerzoni, M. E. (2014). Eucalyptus Essential Oil as a Natural Food Preservative In Vivo and In Vitro Antiyeast Potential. BioMed Research International.

Ultee, A., Bennik, M. H., & Moezelaar, R. (2002). The phenolic hydroxyl group of carvacrol is essential for action against the food-borne pathogen *Bacillus cereus*. *Applied and Environmental Microbiology*, *68*(4), 1561–1568. doi:10.1128/AEM.68.4.1561-1568.2002 PMID:11916669

Ultee, E., & Smid, J. (2001). Influence of carvacrol on growth and toxin production by *Bacillus cereus*. *International Journal of Food Microbiology*, *4*(3), 373–378. doi:10.1016/S0168-1605(00)00480-3 PMID:11294360

UNIDO & FAO. (2005). *Herbs, spices and essential oils:post-harvest operations in developing countries*. Vienna: United Nations Industrial development Organization & Food and Agriculture organization of United Nations (UNIDO).

Valko, M., Izakovic, M., Mazur, M., Rhodes, C. J., & Telser, J. (2004). Role of oxygen radicals in DNA damage and cancer incidence. *Molecular and Cellular Biochemistry*, *266*(1/2), 37–56. doi:10.1023/B:MCBI.0000049134.69131.89 PMID:15646026

Van Boekel, M.A.J.S. (2006). *Formation of flavour compounds in the Maillard reaction*. Academic Press.

Van Guilder, G. P., Hoetzer, G. L., Greiner, J. J., Stauffer, B. L., & Desouza, C. A. (2006). Influence of metabolic syndrome on biomarkers of oxidative stress and inflammation in obese adults. *Obesity (Silver Spring, Md.)*, *14*(12), 2127–2131. doi:10.1038/oby.2006.248 PMID:17189537

Van Meer, G., Voelker, D. R., & Feigenson, G. W. (2008). Membrane lipids: Where they are and how they behave. *Nature Reviews. Molecular Cell Biology*, *9*(2), 112–124. doi:10.1038/nrm2330 PMID:18216768

Van Soest, P. J. (1994). *Nutritional Ecology of the Ruminant* (2nd ed.). Ithaca, NY: Cornell University Press.

Vanamala, J., Reddivari, L., Yoo, K. S., Pike, L. M., & Patie, B. S. (2006). Variation in the content of bioactive flavonoids in different brands orange and grapefruit juices. *Journal of Food Composition and Analysis*, *19*(2-3), 157–166. doi:10.1016/j.jfca.2005.06.002

Váradyová, Z., Kisidayova, S., Siroka, P., & Jalc, D. (2007). Fatty acid profiles of rumen fluid from sheep fed diets supplemented with various oils and effect on the rumen ciliate population. *Czech Journal of Animal Science*, *52*(11), 399.

Varga, J., Rigó, K., Tóth, B., Téren, J., & Kozakiewicz, Z. (2003). Evolutionary Relationships among Aspergillus Species Producing Economically Important Mycotoxins. *Food Technology and Biotechnology*, *41*(1), 29–36.

Varo, P., Veijalainen, K., & Koivistoinen, P. (1984). Effect of heat treatment on the dietary fibre contents of potato and tomato. *Journal of Food Technology*, *19*(4), 485–492. doi:10.1111/j.1365-2621.1984.tb00372.x

Vass, I., Sass, L., Spetea, C., Bakou, A., Ghanatakis, D. F., & Petrouleas, V. (1996). UV-B inhibition of photosystem II electron transport system studied by EPR and chlorophyll florescence. Impairment of donor and acceptor side components. *Biochemistry*, *35*(27), 8964–8973. doi:10.1021/bi9530595 PMID:8688433

Vasta, V., Yáñez-Ruiz, D. R., Mele, M., Serra, A., Luciano, G., Lanza, M., & Priolo, A. (2010). Bacterial and protozoal communities and fatty acid profile in the rumen of sheep fed a diet containing added tannins. *Applied and Environmental Microbiology*, *76*(8), 2549–2555. doi:10.1128/AEM.02583-09 PMID:20173064

Veena, B. (2003). *Nutritional, functional and utilization studies on barnyard millet.* (M. Sc. Thesis). University of Agricultural Sciences Dharwad, Karnataka, India.

Verburgh, K. (2015). Nutrigerontology: Why we need a new scientific discipline to develop diets and guidelines to reduce the risk of aging-related diseases. *Aging Cell*, *14*(1), 17–24. doi:10.1111/acel.12284 PMID:25470422

Viswanath, V., Urooj, A., & Malleshi, N. G. (2009). Evaluation of antioxidant and antimicrobial properties of finger millet polyphenols (*Eleusine coracana*). *Food Chemistry*, *114*(1), 340–346. doi:10.1016/j.foodchem.2008.09.053

Vossenberg, J. L. C. M., & Joblin, K. N. (2003). Biohydrogenation of C18 unsaturated fatty acids to stearic acid by a strain of *Butyrivibrio hungatei* from the bovine rumen. *Letters in Applied Microbiology*, *37*(5), 424–428. doi:10.1046/j.1472-765X.2003.01421.x PMID:14633116

W.H.O. (2003). *Diet, nutrition and the prevention of chronic diseases*. Report of a Joint WHO/FAO Expert Consultation. WHO Technical Report Series 916.

Wachi, Y., Burgess, J. G., Iwamoto, K., Yamada, N., Nakamura, N., & Matsunaga, T. (1995). Effect of ultraviolet-A (UV-A) light on growth, photosynthetic activity and production of biopterin glucoside by the marine UV-A resistant cyanobacterium *Oscillatoria* sp. *Biochimica et Biophysica Acta*, *1244*(1), 165–168. doi:10.1016/0304-4165(94)00219-N PMID:7766653

Wakelin, , & White, . (1999). Natural rubber latex allergy. *Clinical and Experimental Dermatology*, *24*(4), 245–248. doi:10.1046/j.1365-2230.1999.00470.x PMID:10457121

Walker, C. L. F., & Black, R. F. (2007). Functional Indicators for Assessing Zinc Deficiency. *Food and Nutrition Bulletin*, *23*(3), 454–479. doi:10.1177/15648265070283S305

Wallace, R. J., McKain, N., Shingfield, K. J., & Devillard, E. (2007). Isomers of conjugated linoleic acids are synthesized via different mechanisms in ruminal digesta and bacteria. *Journal of Lipid Research*, *48*(10), 2247–2254. doi:10.1194/jlr.M700271-JLR200 PMID:17644775

Walters, D. R., Walker, R. L., & Walker, K. C. (2003). Lauric Acid exhibits antifungal activity against plant pathogenic fungi. *Journal of Phytopathology*, *151*(4), 228–230. doi:10.1046/j.1439-0434.2003.00713.x

Wang, H., Hui, K. M., Xu, S., Chen, Y., Wong, J. T., & Xue, H. (2002). Two flavones from Scutellaria baicalensis Georgi and their binding affinities to the benzodiazepine site of the GABAA receptor complex. *Die Pharmazie*, *57*(12), 857–858. PMID:12561253

Wang, L. M., Lv, J. P., Chu, Z. Q., Cui, Y. Y., & Ren, X. H. (2007). Production of conjugated linoleic acid by *Propionibacterium freudenreichii*. *Food Chemistry*, *103*(2), 313–318. doi:10.1016/j.foodchem.2006.07.065

Welch, R. M., & Graham, R. D. (2004). Breeding for micronutrients in staple food crops from a human nutrition perspective. *Journal of Experimental Botany*, *55*(396), 353–364. doi:10.1093/jxb/erh064 PMID:14739261

WHO. (2015). *Food Safety Program updates*. Retrieved from. http://www.who.int/mediacentre/factsheets/fs225/en/

Wicher, K., & Reisman, R. (1980). Anaphylactic reaction to penicilin (or penicilin-like substantce) in soft drink. *The Journal of Allergy and Clinical Immunology*, *66*(2), 640. doi:10.1016/0091-6749(80)90063-9 PMID:6967496

Wiedenfeld, H., & Edgar, J. (2011). Toxicity of pyrrolizidine alkaloids to humans and ruminants. *Phytochemistry Reviews*, *10*(1), 137–151. doi:10.1007/s11101-010-9174-0

Wilcox, L. J., Borradaile, N. M., de Dreu, L. E., & Huff, M. W. (2001). Secretion of hepatocyte apoB is inhibited by the flavonoids, naringenin and hesperetin, via reduced activity and expression of ACAT2 and MTP. *Journal of Lipid Research*, *42*(5), 725–734. PMID:11352979

Wilde, P. F., & Dawson, R. M. C. (1966). The bihydrogenation of alpha- linoleic and oleic acid by rumen micro- organisms. *The Biochemical Journal*, *98*(2), 469–475. doi:10.1042/bj0980469 PMID:4287407

William, A. G., & Coleman, G. S. (1997). The rumen protozoa. In The rumen microbial ecosystem (pp. 73-139). Springer.

Williams, C. H. Jr. (1976). Flavin containing dehydrogenases. In P. D. Boyer (Ed.), *The Enzymes* (pp. 89–173). New York: Academic Press.

Williamson, E., Driver, S., & Baxter, K. (2009). *Interações medicamentosas de Stockley*. Porto Alegre, Rio Grande do Sul, Brasil: Artmed.

Wink, M., & Van Wyk, B. E. (2008). Mind-altering and poisonous plants of the world. Timber Press.

Wink, D. A., Hanbauer, I., Krishna, M. C., DeGraff, W., Gamson, J., & Mitchell, J. B. (1993). Nitric oxide protects against cellular damage and cytotoxicity from reactive oxygen species. *Proceedings of the National Academy of Sciences of the United States of America*, *90*(21), 9813–9817. doi:10.1073/pnas.90.21.9813 PMID:8234317

Woodside, J. V., McGrath, A. J., Lyner, N., & McKinley, M. C. (2015). Carotenoids and health in older people. *Maturitas*, *80*(1), 63–68. doi:10.1016/j.maturitas.2014.10.012 PMID:25466302

Wright, A. D. G. (2009). The rumen ciliates. In R. Röttger, R. Knight, & W. Foissner (Eds.), *Protozoological Monographs* (Vol. 4, pp. 202–210). Shaker Verlag Achen, Germany.

Wright, A. D. G., & Klieve, A. V. (2011). Does the complexity of the rumen microbial ecology preclude methane mitigation? *Animal Feed Science and Technology*, *166*, 248–253. doi:10.1016/j.anifeedsci.2011.04.015

Wu, S., Patel, K.B., Booth, L.J. Metcalfb, J.P., Lin, H.K., & Wu, W. (2010). *Protective essential oil attenuates influenza virus infection: An in vitro study in MDCK cells*. Academic Press.

Wu, J. J., Liu, J., Chen, E. B., Wang, J. J., Cao, L., Narayan, N., & Finkel, T. et al. (2013). Increased mammalian lifespan and a segmental and tissue-specific slowing of aging after genetic reduction of mTOR expression. *Cell Reports*, *4*(5), 913–920. doi:10.1016/j.celrep.2013.07.030 PMID:23994476

Wullschleger, S., Loewith, R., & Hall, M. N. (2006). TOR signaling in growth and metabolism. *Cell*, *124*(3), 471–484. doi:10.1016/j.cell.2006.01.016 PMID:16469695

Wu, S. L., Pan, C. E., Yu, L., & Meng, K. W. (2005). Immunosuppression by combined use of cyclosporine and resveratrol in a rat liver transplantation model. *Transplantation Procedures*, *37*(5), 2354–2359. doi:10.1016/j.transproceed.2005.03.112 PMID:15964415

Wu, S. L., Yu, L., Meng, K. W., Ma, Z. H., & Pan, C. E. (2005). Resveratrol prolongs allograft survival after liver transplantation in rats. *World Journal of Gastroenterology, 11*(30), 4745–4749. doi:10.3748/wjg.v11.i30.4745 PMID:16094722

Xiao, Z., Liu, W., Zhu, G., Zhou, R., & Niu, Y. (2014). A review of the preparation and application of flavour and essential oils microcapsules based on complex coacervation technology. *Journal of the Science of Food and Agriculture, 94*(8), 1482–1494. doi:10.1002/jsfa.6491 PMID:24282124

Yanez-Ruiz, D. R., Scollan, N. D., Merry, R. J., & Newbold, C. J. (2006). Contribution of rumen protozoa to duodenal flow of nitrogen, conjugated linoleic acid and vaccenic acid in steers fed silages differing in their water-soluble carbohydrate content. *The British Journal of Nutrition, 96*(05), 861–869. doi:10.1017/BJN20061927 PMID:17092374

Yang, L., Huang, Y., Wang, H. Q., & Chen, Z. Y. (2002). Production of conjugated linoleic acids through KOH-catalyzed dehydration of ricinoleic acid. *Chemistry and Physics of Lipids, 119*(1), 23–31. doi:10.1016/S0009-3084(02)00052-X PMID:12270670

Yan, J., Tsuichihara, N., Etoh, T., & Iwai, S. (2007). Reactive oxygen species and nitric oxide are involved in ABA inhibition of stomatal opening. *Plant, Cell & Environment, 30*(10), 1320–1325. doi:10.1111/j.1365-3040.2007.01711.x PMID:17727421

Yankah, V. V. (2006). Lipids phytosterols and human healtl. In *AKOH, Casimir C. Handbook of functional lipids* (pp. 403–418). New York, NY: CRC.

Yao, S.-L., Xu, Y., Zhang, Y.-Y., & Lu, Y.-H. (2013). Black rice and anthocyanins induce inhibition of cholesterol absorption in vitro. *Food & Function, 4*(11), 1602–1608. doi:10.1039/c3fo60196j PMID:24056583

Yenagi, N. B., Naik, & Josna. (2011). Knowledge, Attitude and Practice of Farm Women of Millet Growing Areas Towards Millet Consumption. *National symposium on recapturing of nutritious millets for Health and Management of diseases*. NAIP Project.

Young, E., & Stoneham, M. D. (1994). A population study of food intolerance. *Lancet, 343*(8906), 1127–1130. doi:10.1016/S0140-6736(94)90234-8 PMID:7910231

Yu, C., Shin, Y. G., Chow, A., Li, Y., Kosmeder, J. W., Lee, Y. S., & Van Breemen, R. B. et al. (2002). Human, rat and mouse metabolism of resveratrol. *Pharmaceutical Research, 19*(12), 1907–1914. doi:10.1023/A:1021414129280 PMID:12523673

Zatta, L., Nepel, A., Barison, A., & Wypych, F. (2012). Montmorilonita modificada como catalisador heterogêneo em reações de esterificação (m)etílica de ácido láurico. *Quimica Nova, 35*(9), 1711–1718. doi:10.1590/S0100-40422012000900002

Zeng, H. J., Hu, G. H., You, J., Yang, R., & Qu, L. B. (2015). Spectroscopic and molecular modeling investigation on theinteractions between hyaluronidase and baicalein and chrysin. *Process Biochemistry, 50*(5), 738–745. doi:10.1016/j.procbio.2015.02.007

Zhang, B., Rong, C., Chen, H., Song, Y., Zhang, H., & Chen, W. (2012). De novo synthesis of trans-10, cis-12 conjugated linoleic acid in oleaginous yeast *Yarrowia lipolytica. Microbial Cell Factories, 11*(1), 51. doi:10.1186/1475-2859-11-51 PMID:22545818

Zhang, J., Cao, Y. L. K. B., Wu, L., & Xu, S. (2012). Iron and Zinc accumulation trend in a Japonica rice grains after anthesis. *Afr. J. Agric. Res., 7*(8), 1312–1316.

Zhang, L., Lin, G., Kovács, B., Jani, M., Krajcsi, P., & Zuo, Z. (2007). Mechanistic study on the intestinal absorption and disposition of baicalein. *European Journal of Pharmaceutical Sciences, 31*(3-4), 221–231. doi:10.1016/j.ejps.2007.04.001 PMID:17507208

Zhang, M. W., Guo, B. J., & Peng, Z. M. (2005). Genetic effects of grain characteristics of *indica* black rice and their uses on indirect selections for some mineral element content in grains. *Genetic Resources and Crop Evolution, 52*(8), 1121–1128. doi:10.1007/s10722-004-6114-0

Zheng, H. C., Liu, J. X., Yao, J. H., Yuan, Q., Ye, H. W., Ye, J. A., & Wu, Y. M. (2005). Effects of dietary sources of vegetable oils on performance of high-yielding lactating cows and conjugated linoleic acids in milk. *Journal of Dairy Science, 88*(6), 2037–2042. doi:10.3168/jds.S0022-0302(05)72880-0 PMID:15905434

Zhong, W., Liu, N., Xie, Y., Zhao, Y., Song, X., & Zhong, W. (2013). Antioxidant and anti-aging activities of mycelial polysaccharides from *Lepista sordida. International Journal of Biological Macromolecules, 60*, 355–359. doi:10.1016/j.ijbiomac.2013.06.018 PMID:23811078

Zhou, Q. M., Wang, X. F., Liu, X. J., Zhang, H., Lu, Y. Y., & Su, S. B. (2011). Curcumin enhanced antiproliferative effect of mitomycin C in human breast cancer MCF-7 cells *in vitro* and *in vivo. Acta Pharmacologica Sinica, 32*(11), 1402–1410. doi:10.1038/aps.2011.97 PMID:21986579

Zhou, Z. P., Liu, L. N., Chen, X. L., Wang, J. X., Chen, M., Zhang, Y. Z., & Zhou, B. C. (2005). Factors that affect antioxidant activity of C-phycocyanins from Spirulina platensis. *Journal of Food Biochemistry, 29*(3), 313–322. doi:10.1111/j.1745-4514.2005.00035.x

Zhu, R., Wang, Y., Zhang, L., & Guo, Q. (2012). Oxidative stress and liver disease. *Hepatology Research, 42*(8), 741–749. doi:10.1111/j.1872-034X.2012.00996.x PMID:22489668

Zukiewicz-Sobczak, W. (2013). The role of fungi in allergic diseases. *Postep Derm Alergol, 1*, 42–45. doi:10.5114/pdia.2013.33377 PMID:24278044

About the Contributors

Sailas Benjamin, a renowned industrial and environmental biotechnologist, has served University of Calicut as the Director of Research. Being a leader of several research projects, Prof. Benjamin has published several research papers in international and national journals of high repute, and several industrially-significant novel strains of bacteria/fungi were discovered and characterized; apart from 5 patents and 1 book to his credit. He is one of the pioneering researchers pertaining to the bioremediation of hazardous phthalates. Having completed his M.Sc. Degree (University of Kerala), he secured his M.Phil Degree (Cytogenetics) from the same University. In 1998, he secured his Ph.D. Degree (Biotechnology, Cochin University of Science and Technology, Kerala; CUSAT) under the supervision of the world renowned biotechnologist, Prof. Ashok PANDEY at National Institute for Interdisciplinary Science and Technology (NIIST), Thiruvananthapuram. In between, Prof. Benjamin also secured Post-graduate Diploma in Public Relations and Journalism (PGDPRJ), from the Public Relations Society of India. He is the recipient of many national and international awards/fellowships, serving as Member of Editorial Board of prestigious International Journals such as Advances in Enzyme Research, SM Journal of Nutrition and metabolism, and also the recipient of prestigious PDFs from Japan (JST, worked at National Food Research Institute under renowned scientist Dr. Chikafusa FUKAZAWA); Germany (DFG worked at University of Muenster under renowned Professor Dr. Friedrich SPENER); Research Fellowship from India (CSIR), Fellow of the International Society of Biotechnology (FIBST), Invitation Fellowship from JSPS, Government Japan, etc.

* * *

Tripti Malik Ahuja is currently Associate Professor in Microbiology at Dolphin (P.G) Institute of Biomedical & Natural Sciences, affiliated to HNB Garhwal Central University, Uttrakhand. She has a profound experience of teaching and research accounting to 14 years. She has secured her doctoral degree in Microbiology from Gurukul Kangri University, Haridwar. Her research interests include antimicrobial natural products, essential oils and host pathogen interactions. She has been investigated a number of research projects funded by state and central government agencies. She has authored many book chapters and research articles in peer reviewed journals of both national and international repute. She has participated in many national and international seminars and conferences. She is also an active reviewer for a number of journals.

Hrideek T. K. has fifteen years research experience in the field of Plant breeding. A doctorate from University of Calicut with specialization in Genetics and Plant breeding and currently working in Genetic improvement of trees. Developed Clonal evaluation plots of tree species at KFRI, protocols for propagation and reproductive biology studies of several important Rare Endangered and Threatened species. Has also worked in MSSRF and actively involved in the genetic improvement of Millets.

Nampoothiri Ku K. specializes in Genetics and Plant breeding. Has five decades of experience in plantation crop research and management. Developed high yielding coconut and pepper varieties. Retired as Director, Central plantation Crops Research Institute (ICAR) and Director, M.S.Swaminathan Research Foundation. Involved in developing millet varieties suitable for the rural communities. FAO consultant.

Ravi-Kumar Kadeppagari has obtained his education from the premier organizations of India like Regional Institute of Education (Constituent of NCERT, New Delhi), Pondicherry University (A Central University), Central Food Technological Research Institute (Unit of CSIR, New Delhi). He had extensively worked with post-translational processing of the industrially relevant enzymes from microbes. Then he moved to Northwestern University, Chicago, USA to pursue his post-doc, where he found alternate pathway used by the Adeno viral oncoprotein E1A to induce cells to proliferate. This led to new targets for inhibiting the cancer cells. During his second post-doc at Lousiana State University Health Sciences Center, USA, he worked with the molecular and cellular mechanisms used by the Herpes Simplex Virus 2 to subvert host defense against the virus. This study led to new targets for developing the vaccine against herpes. Currently at Jain University his lab works with the problems related to the water, food, health, energy and surveillance. Specifically, the following research areas were focused. Biomolecules for decontaminating and decolorisation of water; Nutraceuticals, food related enzymes and nano-fertilizers; Therapeutic enzymes from the microbial sources; Bioactive molecules- enzyme inhibitors, anti-microbial and anti-cancerous metabolites; Nano-delivery systems; Enzymatic biofuel cells, microbes as energy sources; Nanobiosensor for ammonia detection; Immunosensors for pathogen detection.

Swarna Kanchan (PhD thesis submitted, BITS Pilani India) is currently working as Assistant Professor at Shridhar University, Pilani. He has worked as Research Associate at Amity Institute of Biotechnology, Amity University, Noida before joining BITS, Pilani. He has also qualified CSIR-UGC National Eligibility Test (NET) for Lectureship in "Life sciences" category twice. He has published many books/book chapters/research articles in peer reviewed journals of national and International repute. His research interest includes Molecular evolution, Molecular modeling, Genomics, Structural bioinformatics and Biotechnology.

Minu Kesheri has received her PhD degree from Banaras Hindu University, Varanasi, India and is currently working as Assistant Professor, Department of Life Sciences & Head, Research and Consultancy, Shridhar University, Pilani, Rajasthan India. She has published many books/book chapters /research articles in peer reviewed journals of national and International repute. Her research interest includes Proteomics, Phycology, Cyanobacterial Stress, Biochemistry, Physiology and Biotechnology.

Miguel Angel Lopez is a Veterinary Graduate, Ms in Public Health, Gouvernamental Audithor of Health and Food Safe. Now professor of critic point health analisys at Basque Culinary Center.

Jose Iñaki Alava Marquinez obtained his first degree in Chemistry (MSc) at the University of Basque Country (Spain) in 1981. He moved in 1982 to the Research & Development at the Ramon y Cajal Hospital (Madrid -Spain), performing toxicology research granted by the Spanish Research Council. During the period of 1983 to 1986, he worked in the pharmaceutical company ALTER as a research scientist, participating in the development of new pharmaceutical products. He continued research at the Cell Culture Unit in the Haematology Dpto., in the Ramon y Cajal Hospital (Madrid - Spain) for a period of 3 years. He obtained a doctorate (PhD) in Biochemistry by the University of Alcalá de Henares (Madrid) in 1989. During the period from 1988 to 1991 he was Technical manager of the consultant Company SEIC. Since 1991, Dr. Alava is a member of the research staff of Health Unit at INASMET first and Tecnalia until 2010. As part of the research staff, has participated and led a relevant number of international projects in Biomaterials and foods fields and is author of more than 40 scientific papers and member of many scientific societies. Then pass to manage the research area of Basque Culinary Center and now work as Professor of Culinary Sciences.

Murlidhar Meghwal has received his B. Tech. degree (Agricultural Engineering) in 2008 from College of Agricultural Engineering Bapatla, Acharya N. G. RANGA Agricultural University, Hyderabad, India; Dr. Meghwal has received his M. Tech. degree (Dairy and Food Engineering) in 2010 and PhD degree (Food Process Engineering) in 2014 from Indian Institute of Technology Kharagpur, West Bengal, India. He worked for one-year as research associate at INDUS Kolkata, (rice parboiling, milling and processing industry) for development of a quicker and industrial level parboiling system for paddy and rice milling. In his PhD research, he has worked on ambient and cryogenic grinding of fenugreek and black pepper by using different grinders to select a suitable grinder. Currently, Dr. Meghwal is working on: Developing inexpensive, disposable and biodegradable food containers using agricultural wastes; and Freeze drying of milk. At present, he is actively involved in research and teaching at the Food Science and Technology Division, Jain University Bangalore, India. He has written one book and many research publications in food engineering. He has attended many national and international seminars and conferences. He is reviewer and member of editorial boards of reputed journals. He is recipient of Bharat Scout award from President of India as well as Bharat Scouts award from Governors. He has received meritorious "Foundation for Academic Excellence and Access (FAEA - New Delhi) Scholarship" for his full undergraduate studies from 2004 to 2008. He has received Senior Research Fellowship awarded by Ministry of Human Resources Development (MHRD), Government of India, during 2011-14, also has received Scholarship of Ministry of Human Resources Development (MHRD), Government of India during M. Tech. studies and research during 2008-2010. Dr Meghwal is a good sport person, mentor, social activist, critical reviewer, thinker, fluent writer and well-wishing friend to all.

Prakasan Priji is a post graduate in Biotechnology from Anna University, Tamilnadu, India with III rank and also secured 97 percentile in GATE 2010, a national level test. She has secured Doctor of Philosophy Degree in Biotechnology from the University of Calicut, Kerala, India under the supervision of Prof. Sailas Benjamin, Professor, Enzyme Technology Laboratory, Biotechnology Division, School of Biological Sciences, University of Calicut. During her Ph.D. programme, he has published three papers in international journals as first author, co-authored more than a dozen papers in international journals with good impact factors, and also presented many papers in international/ national conferences/ Seminars. During this time, she had been well trained in Microbiology, Biochemistry and Biotechnology.

Abishek Santhakumar is currently an academic and clinical researcher at the School of Medical and Applied Sciences, CQUniversity, Australia. Abishek obtained his Bachelor degree in Medical Science in SRM University, India in 2008. Abishek then completed his Masters in Laboratory Medicine at RMIT University, Australia in 2010. Linking up isolated facts into comprehensive understandings to discover something is what science is described as and this cognitive process fascinated Abishek to pursue a PhD in Haematology at Griffith University, Australia (2011-2014). His current research interest is to get cogent evidence on how natural dietary antioxidant functional foods may help alleviate the risk of thrombosis and its potential as anti-platelet therapy. He has published a number of peer-reviewed journal articles, reviews and successful in research grants. He is a fellow of the Institute of Biomedical Science, UK and an active member in a number of societies such as AIMS, ASTH, HSANZ, ASMR. He is also an active reviewer for a number of journals.

P. Savitha was awarded in PhD (2014) Plant Breeding and Genetics, Tamil Nadu Agricultural University, Coimbatore, India. Her major area of research work on finger millet and rice. She had published eight research article in National and International Journals and presented research paper in National and International seminars.

Indu Singh is the Program Director of Medical Laboratory Science at Griffith University with significant experience in supervision and education of Laboratory Medicine and post graduate research students. She has more than 30 years of clinical experience as practicing medical scientist. As an academic, she has more than 15 years of haematology and immunohaematology teaching experience at universities and her research focuses on mechanisms and pathology of haemostasis and platelet function in response to life style induced oxidative stress and role of antioxidants as possible anti-platelet therapy.

R. P. Sinha is Professor and Coordinator (Industrial Microbiology) at Centre of Advanced Study in Botany Banaras Hindu University Varanasi-221005 India.

Hafiz Ansar Rasul Suleria is currently working as RHD Fellow in School of Medicine, The University of Queensland, Australia funded by Australian Government. He is also working as Postgraduate Research Fellow with Commonwealth Scientific and Industrial Research Organization (CSIRO, Australia). In May 28th 2014, he has been awarded the Early Career Research Award, 2014 (CSIRO, University of Adelaide, Australia) on cutting edge Science Symposium funded by Australian Government. He has been working as Lecturer in Department of

Food Science, Government College University Faisalabad, Pakistan. Recently, he has been awarded IUTOX Junior Fellowship for Young Scientist (International Union of Toxicology) for the XIII International Congress of Toxicology, June 30-July 4, 2013 in Seoul, South Korea. He has also been awarded International Postgraduate Research Scholarship (IPRS) and Australian Postgraduate Award (APA) funded by Australian Government for his PhD studies in University of Queensland Australia. He has visited in different International Universities during Student Exchange Program funded by Higher Education Commission (HEC) and Ministry of Foreign Affairs, Pakistan and Bangladesh. Mr. Suleria has been working as Research Associate in PAK-US Joint Project funded by HEC and Department of State, USA with collaboration of University of Massachusetts, USA and National Institute of Food Science and Technology, University of Agriculture Faisalabad, Pakistan. His research expertise is on Natural product phytochemistry, Functional & Nutraceutical foods, Food Nutrition & Metabolic Syndromes. He has got various trainings on advance analytical techniques. He has awarded various International Travel Grant Awards to attend International Conferences, Seminars and Workshops as Speaker, Co-Chair, and Mediator. He is member of various National and International Organizations like IFT, European Federation of Food Science and Technology, International Society of Food and Hygiene and PSFST, IUTOX and SOT. Mr. Suleria has published more than 20 International Research and Review Articles in various high reputed/impacted journals. He is also a potent reviewer of International Journals like International Journal of Food Science and Nutrition, Critical Reviews of Food Science and Nutrition and International Journal of Food Science & Technology.

Kizhakepowathil Nair Unni is a post graduate in Biotechnology from Periyar University, Tamilnadu, India. He has secured his Doctor of Philosophy Degree in Biotechnology from the University of Calicut, Kerala, India under the supervision of Prof. Sailas Benjamin, Professor, Enzyme Technology Laboratory, Biotechnology Division, School of Biological Sciences, University of Calicut. During his Ph.D. programme, he has published several papers in international journals with good impact factors as first author and co-author. During this time, he has well trained in Microbiology, Biochemistry and Biotechnology.

André-Denis Wright is Professor and Director of the School of Animal and Comparative Biomedical Sciences at the University of Arizona (UA). Dr. Wright holds the Carl and Patricia Weiler Endowed Chair for Excellence in Agriculture & Life Sciences and is a BIO5 Research Fellow. Before coming to UA in Nov. 2014, Dr. Wright was Professor and Department Chair of Animal Science at the University of Vermont, and Director of the University of Vermont's Dairy Center of Excellence.

For nearly two decades, Dr. Wright has been developing strategies to increase the efficiency of nutrient utilization in livestock and to raise the level of production of food in an ecologically sustainable way (i.e., decrease enteric methane). Several years ago, his research interests expanded to also include human gut microbiology. Dr. Wright's internationally recognized research uses next-generation sequencing and bioinformatics to examine the gut microbiome of animals, including humans, to better understand the interactions between host genetics, immune responses, and the gut microbiota, which are largely unexplored. Dr. Wright received his Ph.D. from the University of Guelph in Canada, has published over 100 peer-reviewed papers and 16 book chapters, and has given 30 plenary lectures in 10 different countries. Dr. Wright currently serves on the Editorial Boards for 5 journals, and has served on review panels for the USDA, NSF, and NASA.

Index

E

F

G

H

I

K

M

N

O

P

R

S

T

U

www.ingramcontent.com/pod-product-compliance
Lightning Source LLC
LaVergne TN
LVHW080557300926
849162LV00005B/977